T0348602

Updates in Tropical Medicine

Editors

MICHAEL LIBMAN
CÉDRIC P. YANSOUNI

INFECTIOUS DISEASE CLINICS
OF NORTH AMERICA

www.id.theclinics.com

Consulting Editor
HELEN W. BOUCHER

March 2019 • Volume 33 • Number 1

ELSEVIER

1600 John F. Kennedy Boulevard • Suite 1800 • Philadelphia, Pennsylvania, 19103-2899.
http://www.theclinics.com

INFECTIOUS DISEASE CLINICS OF NORTH AMERICA Volume 33, Number 1
March 2019 ISSN 0891–5520, ISBN-13: 978-0-323-65511-8

Editor: Kerry Holland
Developmental Editor: Donald Mumford

Infectious Disease Clinics of North America (ISSN 0891–5520) is published in March, June, September, and December by Elsevier Inc., 360 Park Avenue South, New York, NY 10010-1710. Periodicals postage paid at New York, NY and additional mailing offices. Subscription prices are $330.00 per year for US individuals, $660.00 per year for US institutions, $100.00 per year for US students, $396.00 per year for Canadian individuals, $824.00 per year for Canadian institutions, $432.00 per year for international individuals, $824.00 per year for international institutions, and $200.00 per year for Canadian and international students. To receive student rate, orders must be accompanied by name of affiliated institution, date of term, and the *signature* of program/residency coordinator on institution letterhead. Orders will be billed at individual rate until proof of status is received. Foreign air speed delivery is included in all *Clinics* subscription prices. All prices are subject to change without notice. **POSTMASTER**: Send address changes to *Infectious Disease Clinics of North America,* Elsevier Health Sciences Division, Subcription Customer Service, 3251 Riverport Lane, Maryland Heights, MO 63043. **Customer Service: 1-800-654-2452 (US). From outside of the US and Canada, call 1-314-447-8871. Fax: 1-314-447-8029. E-mail: JournalsCustomerService-usa@elsevier.com (print support) or JournalsOnlineSupport-usa@elsevier.com (online support).**

Infectious Disease Clinics of North America is also published in Spanish by Editorial Inter-Médica, Junin 917, 1er A 1113, Buenos Aires, Argentina.

Reprints. For copies of 100 or more, of articles in this publication, please contact the Commercial Reprints Department, Elsevier Inc., 360 Park Avenue South, New York, New York 10010-1710. Tel. 212-633-3874, Fax: 212-633-3820, E-mail: reprints@elsevier.com.

Infectious Disease Clinics of North America is covered in *MEDLINE/PubMed (Index Medicus), Current Contents/Clinical Medicine, Science Citation Alert, SCISEARCH,* and *Research Alert.*

Contributors

CONSULTING EDITOR

HELEN W. BOUCHER, MD, FIDSA, FACP
Director, Infectious Diseases Fellowship Program, Division of Geographic Medicine
and Infectious Diseases, Tufts Medical Center, Associate Professor of Medicine,
Tufts University School of Medicine, Boston, Massachusetts, USA

EDITORS

MICHAEL LIBMAN, MD, FRCPC
JD MacLean Centre for Tropical Diseases (Director), Division of Infectious Diseases,
Professor of Medicine, Department of Microbiology, McGill University Health Centre,
Montréal, Quebec, Canada

CÉDRIC P. YANSOUNI, MD, FRCPC, DTM&H
Associate Director, JD MacLean Centre for Tropical Diseases, Division of Infectious
Diseases, Assistant Professor, Department of Medical Microbiology, McGill University
Health Centre, Montréal, Quebec, Canada

AUTHORS

NEILL K.J. ADHIKARI, MDCM, MSc
Staff Physician, Department of Critical Care Medicine, Sunnybrook Health Sciences
Centre, Assistant Professor, Interdepartmental Division of Critical Care, University of
Toronto, Toronto, Ontario, Canada

NAOMI E. ARONSON, MD
Professor of Medicine, Uniformed Services University of the Health Sciences, Bethesda,
Maryland, USA

LUCAS S. BLANTON, MD
Assistant Professor, Department of Internal Medicine, Division of Infectious Diseases, The
University of Texas Medical Branch at Galveston, Galveston, Texas, USA

EMMANUEL BOTTIEAU, MD, PhD
Professor, Department of Clinical Sciences, Institute of Tropical Medicine, Antwerp,
Belgium

FRANCESCO CASTELLI MD, FRCP (Lond), FFTM RCPS (Glasg), FESCMID
University Department of Infectious and Tropical Diseases, University of Brescia and
ASST Spedali Civili, UNESCO Chair "Training and Empowering Human Resources for
Health Development in Resource-Limited Countries," University of Brescia, Brescia, Italy

CHRISTOPHE CLÉMENT, MD
Staff Physician, Associate Director, Intensive Care Unit, Polyclinique Bordeaux Nord
Aquitaine, Bordeaux, France; Staff Physician, Intensive Care Unit, Mamoudzou Hospital,
Mayotte, France

JAN CLERINX, MD
Department of Clinical Sciences, Institute of Tropical Medicine, Antwerp, Belgium

CHRISTINA M. COYLE, MD, MS
Professor, Department of Medicine, Division of Infectious Disease, Albert Einstein College of Medicine, Bronx, New York, USA

ERMIAS DIRO, MD, PhD
Department of Internal Medicine, University of Gondar, Gondar, Ethiopia

ARJEN M. DONDORP, MD, PhD
Professor of Tropical Medicine, Nuffield Department of Clinical Medicine, University of Oxford, Oxford, United Kingdom; Mahidol-Oxford Tropical Medicine Research Unit (MORU), Faculty of Tropical Medicine, Mahidol University, Bangkok, Thailand

LUIS E. ECHEVERRIA, MD
Grupo de Estudios Epidemiológicos y Salud Pública, Heart Failure and Heart Transplant Clinic, Fundacion Cardiovascular de Colombia, Floridablanca, Santander, Colombia

ERIC J. ECKBO, MD
Department of Pathology and Laboratory Medicine, Division of Medical Microbiology, University of British Columbia, Vancouver General Hospital, Vancouver, British Columbia, Canada

DAVID M. GOLDFARB, MD
Department of Pathology and Laboratory Medicine, Division of Medical Microbiology, Department of Pediatrics, Division of Infectious Diseases, University of British Columbia, Vancouver, British Columbia, Canada

CHRISTINA GREENAWAY, MD, MSc
Division of Infectious Diseases, Jewish General Hospital Centre for Clinical Epidemiology, Lady Davis Institute for Medical Research J.D. MacLean Center for Tropical Diseases at McGill, McGill University, Montreal, Québec, Canada

LOUIS-PATRICK HARAOUI, MD, MSc, FRCP(C)
Hôpital Charles-Le Moyne, Université de Sherbrooke, Longueuil, Québec, Canada

TOM HELLER, MD
Consulting Physician, Lighthouse Clinic, Kamuzu Central Hospital, Lilongwe, Malawi

CHRISTIE A. JOYA, DO
U.S. Naval Medical Research Unit Number 6, Lima, Peru

DANIEL KAMINSTEIN, MD, DTM&H, FACEP
Director of Global Health, Associate Professor, Department of Emergency Medicine, Medical College of Georgia, Augusta University, Augusta, Georgia, USA

HUGH W.F. KINGSTON, BMBCh, MRCP, PhD
Senior House Officer, Nuffield Department of Clinical Medicine, University of Oxford, Oxford, United Kingdom; Research Physician, Malaria Department, Mahidol Oxford Research Unit, Faculty of Tropical Medicine, Mahidol University, Bangkok, Thailand

ALEJANDRO KROLEWIECKI, MD
Instituto de Investigaciones de Enfermedades Tropicales, Universidad Nacional de Salta/CONICET, Oran, Salta, Argentina

FRANÇOIS LAMONTAGNE, MD, MSc
Staff Physician, Department of Medicine, Centre Intégré Universitaire de santé et des Services Sociaux de l'Estrie, Clinician-Scientist, Centre de recherche du CHU de Sherbrooke, Associate Professor, Interdepartmental Division of Critical Care, Université de Sherbrooke, Sherbrooke, Québec, Canada

STIJE J. LEOPOLD, MD, PhD
Research Physician, Malaria Department, Mahidol Oxford Research Unit, Faculty of Tropical Medicine, Mahidol University, Bangkok, Thailand

CARLOS A. MORILLO, MD, FRCPC, FACC, FESC, FHRS
Chief, Division of Cardiology, Professor, Department of Cardiac Sciences, Libin Cardiovascular Institute of Alberta, University of Calgary, Foothills Medical Centre, Calgary, Alberta, Canada

THOMAS B. NUTMAN, MD
Laboratory of Parasitic Diseases, National Institute of Allergy and Infectious Diseases, National Institutes of Health, Bethesda, Maryland, USA

JEFFREY M. PERNICA, MD, DTM&H
Department of Pediatrics, Division of Infectious Diseases, McMaster University, Hamilton Health Sciences Centre, Hamilton, Ontario, Canada

KATHERINE PLEWES, MSc, MD, DPhil, FRCPC
Clinician Investigator, Malaria Department, Mahidol Oxford Research Unit, Faculty of Tropical Medicine, Mahidol University, Bangkok, Thailand; Clinical Assistant Professor, Division of Infectious Diseases, Department of Medicine, University of British Columbia, Vancouver General Hospital, Vancouver, British Columbia, Canada

PRISCILLA RUPALI, MD, DTM&H, FRCP
Professor, Department of Infectious Diseases, Infectious Diseases Training and Research Center, Christian Medical College Hospital, Vellore, Tamil Nadu, India

MAKEDA SEMRET, MSc, MD, FRCP(C)
Antimicrobial Stewardship Program Lead, McGill University Health Centre, JD MacLean Centre for Tropical Diseases, Assistant Professor of Medicine, McGill University, Montreal, Quebec, Canada

FRANCESCA TAMAROZZI, DVM, MD, MSc, PhD
Contract Researcher, Center for Tropical Diseases, IRCSS, Sacro Cuore Don Calabria Hospital, Verona, Italy

JOHAN VAN GRIENSVEN, MD, MSc, PhD
Department of Clinical Sciences, Institute of Tropical Medicine, Antwerp, Belgium

DAVID A. WARRELL, DM, DSc, FRCP, FRCPE, FMedSci
Emeritus Professor of Tropical Medicine, Nuffield Department of Clinical Medicine, University of Oxford, John Radcliffe Hospital, Oxford, United Kingdom

CÉDRIC P. YANSOUNI, MD, FRCPC, DTM&H
Associate Director, JD MacLean Centre for Tropical Diseases, Division of Infectious Diseases, Assistant Professor, Department of Medical Microbiology, McGill University Health Centre, Montréal, Quebec, Canada

Contents

Tropical medicine deals with infectious and noninfectious diseases geographically located between the tropics of Cancer and Capricorn. It encompasses diseases that result from poverty, poor sanitation, infrastructure, and inadequate health resources. Lack of availability of clean water and food made with unhygienic practices add to the morbidity of these diseases. The tropics are reeling under the onslaught of climate change, deforestation, and air, water, and soil pollution, which worsens an already fragile health system. This article provides an overview of the definition, classification, geophysical problems, syndromic approach to common tropical infections, diagnostic challenges in the tropics, and access to medicines.

This article discusses the epidemiology, prevention, clinical features, and treatment of venomous bites by snakes, lizards, and spiders; stings by fish, jellyfish, echinoderms, insects, and scorpions; and poisoning by ingestion of fish, turtles, and shellfish. Invertebrate stings cause fatalities by anaphylaxis, secondary to acquired hypersensitivity (Hymenoptera, such as bees, wasps, and ants; and jellyfish), and by direct envenoming (scorpions, spiders, jellyfish, and echinoderms). Simple preventive techniques, such as wearing protective clothing, using a flashlight at night, and excluding venomous animals from sleeping quarters, are of paramount importance to reduce the risk of venomous bites and stings.

The global burden of malaria remains high, with 216 million cases causing 445,000 deaths in 2016 despite first-line treatment with artemisinin-based combination therapy. Decreasing transmission in Africa shifts the risk for severe malaria to older age groups as premunition wanes. Prompt diagnosis and treatment with intravenous artesunate in addition to appropriate supportive management are critical to reduce deaths from severe malaria. Effective individual management is challenging in settings with limited resources for higher-level care. Adjunctive therapies targeting the underlying pathophysiological pathways have the potential to reduce mortality. Resistance to artemisinin derivatives and their partner drugs threaten malaria management and control.

> Control efforts have considerably reduced the prevalence of human African trypanosomiasis (HAT) due to *Trypanosoma brucei gambiense* in West/Central Africa and to *Trypanosoma brucei rhodesiense* in East Africa. Management of *T brucei gambiense* HAT has recently improved, with new antibody-based rapid diagnostic tests suited for mass screening and clinical care, and simpler treatments, including the nifurtimox-eflornithine combination therapy and the new oral drug fexinidazole to treat the second stage of the disease. In contrast, no major advance has been achieved for the treatment of *T brucei rhodesiense* HAT, a zoonosis that occasionally affects short-term travelers to endemic areas.

> Diagnostic advances in visceral leishmaniasis include the development of the rK39 and rK28 rapid diagnostic test. The direct agglutination test is also increasingly used, as well as conventional and real-time polymerase chain reaction, which also performs well on peripheral blood. The choice of treatment for visceral leishmaniasis depends on the geographic region where the infection is acquired. Liposomal amphotericin B is generally found to be safe and effective in most endemic regions of the world; antimonials still remain to be the most effective in eastern Africa despite its high toxicity. Combination therapy is increasingly explored. Immunosuppressed patients require adapted diagnostic and therapeutic strategies.

> Cutaneous leishmaniasis (CL) is a diverse human disease caused by more than 20 *Leishmania* species transmitted by the bite of an infected sand fly. Diagnostic testing is recommended to confirm infection and determine the infecting species. Treatment decisions are complex and providers should consider infecting species, patient comorbidities, extent and location of lesions, and previous treatments. There is no single universal treatment for CL and some treatment can have toxicity. Treatment should be individualized and factors, such as self-healing nature of this infection, risk of metastatic complications (ie, mucosal leishmaniasis), and patient wishes, need to be included in individual risk-benefit treatment decisions.

> American trypanosomiasis is caused by a parasite endemic of the Americas. Current migration has globalized Chagas disease. Acute infection usually resolves spontaneously. Nonetheless, 20% to 40% develop cardiomyopathy 20 to 30 years later. Progression to cardiomyopathy is devastatingly rapid, manifesting with heart failure and sudden death.

Etiologic treatment is highly effective and recommended in those with acute infections, congenital infections, and parasite reactivation, and women of childbearing age, but in asymptomatic *Trypanosoma* cruzi carriers and patients with early cardiomyopathy remains controversial and under investigation. Progression of heart failure is rapid and accounts for most of the morbidity and related mortality.

Most of the 30 to 100 million people infected with *Strongyloides stercoralis* have subclinical (or asymptomatic) infections. These infections are commonly chronic and longstanding. A change in immune status can increase parasite numbers, leading to hyperinfection syndrome, dissemination, and death if unrecognized. The use of corticosteroids and HTLV-1 infection are most commonly associated with the hyperinfection syndrome. *Strongyloides* adult parasites reside in the small intestine and induce immune responses that are like other nematodes. Definitive diagnosis of *S stercoralis* infection is based on stool examinations for larvae. *S stercoralis* remains largely neglected.

Neurocysticercosis is an infection of the central nervous system by the larval stage of the pork tapeworm *Taenia solium*. The combination of modern diagnostic tests, use of antiparasitic drugs, improved anti-inflammatory treatments, and minimally invasive neurosurgery has improved outcomes in patients with neurocysticercosis. This parasitic infection is complex in both the clinical presentation and the treatment approach, which depends on the number of cysts, location in the brain, stage of degeneration, and host inflammatory response. Therapeutic interventions for each location are different; therefore, principles for managing parenchymal disease cannot be applied to extraparenchymal disease and should be individualized.

 Video content accompanies this article at http://www.id.theclinics. com/.

Ultrasound for diagnosis and staging of schistosomiasis and echinococcosis have paved the way over the past several decades for the application of ultrasound in tropical diseases. Until recently, the size and cost of ultrasound systems limited the application in low-resource settings. The increase in portable ultrasound systems has given more clinicians access to ultrasound, and clinically based protocols for the care of patients have emerged, such as focused assessment with sonography for HIV/TB and tropical cardiac ultrasound. This article explores the history and current use of ultrasound in these diseases and highlights their application in the care of patients.

outcomes. Clinical features include severe volume depletion due to diarrhea and vomiting, shock, rhabdomyolysis, and metabolic disturbances. Overt hemorrhage is uncommon. Point-of-care devices and inexpensive electronic equipment enable better monitoring and record keeping in resource-limited settings.

Migration is increasing and practitioners need to be aware of the unique health needs of this population. The prevalence of infectious diseases among migrants varies and generally mirrors that of their countries of origin, but is modified by the circumstance of migration, the presence of pre-arrival screening programs and post arrival access to health care. To optimize the health of migrants practitioners; (1) should take all opportunities to screen migrants at risk for latent infections such as tuberculosis, chronic hepatitis B and C, HIV, strongyloidiasis, schistosomiasis and Chagas disease, (2) update routine vaccines in all age groups and, (3) be aware of "rare and tropical infections" related to migration and return travel.

Updates in Tropical Medicine

INFECTIOUS DISEASE CLINICS OF NORTH AMERICA

FORTHCOMING ISSUES

June 2019
Management of Infectious Diseases in Stem Cell Transplantation and Hematologic Malignancy
Jo-Ann Young, *Editor*

September 2019
HIV
Paul Edward Sax, *Editor*

December 2019
Emerging and Re-Emerging Infectious Diseases
Alimuddin Zumla and David SC Hui, *Editors*

RECENT ISSUES

December 2018
Device-Associated Infections
Vivian H. Chu, *Editor*

September 2018
Management of Infections in Solid Organ Transplant Recipients
Sherif Beniameen Mossad, *Editor*

June 2018
Overcoming Barriers to Eliminate Hepatitis C
Camilla S. Graham and Stacey B. Trooskin, *Editors*

Preface

What's in a Name and Why "Tropical Medicine" Matters in 2019

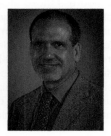

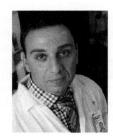

Michael Libman, MD, FRCPC   Cédric P. Yansouni, MD, FRCPC, DTM&H
Editors

This issue of *Infectious Disease Clinics of North America* is titled "Updates in Tropical Medicine." Today, even more than in the past, terms like "tropical medicine" and "tropical diseases" are nearly impossible to define sensibly. Once upon a time, the terms applied to conditions found predominantly in those parts of the world known as the "tropics" (ie, warm and far away from Europe or North America). Clinical parasitology was a dominant component. Over time, new terms meant to refine, expand, subdivide, or amalgamate these groups of illness came into use. Geographic medicine, travel medicine, and migration medicine are a few of these. Many of the illnesses were more properly diseases of poverty, crowding, and poor access to health resources, and so they remain too often today. In recent years, "tropical medicine" has to some extent been subsumed into the broader notion of "global health," a term whose current ubiquity owes much to the fact it means nothing specific.

Yet, in 2019, "tropical diseases," or whatever we choose to call them, still carry a huge burden of illness and are expanding their range in many cases. Several illnesses are now seen more frequently in regions where health care practitioners have little familiarity with their presenting features, diagnosis, or management. Climate change and accelerating urbanization have expanded the range of several geographically restricted pathogens or their vectors in the last decade. Human mobility, via ever-increasing international travel and unprecedented mass migrations between distant corners of the globe, has also entailed the spread of imported exotic diseases. Human intrusions into new habitats can uncover new emerging infections, typically zoonotic, or spread disease into new populations. Already several times in the twenty-first century, unexpected mutations in pathogens or vectors have led to altered transmission, virulence, or clinical presentations of known pathogens. The proliferation of immune suppressive therapies and better survival with immune

Infect Dis Clin N Am 33 (2019) xiii–xiv
https://doi.org/10.1016/j.idc.2018.12.001
0891-5520/19/© 2018 Published by Elsevier Inc.

compromising conditions in middle-income countries have allowed old infections to manifest as new clinical syndromes.

Thus, our aim with this *Infectious Disease Clinics of North America* issue was to provide a state-of-the-art update for infectious diseases clinicians on tropical infections or envenomations rarely seen in most high-resource settings. Our main focus is on the diagnosis and management of these conditions in settings where the availability of resources generally allows the use of technically sophisticated testing and treatment. We have commissioned 15 reviews from leaders in the field to address those areas that have seen the most changes in recent years. The field of medical diagnostics has seen major breakthroughs, especially as molecular technologies have become easier, faster, and cheaper, and this is reflected in almost every one of the articles in this issue. We have also emphasized topics not traditionally regarded as "tropical," such as advances in medical imaging and the crisis of antimicrobial resistance. Kaminstein and colleagues summarize the relevance of accessible ultrasound equipment to tropical diseases, while Semret and colleagues summarize emerging data on antimicrobial resistance in low-resource settings and its implications for local populations as well as for the spread of resistance around the world.

In summary, we hope this issue will equip clinicians to provide the best possible care for tropical diseases, wherever they are encountered.

Michael Libman, MD, FRCPC
McGill University Health Centre
1001 Boulevard Décarie
Glen Site, Office #E05.1830
Montréal, QC H4A 3J1, Canada

Cédric P. Yansouni, MD, FRCPC, DTM&H
McGill University Health Centre
1001 Boulevard Décarie
Glen Site, Office #EM3.3242
Montréal, QC H4A 3J1, Canada

E-mail addresses:
michael.libman@mcgill.ca (M. Libman)
cedric.yansouni@mcgill.ca (C.P. Yansouni)

Website:
http://www.mcgill.ca/tropmed

Introduction to Tropical Medicine

Priscilla Rupali, MD, DTM&H, FRCP

KEYWORDS

• Introduction • Classification • History • Tropical medicine • Fever • Diarrhea

KEY POINTS

- Tropical medicine is the practice of medicine in the tropics between the tropic of Cancer and Capricorn.
- It includes common infections, such as HIV, tuberculosis, malaria, and various other neglected tropical diseases, and noninfectious causes, such as snakebites, cancers, malnutrition, and nutrient deficiencies.
- It also deals with diseases that are indirectly or directly caused by climate change, air, water, and soil pollution.
- Access to medicines and health infrastructure impacts patient care in these areas leading to high mortality and morbidity.

INTRODUCTION

Tropical medicine is a branch of medicine that deals with communicable and noncommunicable diseases in the tropics. Most of the communicable diseases are infections that are endemic to the tropics contributing to significant morbidity and mortality. The three major infections in the tropics are human immunodeficiency virus (HIV)/AIDS, malaria, and tuberculosis. Tropical medicine involves rare and exotic parasitic and bacterial diseases but in addition involves variety of noncommunicable diseases, such as vitamin deficiencies, snakebites, scorpion stings, and toxin-related cardiac and neurologic manifestations. Hence this field involves not just microbiology, virology, parasitology, and epidemiology but also a fair bit of internal medicine.

HISTORY

Sir Patrick Manson (1844–1922) was a Scottish physician who graduated from the University of Aberdeen with degrees in surgery, medicine, and law. His medical career

The author has no financial conflicts of interests to declare and did not receive any funding to complete this article.

Department of Infectious Diseases, Infectious Diseases Training and Research Center, Ida Scudder Road, Christian Medical College Hospital, Vellore, Tamilnadu 632004, India

E-mail address: prisci@cmcvellore.ac.in

spanned many decades in China, Hong Kong, and Taiwan (then called Formosa). He eventually came back to London where he lectured on tropical diseases at the St. George's hospital. He then became the chief medical officer to the Colonial Office. At this point he used his considerable influence to found a school for tropical medicine at the Albert Dock Seamen's Hospital. The London School of Hygiene and Tropical Medicine was formally inaugurated on October 2, 1899. He eventually went on to become the first president of the Royal Society of Tropical Medicine and Hygiene in 1907. He also made numerous contributions to parasitology, such as (1) the establishment of mosquito as the intermediate host of *Wuchereria bancrofti*, the causative agent of filariasis; (2) proposed the mosquito-malaria theory, which eventually spurred Sir Ronald Ross to discover that a mosquito was the definitive host for malaria; and (3) the discovery of a new species of *Schistosoma* (*Schistosoma mansoni*) and a new parasite, *Spirometra* or *Sparganum mansoni* and *Spirometra mansonoides*. A species of mosquito *Mansonia* spp and a filarial worm *Mansonella* spp were so named to honor him. He is hence known as the "Father of Tropical medicine."

PHYSICAL GEOGRAPHY

The tropics are regions of the earth that lie on either side of the equator between the tropics of Cancer and Capricorn (**Fig. 1**). The tropics include parts of Central and South America, Australia, Africa, India, and Oceania. The tropics account for 36% of the Earth's landmass, and are home to a third of the world's people.[1] The tropics are warm throughout the year with temperatures ranging from 25°C to 28°C (77°F–82°F) because they are close to the equator with direct sunlight most of the year. However, rainfall does vary remarkably from one area to another with the Amazon basin recording a high rainfall and North Africa being an arid area recording little to no rainfall most of the year. These climatic conditions often influence the flora, fauna, and insect wildlife in these areas.

ENVIRONMENTAL FACTORS

Tropical regions are dominated by equatorial climates with a mean temperature greater than 18°C, and arid zones are characterized by general lack of water, which

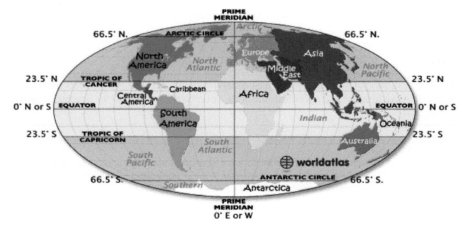

Fig. 1. Map of the tropics. (*From* WorldAtlas.com. Used with permission.)

harms plant and animal life. They host 80% of the world's biodiversity. Environmental factors include the following:

- Climate: Climate change has a wide-ranging impact on habitats, species distribution, human health, agriculture, sea levels, and the frequency/intensity of extreme weather events. Changing rainfall patterns and increased temperatures have also led to increase in vector borne diseases, such as dengue and malaria, because of increased vector distributions and decreased vector and parasite incubation periods.
- Air pollution: Among the tropical regions, Southeast Asia reported the greatest increase in CO2 emissions leading to a decreased air quality followed by South Asia and South America, which has significantly impacted the climate and led to higher weather-related mortality and morbidity, infectious disease rates, and respiratory illnesses.
- Land degradation: Although land productivity has gone up because of increased livestock and cereal production, land degradation caused by poor agricultural practices and deforestation has led to altered ecosystems and has not changed the fact that more people in the tropics experience undernourishment compared with the rest of the world.
- Water scarcity: The tropics have more than 54% of the world's renewable water sources, yet more than half of these areas are considered vulnerable to water stress because of the inequality of water distribution, with Southeast Asia having the highest pollution discharge in the world. Overexploitation of wild marine food resources has led to the coral reef systems to be at high or medium risk of damage.
- Biodiversity: Tropical biodiversity is being threatened across all taxonomic groups with a rapid loss of primary forests. Protection and maintenance of these fragile ecosystems will have a long-term impact on human health and requires cooperation at global, regional, and international levels.

SOCIAL CONDITIONS

Health is defined by the World Health Organization (WHO) as a "state of complete physical, mental and social well-being not merely the absence of disease or infirmity." However, there are many social determinants of health that affect a person's disease burden or longevity and these are often underemphasized or overlooked because the impact is often unmeasurable. Climate and other environmental factors and such social factors as poverty, overcrowding, undernutrition, and limited access to appropriate health care coupled with the lack of education and poor governance contribute to a higher prevalence of communicable and noncommunicable diseases.

According to the State of Tropics report 2014,[2] globally extreme poverty has declined by almost 50% since the 1980s but almost two-thirds of the poorest people in the world continue to live in the tropics. Poverty reduction has taken place mostly in Southeast Asia and Central America coupled with a rapid increase in urbanization in these areas. The urbanization rate in the tropics has increased disproportionately to almost 45% by 2010, in turn giving rise to large populations of slum dwellers as compared with the temperate regions, which in turn brings with it diseases of hygiene and sanitation.

POPULATION INDICES

About 40% of the world's population and 55% of children younger than age 5 also live in the tropics. By 2050, this is expected to increase to 50% and 60%, respectively.

Between 1950 and 2010, the life expectancy in the tropics increased by 22.8 years to 64.4 years and infant mortality reduced by 36%. Despite these enormous strides in the improvement of mortality, 6.9 million children younger than age 5 died in 2011, of which 99% were in low- and low-middle-income countries.

TRANSMISSION

Infectious agents and toxins are transmitted through water, soil, food, vectors, plants, and animals.

Water Sanitation and Hygiene

Freshwater constitutes only 2.5% of the total water resources on the planet. Of this only 0.3% is available as surface water, whereas the rest is in polar ice sheets, snow cover, and underground aquifers. Water scarcity is defined as less than 2000 cubic meters of water available per person per year. In the tropics the number of nations with water scarcity has tripled since 1962. This scarcity is most acute in South Asia, where 90% of the population is considered vulnerable, followed by North Africa and the Middle East at 62%.

Statistics gathered by United Nations show that 900 million people lack access to safe drinking water and 2500 million live without appropriate sanitation. Hence access to safe water and sanitation were recognized as human rights in 2010 by the United Nations General assembly.

Waterborne or water-related diseases[3] encompass illnesses resulting from indirect and direct exposure to water. The four main routes of transmission include (1) waterborne, (2) water washed, (3) water based/insect vector, and (4) water related.

Waterborne

These diseases are transmitted through the direct drinking of water contaminated with pathogenic microorganisms. Contamination of drinking water often occurs through fecal contamination, caused by poor sewage disposal and improper sanitation. If contamination levels are high, the young, the old, and the immunocompromised are at significant risk of diarrheal diseases and some others. Some of the pathogenic organisms and diseases they cause are as follows:

Protozoa
  Entamoeba histolytica: Amebic dysentery
  Cryptosporidium spp: Explosive watery diarrhea
  Giardia lamblia: Chronic diarrhea
  Balantidium coli: Persistent and occasionally invasive diarrhea
  Naegleria fowleri: Acute meningoencephalitis
  Acanthamoeba spp: Granulomatous amebic encephalitis

Bacteria
  Salmonella typhi, *Salmonella paratyphi* A, B, C: typhoid fever
  Campylobacter jejuni: acute invasive diarrhea
  Shigella spp: bacillary dysentery
  Escherichia coli: acute watery or invasive diarrhea
  Leptospira interrogans: leptospirosis
  Vibrio cholera: cholera

Viruses
  Rotavirus
  Hepatitis A
  Poliomyelitis

Waterwashed

These are also known as water-scarce diseases, which thrive in water scarcity and poor sanitation. This depends more on water quantity than quality.

a. Soil-transmitted helminths: Diseases of poor sanitation transmitted through contaminated soil. Most prevalent helminths include *Ascaris* spp, *Trichuris trichura*, *Ancylostoma duodenale*, or *Necator Americanus*.
b. Acute respiratory infections: They are responsible for 19% of the total child deaths every year and good hygienic practices including hand washing with soap can significantly reduce the transmission of acute respiratory infections.
c. Skin and eye diseases: Scabies, impetigo, trachoma, yaws, conjunctivitis, and skin ulcers.
d. Fleas, ticks, and lice: Typhus, scabies, relapsing fever.

Water-based diseases

These are infections caused by parasitic pathogens found in aquatic host organisms. Humans become infected either through skin penetration (schistosomiasis) or by ingesting the infective forms (dracunculiasis [ingestion of larvae in crustacean], paragonimiasis [metacercariae ingested in crab or crayfish], clonorchiasis [metacercariae ingested in fish]).

Water-related or vector-transmitted diseases

These are diseases caused by the insect vectors breeding in and around water bodies. Malaria is one of the water-related diseases endemic in 117 countries with 3.2 billion people at risk. About 59% cases occur in Africa, 38% in Asia, and 3% in Americas. Mosquito-borne diseases include malaria, yellow fever, dengue fever, and filariasis. Fly-borne diseases include onchocerciasis and loiasis.

Food Borne

Foodborne illnesses are defined by the WHO as diseases of infectious or toxic nature caused by the consumption of contaminated food or water. They are classified into two broad groups: intoxication and infection. Intoxication is caused by ingestion of toxin produced by pathogens, whereas infection is caused by ingestion of food containing viable pathogens. Intoxication is also possible by eating animals that have consumed toxin-producing organisms. Foodborne diseases result in considerable morbidity and mortality, and contribute to significant costs in tropical countries. Many of these are caused by bacteria, viruses, parasites, chemicals, and prions through contaminated food. The WHO estimates from 1990 to 2012 data that 582 million cases were caused by contaminated food resulting in 25.2 million DALYs (Disease adjusted life years).[4,5] Norovirus is a leading cause of foodborne illness (125 million) followed by *Campylobacter* spp with 96 million cases. In addition, nontyphoidal *Salmonella* diarrheal and invasive infections result in a high burden of 4.07 million DALYs in the African region followed by the Southeast Asian region in children less than 5 years.

The main pathogens of foodborne illnesses are bacteria (66%), viruses (4%), chemicals (26%), and parasites (4%). Bacteria cause 66% of the foodborne illnesses and botulism, *Clostridium perfringens* gastroenteritis, *E coli* infection, salmonellosis, and staphylococcal food poisoning. The most common clinical symptoms are diarrhea, vomiting, abdominal cramps, headache, and nausea.

Foodborne parasitic diseases excluding enteric protozoa cause an estimated 23.2 million cases and 45,927 deaths annually resulting in an estimated 6.64 million DALYs.[5] Among these foodborne ascariasis and toxoplasmosis were common contributing to 12.3 and 10.3 million cases respectively. Human cysticercosis with 2.78 million, foodborne trematodiasis with 2.02 million, and toxoplasmosis with 825,000 DALYs resulted in a high burden of disease. Foodborne enteric protozoa resulted in an additional 67.2 million illnesses. Clinically foodborne pathogens can cause diarrhea, intoxications, and invasive enteric diseases.

Bacteria
Bacteria producing acute diarrheas include *Campylobacter, Salmonella* spp, *Shigella* spp, *Staphylococcus aureus*, nontyphoidal *Salmonella*, enteropathogenic *E coli*, and *V cholerae*.[6]

Bacteria causing intoxications include *Clostridium botulinum, C perfringens, Bacillus cereus*, and enterotoxigenic *E coli*.

Bacteria causing chronic diarrheas include *Brucella* spp, *Listeria* spp, and *Mycobacterium tuberculosis* in immunocompetent hosts and nontuberculous mycobacteria in immunocompromised hosts.

Viruses
Most of the burden of foodborne illness caused by viruses is transmitted by poor hygienic practices either during food handling or food production.[7] They are transmitted by the fecal-oral route infecting their host after ingestion, followed by invasion of cells in the epithelial lining of the gut and replication at the same site or elsewhere in the body.

Food handling and food contamination
  Norovirus and hepatitis A are considered priority pathogens by the WHO and FAO (Food and Agriculture Organization of United Nations). Increasingly hepatitis E is a pathogen that is assuming increasing importance.

Zoonotic food borne viruses
  Severe acute respiratory syndrome, monkey pox, and Nipah virus have been transmitted through various food-related incidents.

Parasites
Numerous parasites are transmitted by food including protozoa and helminths. However, some of these can also be transmitted by water, soil, or person to person contact. A wide variety of helminthic roundworms, tapeworms, and flukes are transmitted in foods, such as undercooked fish; crabs and mollusks; meat; raw aquatic plants, such as watercress; and raw vegetables contaminated by human feces.

Protozoa
  Cryptosporidium spp, *Giardia intestinalis, Cyclospora cayetenensis*, and *Toxoplasma gondii*

Roundworms
  Trichinella spp and *Anisakis* spp

Tapeworms
  Diphyllobothrium spp and *Taenia* spp

Chemicals and toxins
Insecticides used in crops, alcoholic beverages containing methanol, poisonous plants (eg, mushrooms, raw cassava roots), oysters, mussels, and clams (which ingest dinoflagellates producing saxitoxin), large reef fish (which ingest marine algae producing ciguatera toxin), finfish spoiled by bacteria leading to scombroid poisoning, and ingestion of puffer fish containing tetrodotoxin all can contribute to significant morbidity.

Vector Borne

Vector-borne diseases impose heavy economic and health burdens leaving many people who survive the infection permanently debilitated, disfigured, maimed, or blind. Vectors thrive in conditions where housing is poor, water is unsafe, and environment is contaminated with filth exacting their toll on the poor in developing countries **(Table 1)**.

Malaria is the vector-borne disease that causes the largest amount of morbidity and mortality. Dengue, yellow fever, and Zika are diseases that cause large outbreaks paralyzing health systems and contributing to considerable social and economic disruption. Onchocerciasis causes blindness, chikungunya severe arthritis, Japanese encephalitis permanent neurologic damage, Chagas heart failure and early death, and schistosomiasis poor nutritional status and school performance.

Other Tropical Diseases

Insect bites

Insect bites can cause problems and are venomous or nonvenomous. Venomous insects attack as a defense mechanism injecting painful toxic venom through their stings. Nonvenomous insects bite to feed on the blood of mammals (http://www.traveldoctor.co.uk/stings.htm).[8]

Snakebites and scorpion stings

Snakes are common in rural areas of tropical countries. Snakebites are a serious occupational hazard for agricultural laborers and fishermen. Generally, the two main families with maximum morbidity and mortality include Viperidae and Elapidae. Snakebites have now been included as a neglected tropical disease with one of the highest rates of mortality as demonstrated by the million deaths study.

Cancers

About 16% of cancers worldwide are caused by infectious agents in the developing world, and the most important cause after tobacco. If infections are controlled up to 1 in 10 cancers in the developing world can be prevented. Human papilloma virus is the most common infectious agent, followed by hepatitis B and Epstein-Barr virus contributing to cancers worldwide.

Table 1
List of common vectors and transmitted diseases

Vectors	Diseases Transmitted
Mosquitoes	
Aedes aegypti	Dengue, yellow fever, chikungunya, Zika
Aedes albopictus	Chikungunya, dengue, West Nile virus
Culex quinquefasciatus	Lymphatic filariasis
Anopheles spp	Malaria, lymphatic filariasis
Haemagogus spp	Yellow fever
Sandflies	Leishmaniasis
Triatomine bugs	Chagas disease
Ticks	Crimean-Congo hemorrhagic fever, tick-borne encephalitis, typhus, Lyme disease
Fleas	Plague, murine typhus
Flies	Human African trypanosomiasis, onchocerciasis

Malnutrition and related nutrient deficiencies

Protein energy malnutrition and micronutrient deficiencies of vitamins and minerals are common in tropical countries and these often contribute to delayed childhood growth and poor child health indices. Although universal immunization and nutrient supplementation at child care centers through mid-day meal schemes have played a major role in mitigating this problem, these are often encountered in many poverty-stricken or famine-ridden countries.

CLASSIFICATION OF TROPICAL DISEASES

Tropical diseases are classified as communicable and noncommunicable diseases. Communicable diseases by definition include diseases that are transmitted to humans and in turn are further classified as those caused by bacteria, viruses, protozoa, parasites, and fungi. Noncommunicable diseases are diseases caused by genetic and lifestyle factors, such as cancers, cardiovascular diseases, diabetes, and chronic respiratory diseases. In addition, snakebites, scorpion stings, and marine and terrestrial envenomations are also management dilemmas. It is important to note that because of constraints of poverty in the tropics, often unsafe food practices are condoned leading to high morbidity among individuals. Air and water pollution can lead to a myriad of respiratory, gastrointestinal, skin, and neurologic disorders along with serving as carriers of infectious pathogens. Although it is impossible to list all the causative pathogens of disease in the tropics, a syndromic approach and a region-wise probability of common tropical diseases is most helpful when dealing with a patient in the tropics or even a returned traveler.

Fever in the Tropics

Each area of the world is unique and endemic for specific tropical diseases. There is now through the Geosentinel network a large amount of data about the causes of fever in travelers in contrast with data from the tropical regions. Studies that are available use inconsistent definitions about "acute undifferentiated febrile illnesses" and diagnoses are not often confirmed. Fever in the tropics is often syndromic and in the absence of appropriate and accurate diagnostics, common diseases are vastly overdiagnosed, such as malaria in Africa and typhoid fever in South Asia. The advent of rapid diagnostic testing has led to the recognition of other important causes of acute febrile illnesses in the tropics (**Table 2**).

Neurologic Syndromes

Neurologic diseases in the tropics, although rare, are a cause of considerable morbidity and mortality. A history of travel including geographic locale and activities indulged in, possible exposures encountered, vaccines, prophylaxis and protective measures taken, along with the immune status of the host could help determine the etiologic organism of a particular neurologic syndrome. The neurologic syndromes are divided into global and focal syndromes (**Table 3**).

Dermatologic Syndromes

Skin lesions are a common problem in the tropics and they could be a primary problem or secondary to an underlying systemic condition. It is important to focus on infections that are treatable, transmissible, and have a high morbidity or mortality. The history must include details of previous travel, previous skin lesions, activities indulged in, immune status of the host, vaccinations, and prophylaxis. Exposures to fresh or sea water, animals, arthropods, plants, breaks in skin including tattoos, sexual activities, and

Table 2
Classification of common causes of fever by geographic area

Syndrome	Causative Pathogen	Disease	Region Where it Is Common
Acute undifferentiated fever	*Orientia tsutsugamushi*	Scrub typhus[13]	South and Southeast Asia North Asia Africa Oceania
	Plasmodium falciparum and *vivax*	Malaria[14]	Africa and the Middle east South and Southeast Asia Oceania South and Central America
	Dengue virus	Dengue	Southeast Asia India Oceania Central and South America Central Africa
	Leptospira spp	Leptospirosis[15]	Southeast Asia South and Central America Africa India
	Salmonella typhi	Typhoid fever[16]	South and Southeast Asia South Central Asia Oceania Africa
	Bartonella bacilliformis	Oroya fever	South America
Prolonged fever syndromes	*Burkholderia pseudomallei*	Melioidosis	Southeast Asia India Oceania Western Australia
	Brucella spp	Brucellosis	India Parts of Africa Mongolia Syria Peru Central America
	Leishmania donovani	Visceral leishmaniasis	India Africa South America
	Penicillium marneffei	Penicilliosis	Southeast Asia Southeast India
	Histoplasma capsulatum	Histoplasmosis	Southeast India Southeast Asia Parts of North America South and Central America
	Paracoccidiodes brasiliensis	Paracoccidiodomycosis	South America

Data from Refs.[13–16]

Table 3
Predominant neurologic syndromes and its clinical presentation

	Clinical Presentation	Etiologic Organism
Global syndromes	Febrile confusion or encephalopathy	Malaria, typhoid, scrub typhus, leptospirosis, dengue
	Meningitis	Streptococcus pneumoniae, Haemophilus
	Acute	influenzae, Neisseria meningitidis, herpes
	Chronic	simplex, Enterovirus, mumps, Naegleria fowleri Mycobacterium tuberculosis, Brucella, Treponema pallidum, Borrelia burgdoferi, Cryptococcus spp, Histoplasma capsulatum, Toxoplasma gondii, Taenia solium
	Encephalitis	Herpes simplex, Enterovirus 70,71, poliovirus, measles, varicella zoster, HIV, rabies, Lassa fever, Lyssa virus, Nipah, West Nile virus, Western equine encephalitis, Eastern equine encephalitis
	Cognitive decline	Subacute sclerosing panencephalitis, T pallidum, HIV
	Movement disorders	Streptococcus pyogenes, Japanese encephalitis, scrub typhus, rabies
Focal syndromes	Hemiparesis/seizures	T gondii, M tuberculosis, C neoformans, bacterial abscess, JC virus
	Paraparesis	Human T-cell lymphotropic virus type 1, HIV,
	Spastic	Campylobacter, lathyrism, polio
	Flaccid	
	Polyneuropathies	Diphtheria, snakebite, botulism

medications are important. Time of onset of skin lesions, their evolution, and associated symptoms, such as itching, pain, or fevers, are important clues to the diagnosis. Although tropics are often considered exotic locations skin problems can often be from cosmopolitan causes. Sunburn, scabies, and prickly heat are common and chronic skin problems, such as atopic dermatitis, may exacerbate in a tropical environment. Tropical biodiversity also results in a wide variety of plants and hence hypersensitivity to plants, plant products, and drugs may also occur. It is important not to forget mundane causes, such as pyoderma and folliculitis. Because skin manifestations are myriad a syndromic approach does help to narrow down a definite diagnosis (**Table 4**).

Diarrheal Syndromes

Diarrhea as a syndrome in the tropics has been described as "Montezuma's revenge" and "Delhi belly" because of the associated morbidity. It also is the second most important cause of child deaths younger than the age of 5 years contributing to almost 500,000. In the Global Burden of Disease Study[9] diarrhea was a leading cause of death among all ages contributing to 1.31 million deaths. Most of the deaths in children and adults were attributable to *Rotavirus*, *Shigella* spp, and *Salmonella* spp. However, deaths on the whole have been reduced by 20.8% from 2005 to 2015. In the Global Enteric Multicenter Study[10] done in children younger than age 5, interventions to reduce deaths should be directed against five pathogens: stable enterotoxigenic *E coli*, enteropathogenic *E coli*, *Cryptosporidium* spp, *Rotavirus*, and *Shigella* spp. Different clinical syndromes of diarrhea have been defined, each reflecting different etiology and pathogenesis. These are briefly described in **Tables 5** and **6**.

Table 4
Dermatologic syndromes and etiology

Syndrome	Important Points	Differential Diagnoses
Fever with rash	Duration of fever, associated symptoms, type and pattern of rash, exposure to sick contacts, mosquitoes, geographic area	Dengue fever, chikungunya, measles, rubella, mumps, typhoid, Katayama fever
Migratory rashes	Exposures, travel, and eosinophilia	Cutaneous larva migrans, gnathostomiasis, Larva currens
Fever with papules	Systemic symptoms, immunocompromise	Histoplasmosis, penicilliosis, nocardiosis, coccidiodomycosis, paracoccidiodomycosis
Nodules	Geographic locale, occupation, exposures	Myiasis, onchocercomas, cutaneous leishmaniasis
Vascular nodules	Immune status, exposure to brackish water and sandfly bites	Rhinosporidiosis, chronic bartonellosis
Ulcers, cutaneous and mucosal	Vaccination and nutrition status, exposures to cattle or pets, occupation, proximity to the jungle	Buruli ulcer, cutaneous leishmaniasis, cutaneous diphtheria, tropical ulcer, atypical mycobacteria, paracoccidiodomycosis, sporotrichosis
Eschars	Insect bites painful or painless, surrounding induration, exposures, systemic symptoms	Scrub typhus, anthrax, Loxosceles spider bite, trypanosomiasis, plague, tularemia, African tick typhus
Nodules with sinuses	Occupation, trauma, color of grains	Mycetoma, actinomycetoma, botryomycosis

DIAGNOSTIC CHALLENGES IN THE TROPICS

Various challenges exist in the diagnosis of tropical infections. The challenges are multiple and are divided as discussed next.

Disease Related

The burden of disease and the kind of setting where the disease is being diagnosed often determines the need of an appropriate diagnostic test. In a high-prevalence, low-resource setting a test that is low cost, point of care, requiring little technical expertise, with a high positive predictive value is required. In contrast in a low-prevalence, low-resource setting, additional tests may need to be performed to confirm the diagnosis. Subclinical and asymptomatic manifestations of a tropical disease may also make it difficult for a diagnostic test to distinguish between clinical disease and the former. In addition, if a test is serology-based in an endemic setting it may be difficult to establish causality for the clinical manifestations of the disease if baseline antibody titers is high.

Test Related

Although there are obvious infrastructural and financial challenges in low-resource settings there are also impediments with the lack of trained laboratory staff and quality assurance of available laboratory diagnostics. In addition, an ideal laboratory test needs to be rapid, point of care, requiring minimal technical expertise, following norms

Table 5
Etiologic classification of diarrhea based on stool appearance

Stool Appearance	Small Bowel	Large Bowel
Appearance and volume	Watery and large volume	Mucoid or bloody and small volume
pH and reducing substance	<5.5 and positive for reducing substances	>5.5 and negative for reducing substances
Serum and stool WBC	No bandemia and WBCs in stool <5/hpf	Bandemia and WBCs in stool >10/hpf
Organisms	*Rotavirus, Astrovirus, Calicivirus, Norovirus,* adenovirus	*Escherichia coli* (EIEC, EHEC), *Shigella, Salmonella, Campylobacter, Aeromonas, Yersinia, Plesiomonas*

Abbreviations: EHEC, Enterohaemorrhagic *E coli*; EIEC, Enteroinvasive *E coli*; hpf, high-powered field; WBC, white blood count.

of good clinical laboratory practice and health and safety measures in the workplace. The advent of molecular techniques has made this a reality and the need of the hour is an accurate rapid diagnostic test. Today the high burden diseases, such as tuberculosis, HIV infection, and malaria, all have rapid diagnostic tests, which has been a revolution with regard to appropriate case management of these diseases. A definite challenge has been to find similar easy diagnostic test strategies for diagnosis and epidemiologic surveillance for other tropical infections associated with high morbidity and mortality.

Table 6
Etiologic classification based on symptomatology

Symptoms and Signs	Pathophysiology	Possible Etiology
Large watery stools	Secretory small bowel	ETEC, EPEC, *Salmonella, Vibrio parahemolyticus*
Large volume watery	Enterotoxin mediated	*Vibrio cholera*, ETEC, *Cryptosporidium* spp
Many small volume stools	Large bowel irritation	*Shigella, Salmonella, Campylobacter, Yersinia enterocolitica, Entamoeba histolytica, Clostridium perfringens*
Tenesmus, fecal urgency, dysentery	Colitis	*E histolytica*, EIEC, EHEC, *Shigella, Campylobacter, Y enterocolitica, Clostridium difficile*
Diarrhea and vomiting	Toxin-mediated gastroenteritis	*Calicivirus, Rotavirus, Bacillus cereus, Staphylococcus aureus*
Fever and diarrhea	Mucosal invasion	*E histolytica*, EHEC, EIEC, *Shigella, Salmonella, C difficile, Campylobacter, Norovirus*
Persistent diarrhea	Secondary malabsorption, invasion	*Giardia, Cryptosporidium, E histolytica, Aeromonas, Isopsora belli, Microsporidium*

Abbreviations: EHEC, Enterohaemorrhagic *E coli*; EIEC, Enteroinvasive *E coli*; EPEC, Enteropathogenic *E coli*; ETEC, Enterotoxigenic *E coli*.

ACCESS TO MEDICINES

The WHO constitution dictates, "All people share the right to the highest attainable standard of health." Huge advances are being made toward internationally agreed global health targets, some of which include a reduction in child mortality by 50% between 1990 and 2013 and a 48% decline in AIDS related deaths since the peak of the HIV/AIDS epidemic in 2005 with at least half the infected people being able to access antiretroviral therapy. Many international agencies, such as the WHO and UNAID (Joint United Nations Programme on HIV/AIDS), pharmaceutical companies and Combating Antibiotic Resistant Bacteria Biopharmaceutical Accelerator and the Global Antibiotic Research and Development Partnership have incessantly campaigned for increased access to medicines leading to an achievement of many of the health-related millennium development goals.[11]

NEGLECTED TROPICAL DISEASES

Controlling, eliminating, and eradicating neglected tropical diseases has been a major focus for the WHO since 2003 as it moved away from specific diseases to the health needs of poor communities. Over the years many disease conditions that were believed to require a concerted effort by the WHO were included. These were identified as follows (**Table 7**)[12]

This has led the WHO to adopt five major strategies to combat these diseases:

1. Preventive chemotherapy: Optimum large-scale use of safe, single-dose medicines against four different helminthiasis: lymphatic filariasis, onchocerciasis, schistosomiasis, and soil-transmitted helminthiasis. Azithromycin administration for treatment of trachoma.
2. Intensified disease management: Improved case detection and decentralized clinical management of human African trypanosomiasis, Chagas disease, leishmaniasis, and Buruli ulcer.
3. Vector and intermediate host control: Integrated vector and intermediate host management uses efficient, ecologically sound, and sustainable interventions to control vector-borne and intermediate host-mediated neglected tropical diseases.
4. Veterinary public health at the human animal interface: An integrated human and animal health approach is required for such diseases as cysticercosis, echinococcosis, and rabies, which involve vertebrate hosts.
5. Provision of safe water, sanitation and hygiene: Better sanitation and improved safe water supply coupled with vector control is being looked at for long-term economic growth and food production.

Table 7
List of neglected tropical diseases – WHO 2017

Dengue	Rabies	Trachoma	Buruli ulcer
Yaws	Leprosy	Chagas disease	Echinococcosis
Human African trypanosomiasis		Cysticercosis	Schistosomiasis
Soil-transmitted helminths		Foodborne trematodiasis	Onchocerciasis
Lymphatic filariasis		Snakebite envenoming	Mycetoma
Chromoblastomycosis and other deep mycoses			Scabies

SUMMARY

Tropical medicine is an amalgamation of infectious and noninfectious diseases and deals with many important issues, such as water, hygiene, and sanitation, which is out of reach for many low- and middle-income tropical countries. As a result, the health indices for these countries often suffer necessitating global and local public health interventions. Research, development, global support, and funding along with access to major health interventions has empowered many of these countries to overcome the challenges faced by them while combating tropical diseases.

REFERENCES

1. Tropics. Available at: https://www.nationalgeographic.org/encyclopedia/tropics/. Accessed May 24, 2018.
2. 2014 Report. State of the Tropics. James Cook University. Available at: https://www.jcu.edu.au/state-of-the-tropics/publications/2014. Accessed May 24, 2018.
3. Forstinus NO, Ikechukwu NE, Emenike MP, et al. Water and waterborne diseases: a review. IJTDH 2016;12(4):1–14.
4. Kirk MD, Pires SM, Black RE, et al. World Health Organization estimates of the global and regional disease burden of 22 foodborne bacterial, protozoal, and viral diseases, 2010: a data synthesis. PLoS Med 2015;12(12): e1001921.
5. Torgerson PR, Devleesschauwer B, Praet N, et al. World Health Organization estimates of the global and regional disease burden of 11 foodborne parasitic diseases, 2010: a data synthesis. PLoS Med 2015;12(12):e1001920.
6. Addis M, Sisay D. A review on major food borne bacterial illnesses. J Trop Dis 2015;3:176.
7. Institute of Medicine. Improving food safety through a one health approach. Washington, DC: The National Academies Press; 2012.
8. Insect bites and stings. Available at: http://www.traveldoctor.co.uk/stings.htm. Accessed June 25, 2018.
9. GBD Diarrhoeal Diseases Collaborators. Estimates of global, regional, and national morbidity, mortality, and aetiologies of diarrhoeal diseases: a systematic analysis for the Global Burden of Disease Study 2015. Lancet Infect Dis 2017; 17:909–48.
10. Kotloff KL, Nataro JP, Blackwelder JC, et al. Burden and aetiology of diarrhoeal disease in infants and young children in developing countries (the Global Enteric Multicenter Study, GEMS): a prospective, case-control study. Lancet 2013;382: 209–22.
11. Access to Medicine index 2018 –methodology report. Available at: http://apps.who.int/medicinedocs/documents/s23336en/s23336en.pdf. Accessed June 25, 2018.
12. WHO. Accelerating work to overcome the global impact of neglected tropical diseases. A roadmap for implementation. Available at: www.who.int/neglected_diseases/en. Accessed June 25, 2018.
13. Xu G, Walker DH, Jupiter D, et al. A review of the global epidemiology of scrub typhus. PLoS Negl Trop Dis 2017;11(11):e0006062.
14. World malaria map. Available at: https://www.cdc.gov/malaria/travelers/about_maps.html. Accessed June 25, 2018.

15. Costa F, Hagan JE, Calcagno J, et al. Global morbidity and mortality of leptospirosis: a systematic review. PLoS Negl Trop Dis 2015;9(9):e0003898.
16. Mogasale V, Maskery B, Ochiai RL, et al. Burden of typhoid fever in low-income and middle-income countries: a systematic, literature-based update with risk-factor adjustment. Lancet Glob Health 2014;2:e570–80.

Venomous Bites, Stings, and Poisoning: An Update

David A. Warrell, DM, DSc, FRCP, FRCPE, FMedSci

KEYWORDS

- Snake bite • Lizard bite • Fish sting • Jellyfish sting • Seafood poisoning
- Scorpion sting • Spider bite • Antivenom

KEY POINTS

- Snakebite, largely an occupational disease of impoverished agricultural workers and their families in rural areas of tropical developing countries, causes more than 100,000 deaths each year and, among survivors, great physical and psychological morbidity.
- Serious clinical effects of snakebite envenoming include hemorrhage, shock, acute kidney injury, generalized rhabdomyolysis, descending paralysis, and local tissue damage for which the treatment is antivenom and supportive therapy.
- Invertebrate stings cause fatalities by anaphylaxis, secondary to acquired hypersensitivity (Hymenoptera, such as bees, wasps, and ants, and jellyfish); and by direct envenoming (scorpions, spiders, and jellyfish).
- Simple preventive techniques, such as wearing protective clothing, using a flashlight at night, and excluding venomous animals from sleeping quarters, are of paramount importance to reduce the risk of venomous bites and stings.
- Common and geographically widespread ciguatera, scombroid, and tetrodotoxic fish poisonings and paralytic and amnesic shellfish poisonings, are treated symptomatically and prevented by avoiding eating high-risk species and being aware of danger signals, such as red tides.

VENOMOUS SNAKES

Of the five families of snakes that contain species capable of envenoming humans, the Elapidae and Viperidae are by far the most important from the medical point of view. Elapidae include cobras, kraits, mambas, coral snakes, Austro-Oceanian snakes, and sea snakes (Laticauda and Hydrophiinae). Viperidae comprise old world vipers and adders (Viperinae) and pit vipers (rattlesnakes, moccasins, lance-headed vipers, mamushis, habus, and other Euro-Asian pit vipers). The less important groups are

No funding.
The author has nothing to disclose.
Nuffield Department of Clinical Medicine, University of Oxford, John Radcliffe Hospital, Headington, Oxford OX3 9DU, UK
E-mail address: david.warrell@ndm.ox.ac.uk

Infect Dis Clin N Am 33 (2019) 17–38
https://doi.org/10.1016/j.idc.2018.10.001
0891-5520/19/© 2018 Elsevier Inc. All rights reserved.

id.theclinics.com

Lamprophiidae (Atractaspidinae; African/Middle Eastern burrowing asps) and "Colubridae" (now divided; rear-fanged snakes).[1]

In most parts of the globe, except for some islands in the Caribbean, Eastern Mediterranean, and Eastern Pacific, venomous snakes are an environmental and occupational danger.

Importance and Epidemiology

In Brazil, 26,000 snakebites were reported in 2016, with 109 deaths. Well-designed surveys have estimated annual snakebite mortalities of 46,000 in India,[2] 6000 in Bangladesh,[3] and 400 in Sri Lanka.[4] Community-based studies in selected areas of Africa and Asia revealed incidences of snakebite mortality ranging from 4 to 162 per 100,000 population per year.[5] Global estimates of almost 3 million bites and up to 140,000 deaths per year have been suggested.[6] Many survivors suffer long-term physical and psychological sequelae. Most bites are inflicted on the legs or feet of agricultural workers or their families. It is an occupational and environmental disease. In India, where 97% of bites occurred in rural areas, the highest incidence of resulting mortality was among children aged 5 to 14 years old in whom it constituted 3% of all deaths in the country.[2] Bites by kraits in South Asia, spitting cobras in Africa, and mulga snakes in Australia are inflicted on people sleeping in their homes, especially on the ground.[7] Snake-bite was accepted by the World Health Organization as a category A neglected tropical disease in 2016, and was discussed at the World Health Assembly in 2018. It may cost more human lives than all other World Health Organization neglected tropical diseases put together. Its neglect has resulted from underestimation of its public health importance. In the rural areas of tropical developing countries in sub-Saharan Africa, Southern Asia, New Guinea, and the Amazon region of South America, access to conventional medical treatment in hospitals is hindered either by difficulties and delays in transporting the victim from remote areas or by a widespread preference for treatment by traditional (herbal) healers.[7] As a result, many patients die outside health care facilities (77% in India) and, therefore, are not recorded in official health ministry returns. In the United States there are less than seven deaths from snakebites each year and in Australia less than three.[8] Exotic species kept as pets are an increasing challenge for poisons centers in Western countries.[9]

Prevention

The risk of snakebite is easily reduced by simple common sense measures, such as wearing protective foot ware, using a light and prodding the ground with a stick after dark, sleeping on a raised bed or hammock or under a well tucked-in mosquito net,[10] avoiding notoriously snake-infested habitats, and being especially vigilant at night and after heavy rains and flooding.

Venom and Venom Apparatus

When a viper strikes its prey, the fangs are erected (**Fig. 1**) and compressor muscles squeeze venom from glands situated behind the eyes through venom ducts and venom canals in the fangs.[11] Elapid fangs are fixed. Snake venoms are composed of hundreds of proteins, polypeptides, and other compounds. Some of the enzymes are digestive hydrolases and other necrotoxins that cause local tissue damage in human bite victims, others (eg, thrombin-like, prothrombin activators) activate blood coagulation and release or enhance endogenous mediators, lowering blood pressure (kininogens, angiotensin-converting enzyme inhibitors, bradykinin-potentiating peptides). Neurotoxins block neuromuscular transmission presynaptically (eg, phospholipase A_2) or post-synaptically (eg, three-finger polypeptides), causing progressive

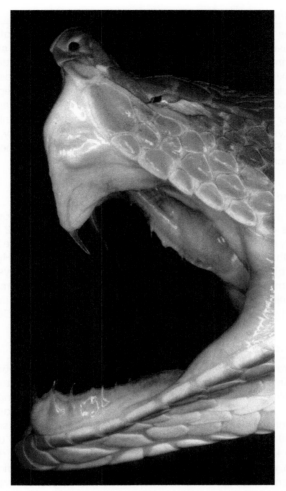

Fig. 1. Fangs of white-lipped green pit viper (*Trimeresurus albolabris*) in Thailand showing erectile fangs. (© 2018 David A. Warrell.)

descending paralysis. Phospholipase A_2 myotoxins cause local and generalized rhabdomyolysis.

Clinical Effects

Bite victims may present with symptoms attributable to their understandable anxiety (eg, tachycardia, sweating, dry mouth, hyperventilation leading to light-headedness, paresthesia, and carpopedal spasms), prehospital treatment (eg, effects of tourniquets, local incisions, suction, topical applications of herbs, chemicals), or to envenoming.[12] Depending on the particular species, between 10% and 80% of patients bitten by venomous snakes are not envenomed (dry bites).[13] Common local symptoms of envenoming include pain, swelling, tenderness and bruising that spread up the bitten limb, bleeding from bite marks, and tender enlargement of draining lymph glands. Systemic envenoming may be announced by nausea, vomiting, and syncope.

Elapid Envenoming

Most elapid bites cause mild or negligible local effects, but venoms of African spitting cobras and Asian cobras, spitting and nonspitting, can induce substantial local swelling, blistering, and necrosis of skin and subcutaneous tissues (**Fig. 2**).[14,15] Classic neurotoxic effects start as early as 15 minutes or as late as 10 hours after the bite. First evidence is bilateral ptosis and external ophthalmoplegia, progressing to descending paralysis affecting muscles innervated by other cranial nerves and eventually bulbar and respiratory muscles (**Fig. 3**). Australian-Oceanian land snakes can cause paralysis, bleeding/coagulation disturbances, myotoxicity, and acute kidney injury (AKI). Sea snake envenoming results in paralysis and generalized rhabdomyolysis complicated by AKI.

Viper, Adder, and Pit Viper Envenoming

Local effects of viperid venoms are generally more severe than those of elapids. If envenoming has occurred, local swelling is usually evident within 2 hours. Swelling and bruising may spread to affect the whole limb, trunk, and the whole body. Blistering may develop within hours and frank tissue necrosis in days (**Fig. 4**). Hypovolemia, hypotension, and bleeding/coagulation abnormalities are common. Systemic bleeding occurs from gums (**Fig. 5**); nose; gastrointestinal and urogenital tracts; lungs; and into the skin, conjunctivae, and brain. Neuromyotoxicity and AKI are common complications of bites by some species, such as Western Russell's viper (*Daboia russelii*).[16]

Laboratory Investigations

A blood count reveals neutrophil leukocytosis, and perhaps thrombocytopenia and anemia. The 20-minute whole-blood clotting test involves placing 2 to 3 mL of freshly drawn venous blood into a new, clean, dry, glass vessel and leaving it undisturbed for 20 minutes. Plastic and detergent-washed vessels do not activate clotting. Failure to clot indicates consumption coagulopathy (plasma fibrinogen concentration <0.5 g/L).[17] Rising serum potassium, creatinine, and urea define AKI. Raised creatine kinase, myoglobin, and potassium levels indicate rhabdomyolysis. Dark red, brown, or black urine may contain erythrocytes, hemoglobin, or myoglobin. Electrocardiogram (EKG) abnormalities include ST–T changes, atrioventricular block, and arrhythmias.

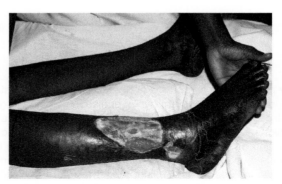

Fig. 2. Areas of superficial necrosis following a bite on the ankle by black-necked spitting cobra (*Naja nigricollis*) bite in Nigeria. (© 2018 David A. Warrell.)

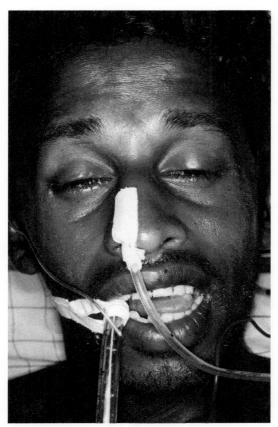

Fig. 3. Bilateral ptosis, external ophthalmoplegia, facial paralysis, inability to open the mouth, and respiratory paralysis in a man bitten by a common krait (*Bungarus caeruleus*) in Sri Lanka. (© 2018 David A. Warrell.)

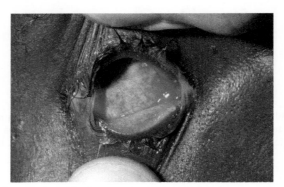

Fig. 4. Painful inflammation, blepharospasm, and leukorrhea caused by venom spat into the eye by a black-necked spitting cobra (*Naja nigricollis*) in Nigeria. (© 2018 David A. Warrell.)

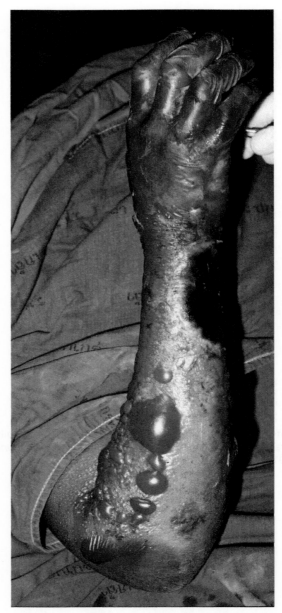

Fig. 5. Swelling, blistering, and severe local tissue destruction that required amputation 5 days after a bite on the wrist by a Malayan pit viper (*Calloselasma rhodostoma*) in Thailand. The patient presented late after being treated by an herbalist. (© 2018 David A. Warrell.)

Management of Snake Bite

First aid

Most traditional first aid methods have proved useless and harmful. Sound princi-ples are reassurance of the frightened victim, immobilization of the whole patient especially the bitten part, application of a pressure pad over the bite site, and urgent but safe transport to medical care. To delay systemic spread of venom toxins from the site of inoculation, local veins and lymphatics draining the site can be com-pressed with a pad of material approximately 6 × 6 × 3 cm, tightly bound directly over the bite site with an inelastic bandage. The bitten limb is immobilized by splint-ing. This is far simpler than the Sutherland compression bandage method and proved effective in a small field trial.[18] In transit to hospital, the patient should, ideally, be placed in the recovery position. Their airway should be guarded and respiration and blood pressure monitored.

Antivenom treatment

Antivenoms (antivenins, antisnakebite sera) are whole or enzyme-digested equine or ovine immunoglobulins that can specifically neutralize the circulating venom toxins against which they were raised. They can correct venom-induced coagulopathies, stop bleeding, and reverse shock and post-synaptic neurotoxicity. Polyspecific (polyvalent) antivenoms cover the venoms of the species of greatest medical impor-tance in a particular geographic area. Monospecific (monovalent) antivenoms are appropriate for areas where only one species exists (eg, adder *Vipera berus* in Scandinavia and parts of Western Europe) or for uncommon bites (eg, boomslang *Dispholidus typus* in Africa and keel-backs *Rhabdophis* sp in South East Asia and Japan). Sadly, these essential drugs are not available in many parts of Africa, Asia, New Guinea, and South America where they are most needed. Indications for antivenom include

1. Evidence of systemic envenoming (hypotension, other signs of cardiovascular toxicity, neurotoxicity, generalized myotoxicity, spontaneous systemic bleeding, uncoagulable blood), supported by peripheral leukocytosis (>20 × 10^9/L), elevated serum enzymes, hemoglobinuria, myoglobinuria, severe anemia/hemoconcentra-tion, uremia, or oliguria.
2. Massive local swelling (more than half of the bitten limb), bites on fingers or toes, and rapidly progressive swelling after bites by species known to cause necrosis.

Intradermal or conjunctival hypersensitivity tests to detect IgE-mediated anaphy-laxis do not predict antivenom reactions reliably and should not be used.

Subcutaneous epinephrine (adrenaline; adult dose 2.5 mL of 0.1% solution) given just before starting antivenom treatment reduces frequency and severity of early reactions.[19]

Antivenom must be given intravenously because it is poorly bioavailable by subcu-taneous or intramuscular routes. Dilution and rate of administration (over 10–60 mi-nutes) seem not to affect the incidence of early reactions.[20] Dosage, the same for children as adults, is usually based on rodent assays or judged empirically. The initial dose is repeated if blood coagulability is not restored after about 6 hours or if there is persistence or progression of shock or paralysis after 1 to 2 hours. Ideally, patients should be monitored for 2 to 3 days after antivenom to detect recurrent systemic enve-noming resulting from continued absorption of venom from the bite site depot or redis-tribution of venom toxins.[21] This has proved to be a particular problem with rapidly cleared Fab fragment antivenoms, such as CroFab, which is used for North American pit viper bites.[22]

Antivenom reactions

The risk of early anaphylactic or pyrogenic reactions, occurring within 10 to 180 minutes of administration, is dose-related and is higher with poorly refined antivenoms that contain complement-activating aggregates of IgG fragments or endotoxins acquired during manufacture. Rarely, patients who have been sensitized to equine/ovine proteins through previous exposure (eg, to equine antitetanus serum or rabies immune globulin) may develop IgE-mediated reactions. At the first sign of an early reaction, which may evolve with frightening speed, epinephrine (adrenaline) should be given intramuscularly (adults 0.5–1.0 mL; children 0.01 mL/kg; of 0.1% solution), together with other appropriate resuscitation.

There is also a dose-related risk of late serum-sickness-type reactions. Between 5 and 24 (mean, 7) days after antivenom, patients may develop fever, pruritus, urticaria, arthralgia with periarticular swellings, lymphadenopathy, mononeuritis multiplex, and albuminuria. Mild reactions may respond to oral histamine H_1 blockers (eg, chlorphenamine: adults 2 mg every 6 hours, children 0.25 mg/kg per day in divided doses), but a 5- to 7-day course of oral prednisolone (adults 5 mg every 6 hours, children 0.7 mg/kg per day in divided doses) is often needed to control the distressing symptoms.

Complicating Organ/System Failures: Supportive Treatment

Bulbar and respiratory paralysis

The risk of aspiration pneumonia, airway obstruction, and respiratory failure is prevented by careful monitoring. As soon as there is pooling of secretions in the pharynx or respiratory distress, a cuffed endotracheal tube or supraglottal airway is inserted. Some patients envenomed by snakes whose neurotoxins act post-synaptically (eg, cobras, Australian-Oceanian death adders *Acanthophis*) respond to anticholinesterase drugs, such as neostigmine, given with atropine to block unpleasant muscarinic side effects of acetylcholine.[23] Responsiveness may be tested by the tensilon test using edrophonium[24] or, more simply in patients with bilateral ptosis, by the ice-pack test.[25]

Cardiovascular disturbances

Hypotension and shock are treated with plasma expanders or vasoconstrictors. Hypotension associated with sinus bradycardia may respond to atropine and other dysrhythmias to appropriate antiarrhythmic drugs, such as verapamil, flecainide, or amiodarone.

Acute kidney injury

If conservative management of AKI fails, renal-replacement therapy or hemoperfusion is needed.

Bite wound infections

These occur in less than 5% of cases. The area of the bite may be hot, red, and tender because of inflammatory effects of the venom and so the term "cellulitis" is misleading. A large variety of bacteria (skin commensals, environmental, and from the snake's mouth) may infect snakebite wounds, but antibiotic prophylaxis is justified only if the wound has been interfered with or there is obvious necrosis. Otherwise, await signs of focal infection, such as an abscess. Aspirate and culture before prescribing. A routine tetanus toxoid booster is justified in all cases of snakebite.

Care of the bitten limb

Nurse the limb in the most comfortable position, avoiding excessive elevation that may increase the risk of intracompartmental ischemia. Blisters and bullae should be left intact to avoid increasing access to infection.

Surgical interventions
Necrotic tissue should be debrided and denuded areas covered with split-skin grafts. Compartment syndrome is grossly overdiagnosed in snakebite victims resulting in many unnecessary, disfiguring, and disabling fasciotomies. Before contemplating any surgery, normal hemostasis must be restored by antivenom and perhaps infusion of clotting factors. Before embarking on fasciotomy, intracompartmental pressure should be measured directly and monitored for at least 1 hour (**Fig. 6**). Only if pressures are sustained at a level that risks ischemic necrosis should fasciotomy be contemplated and, even in these rare cases, results are disappointing because of the underlying venom-induced necrosis.

Spitting elapid ophthalmia
Spitting cobras and the rinkhals (*Hemachatus haemachatus*) eject streams of venom from their fang tips toward the glittering eyes of perceived assailants.[26] Venom causes intensely painful chemical conjunctivitis, edema, and spasms of the eyelids, with profuse purulent secretions (**Fig. 7**). There is a risk of corneal erosion, hypopyon, anterior uveitis, secondary infections, and blindness. First aid treatment is irrigation of the eyes and affected oral/nasal mucosae with generous volumes of water, milk, urine or any other available bland fluid. Pain is relieved with topical anesthetics, such as tetracaine (with caution), or epinephrine/adrenaline (0.1% eye drops). Corneal abrasions are either excluded by fluorescein staining/slit-lamp examination or prevented with topical antimicrobials (eg, tetracycline, chloramphenicol, or fluoroquinolone).

VENOMOUS LIZARDS

Despite wild claims that the giant Komodo dragon (*Varanus komodoensis*) kills by venom rather than brute force, only two lizards are of proven medical importance, the Gila monster (*Heloderma suspectum*) of the south-western United States and

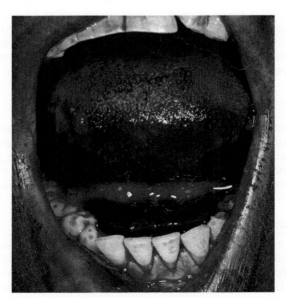

Fig. 6. Severe spontaneous bleeding from the gingival sulci and into the floor of the mouth in a patient bitten by a saw-scaled or carpet viper (*Echis ocellatus*) in Nigeria. (© 2018 David A. Warrell.)

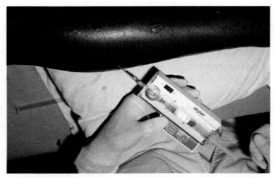

Fig. 7. Direct measurement of pressure in the anterior tibial compartment in a man bitten on the ankle by a puff adder (*Bitis arietans*) in South Africa. Despite the appearances of the tensely swollen, tender, and cold limb, the intracompartmental pressure is only 25 mm Hg. The patient did not require a fasciotomy. (© 2018 David A. Warrell.)

adjacent areas of Mexico and Mexican beaded lizards (*Heloderma horridum*) of western Mexico south to Guatemala.[27] Venom from submandibular glands is conducted along grooves in the lower teeth. It contains peptides, such as exendins-3 and -4, which are glucagon-like peptide-1 analogues that have been developed for treatment of type 2 diabetes mellitus.

Clinical Features and Treatment

Bites are rare and never unprovoked. The powerful jaws are difficulty to disengage. Severe local pain, tender swelling, and regional lymphadenopathy develop rapidly together with systemic symptoms, such as dizziness and hypotensive collapse, angioedema, sweating, rigors, tinnitus, nausea, and vomiting. Leukocytosis, coagulopathy, electrocardiographic changes, myocardial infarction, and AKI are described, but no fatalities are reliably reported. No antivenom is commercially available. Symptomatic treatment includes powerful analgesia, plasma expanders, and epinephrine (adrenaline) or pressor agents.

VENOMOUS FISH

Dangerous but only rarely fatal stings are inflicted by some marine sharks and dogfish, stingrays and mantas, catfish, weever fish, stargazers or stone-lifters, scorpion fish **(Fig. 8)**, stonefish, and lion fish and freshwater stingrays (*Potamotrygon* spp).[28–30] Their venom glands are embedded in grooves in the spines of fins or gill covers or, in the case of stingrays, beneath an integument covering the long barbed precaudal spines.

Incidence and Epidemiology

Each year, there are reports of weever fish (*Trachynis*) stings around the coasts of Britain and the Adriatic. In the United States there are an estimated 1500 stings by rays and 300 by scorpion fish each year. Stings by freshwater rays are common in the Amazon region. Lion, zebra, tiger, turkey, or red fire fish (*Pterois, Dendrochirus* spp) are popular with tropical aquarists whom they sometimes sting. Indo-Pacific *Pterois volitans* and *Pterois miles* have invaded southeastern coastal waters of the United States and Caribbean and the Eastern Mediterranean.

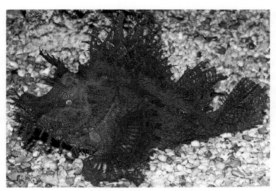

Fig. 8. Weedy scorpionfish (*Rhinopias frondosa*) from the Indian Ocean, capable of inflicting painful stings. (© 2018 David A. Warrell.)

Prevention

The greatest danger is stepping on a stinging fish while wading on the shore or near coral reefs. A shuffling gait, prodding with a stick, and footwear reduce the risk of stings except by stingrays. Divers and fishermen should avoid touching fish unnecessarily.

Venom Composition

Fish venoms contain thermolabile proteins and peptides, enzymes, vasoactive kinins, 5-hydroxytryptamine, histamine, and catecholamines.[31]

Clinical Features

Excruciating pain is associated with tender inflammatory swelling, necrosis, and the risk of secondary infection by marine *Vibrio vulnificus* or freshwater *Aeromonas hydrophila*. Long, barbed stingray spines, up to 30 cm long, lacerate and can penetrate the chest or abdomen, fatally damaging heart, lungs, or viscera as in the case of the famous Australian conservationist, Steve Irwin. Symptoms of systemic envenoming include nausea, vomiting, diarrhea, sweating, hypersalivation, cardiorespiratory disturbances, and generalized convulsions.

Treatment

Rescue the victim from the water, relieve the agonizing pain by immersing the stung part in hot water (<45°C), give supportive care for systemic envenoming, and remove any implanted venomous spines. Australian stonefish (*Synanceja*) antivenom (Seqirus, Melbourne, Australia) covers venoms of some other scorpion fish (Scorpionidae) including Californian *Scorpaena guttata*. Antibiotic treatment of suspected or proven *Vibrio* and *Aeromonas* infections should include doxycycline or cotrimoxazole.

SEAFOOD (FISH AND SHELLFISH) POISONING

Acute nausea, vomiting, abdominal colic, and diarrhea that develop within minutes or a few hours of eating fish or shellfish is more likely to be caused by marine toxins or allergy than bacterial or viral infections. There are two main clinical syndromes: gastroenteritis with neurotoxic symptoms (ciguatera and tetrodotoxic fish poisoning and neurotoxic and amnesic shellfish poisoning) and histamine-like (scombrotoxic) fish poisoning.

Ciguatera Fish Poisoning

This is the commonest cause of seafood poisoning with an estimated annual global incidence of 50,000 to 500,000 cases (case fatality ~0.1%).[32] It is underdiagnosed because of ignorance of its distinctive clinical features and lack of a diagnostic test. Climate change and destruction of coral reef systems have expanded its endemic area from tropical oceans (between ~25–40°N and 30–25°S) to more temperate waters and the increasing appetite for exotic fish in Western countries has led to many sporadic cases. Tropical reef fish, such as groupers, snappers, parrot fish, trigger fish, surgeonfish, mackerel, moray eels, barracudas, and jacks, are most often implicated. Ciguatoxins are polyethers that activate Na^+ or Ca^{2+} channels. Derived ultimately from bacteria in benthic dinoflagellates such as *Gambierdiscus toxicus*, they accumulate in the liver, viscera, and gonads of carnivorous fish at the end of the food chain.

Early symptoms are a burning sensation in the mouth or a metallic taste about 45 minutes after ingestion.[33] Symptoms of acute gastroenteritis follow after about 1 to 6 hours and may persist for a week. After about 24 hours, distinctive neurologic symptoms emerge: generalized pruritus, paresthesia around the mouth and extremities, pain in the teeth, reversed hot-cold sensation (cold allodynia or dysesthesia) especially of the extremities, weakness, ataxia, arthralgia, and myalgia. Neuropsychiatric symptoms may develop within days or weeks. Rarely, cardiovascular disturbances and rashes may occur. Usually, these symptoms last only a few hours, but they may persist for a week, months, or even up to a year as chronic ciguatera in about 5% of cases. Ciguatera-like symptoms after eating turtle flesh (chelonitoxism) are more severe, with higher case-fatality.[34]

Tetrodotoxic ("Fugu") Fish Poisoning

Scaleless puffer, porcupine (**Fig. 9**), toad, and sun fish (Tetraodonitiformes) may become highly poisonous at certain times of year. In Japan, puffer fish ("fugu") is particularly relished for its supposed medicinal properties and, despite stringent regulations, there are still about four deaths each year from tetrodotoxic poisoning. Tetrodotoxins are aminoperhydroquinazolines ultimately derived from *Pseudomonas* bacteria. They produce neurotoxic and cardiotoxic effects by blocking voltage-

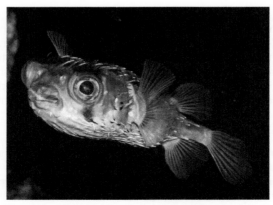

Fig. 9. Long-spined porcupine fish (*Diodon holacanthusa*), a tetrodotoxic fish (Diodontidae) that is extensively distributed in tropical oceans. (© 2018 David A. Warrell.)

gated Na^+ channels. They occur in ovaries, viscera, and skin of tetraodontiform fish but also in some amphibians, octopuses, mollusks, xanthid crabs, and other animals.

Clinical features include nausea and gastro-intestinal symptoms, together with neurotoxic symptoms that evolve within 10 to 45 minutes. Paresthesia of the lips, tongue, and throat, altered taste, dizziness, headache, sweating, hypersalivation, and ataxia are associated with ascending flaccid paralysis with fasciculations that lead to respiratory failure. Hypotension, cardiac bradyarrhythmia and tachyarrhythmia, exfoliative dermatitis, and other rashes are also described. Death occurs within 2 to 6 hours of eating the fish.

Neurotoxic and Paralytic Shellfish Poisoning

Thirty minutes after eating contaminated bivalve mollusks (mussels, clams, oysters, cockles, and scallops), patients develop gastroenteritis, chills, sweats, hypotension, arrhythmias, and ciguatera-like paresthesia, including cold allodynia, with myalgia, muscle spasms, vertigo, and ataxia.[35] Brevetoxins, derived from *Karenia brevis* dinoflagellates, cause harmful algal blooms, sometimes visible as red tides that kill off marine birds, mammals, and fish. In human beings, they cause neurotoxic shellfish poisoning. Symptoms usually last for a few days; paralysis, seizures, and coma are rare complications. However, tetrahydropurine neurotoxins, such as saxitoxin, and gonyautoxins from dinoflagellates, such as *Alexandrium*, *Pyrodinium*, and *Gymnodinium* spp that also produce red tides, can cause, within 12 hours, the descending paralysis of paralytic shellfish poisoning (fatality ~8% in untreated cases).

Amnesic Shellfish Poisoning

Within 24 hours of ingesting bivalve mollusks (scallops, razor clams) and crustaceans, symptoms of gastroenteritis may develop, but in about half the cases, neurotoxic symptoms, such as severe headache, short-term memory loss, agitation, seizures, and coma, may evolve within 48 hours. Amnesia may be permanent. Outbreaks have been reported from North America, Europe, and elsewhere. The causative toxin, domoic acid, is derived from *Pseudo-nitzschia* diatoms.

Histamine-Like (Scombrotoxic) Fish Poisoning

Bacterial decomposition of the histidine-rich dark flesh of scombroid fish (tuna, mackerel, bonito, skipjack) and canned nonscombroid fish (eg, sardines, pilchard) may be decomposed by bacteria releasing histamine and other toxins.[36] First contact of scombrotoxic fish with the lips, tongue, and mouth causes tingling or smarting, a timely warning. Within 20 to 30 minutes of ingestion, histamine-like symptoms may evolve: flushing, burning, sweating, urticaria, pruritis, headache, abdominal colic, nausea, vomiting, diarrhea, bronchial asthma, giddiness, and hypotension.

Treatment of Seafood Poisoning

There are no specific treatments or antidotes. General measures include elimination of gastrointestinal contents, but only if this can be achieved safely within 1 to 2 hours of ingestion, repeated dosing with activated charcoal to bind shellfish toxins to limit their enterohepatic circulation, parenteral fluid replacement, and assisted ventilation where necessary. The value of early mannitol (0.5–1.0 g/kg body weight intravenously over 30–45 minutes within 48–72 hours of exposure) in ciguatera fish poisoning is controversial, but is safe and often recommended.[37] For chronic ciguatera poisoning, amitriptyline and several other psychotropic drugs have been used. Scombroid symptoms respond to epinephrine (adrenaline), anti-H_1 histamine blockers, adrenergic β_2 agonist bronchodilators, and fluid replacement.

Prevention

Seafood toxins resist cooking. Avoid all scaleless fish as potentially tetrodotoxic, avoid very large tropical reef fish because they are more likely to be ciguatera-toxic, and eat only fresh fish to avoid scombroid poisoning. Never eat shellfish during dangerous seasons and red tides.

VENOMOUS MARINE INVERTEBRATES
Cnidarians (Coelenterates, Jellyfish, Portuguese Man O' War, Stinging Corals, Sea Anemones)

Cnidarian tentacles are armed with millions of explosive nematocysts (stinging capsules). Triggered by contact, they fire stinging hairs into the dermis to produce strings of painful, irritant weals.[28–30] Cnidarian venoms contain peptides, vasoactive amines, prostaglandins, kinins, digestive enzymes, and ion channel neurotoxins.[38]

Epidemiology

North Australian box jellyfish or sea wasps (*Chironex fleckeri*) and other cubomedusoids have been responsible for more than 100 recorded fatalities in the Australo-Indo-Pacific region. Portuguese man o' war (*Physalia* spp) and the Chinese jellyfish *Stomolophus nomurai* stings are rarely fatal. In northern Queensland, Florida, the Caribbean, and Thailand, stings by tiny (10 × 30 mm) cubomedusoids, such as Irukandji (*Carukia barnesi*) can be lethal. Stings by North Atlantic *Chrysaora quinquecirrha*, Pacific (*Chrysaora pacifica*) (**Fig. 10**), and Mediterranean *Pelagia noctiluca* are common.

Prevention

Avoid bathing or paddling when warning notices are displayed, or keep to "stinger-resistant" enclosures. Lycra, wetsuits, or nylon pantyhose protect against nematocyst stings. Those with a history of anaphylactic symptoms (eg, after *Physalia* stings) should carry self-injectable epinephrine (adrenaline).

Clinical features

Size and shape of weals may be diagnostic. Pain is immediate and severe. Chirodropid (genera *Chironex* and *Chiropsalmus*) envenoming causes rapidly evolving cough, gastrointestinal symptoms, rigors, myalgias, and profuse sweating that may progress to pulmonary edema, generalized convulsions and cardiorespiratory arrest. Irukandji syndrome comprises immediate severe musculoskeletal pain, delayed and persistent trembling, nausea, vomiting, anxiety, generalized sweating, headache, breathlessness, hypertension, raised troponin levels and EKG T-wave inversion, tachycardia,

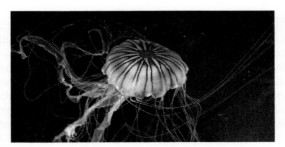

Fig. 10. Japanese sea nettle (*Chrysaora pacifica*), a common cause of jellyfish stings in the Pacific Ocean. (© 2018 David A. Warrell.)

and cardiac failure. *Physalia* envenoming causes vasospasm, nerve entrapment (eg, carpal tunnel syndrome), intravascular hemolysis, peripheral gangrene, and AKI. Those sensitized by previous stings may suffer anaphylaxis when stung again.

Treatment

Save victims from drowning and give cardiopulmonary resuscitation as required. Commercial vinegar or 3% to 10% aqueous acetic acid solution was believed to inactivate nematocysts of *Chironex fleckeri*, Irukandji, and other cubozoans, but this has been questioned. Shave off adherent tentacles using a razor. Hot water immersion relieves the pain of *Chironex* and *Physalia* stings.[39] A slurry of baking soda and water (50% wt/vol) is recommended for stings by *Chrysaora* species. *C fleckeri* antivenom is manufactured in Australia.

Echinodermata (Starfish and Sea Urchins)

Waders can easily impale their feet on echinoderms' long, sharp, venomous spines and grapples, leaving diagnostic blue/black staining at the site of sting. Pain, local swelling, and sometimes syncope, numbness, generalized paralysis, and cardiorespiratory arrest may occur. Penetration of bones and joints leads to secondary infection.

Treatment

Hot water immersion relieves pain. Spines should be removed after softening the skin, usually of the soles of the feet, with 2% salicylic acid ointment or acetone. No antivenoms are available. There is a risk of infection by marine bacteria.

VENOMOUS ARTHROPODS: INSECTS (HYMENOPTERA (BEES, WASPS, YELLOW JACKETS, HORNETS, ANTS)

A single sting by a hymenopteran insect, such as a bee (Apidae), wasp, yellow-jacket, or hornet (Vespidae) (**Fig. 11**), or ant (Formicidae) can cause rapid death from anaphylaxis in someone previously sensitized to its venom.[40] Multiple stings are damaging or even fatal through direct effects of large doses of venom even in unsensitized people. This happened during a recent epidemic of African killer bee attacks in the Americas.[41] Hymenopteran venoms contain amines causing pain and larger molecules that are potential allergens, such as phospholipases A, acid phosphomonoesterases, hyaluronidase, and polypeptide neurotoxins (apamin, melittin).

Epidemiology

Fewer than five people die from identified hymenopteran sting anaphylaxis in England and Wales each year, two to three per year in Australia, and 40 to 50 in the United

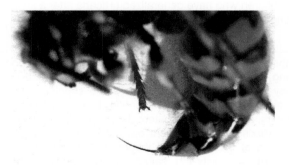

Fig. 11. European wasp (*Vespula germanica*) showing stinger. (© 2018 David A. Warrell.)

States where 4% of the population is susceptible to systemic allergic sting reactions. Beekeepers or their relatives have the highest risk of being sensitized. Imported South American fire ants (*Solenopsis* sp.) are estimated to sting about 2.5 million people each year in the United States, causing systemic allergic reactions in 4 per 100,000 population per year, some of which are fatal. In southern Australia and Tasmania, the prevalence of hypersensitivity to jack jumper ant (*Myrmecia pilosula*) venom is about 2% to 3%. Some reactions are fatal.

Prevention

A history of systemic anaphylaxis following a sting warrants testing for venom-specific IgE in blood (radioallergosorbent test) or by prick skin testing. Those who test positive should be considered for desensitization using purified venoms. After about 2 to 5 years of maintenance desensitization, more than 90% of subjects remain protected against systemic reactions after stopping treatment. Systemic reactions, including anaphylaxis, may complicate desensitization in 5% to 15% of patients. Local reactions are common but usually trivial. Where aggressive hymenopterans (hornets, bees, ants) pose a threat, their nests must be eradicated.

Clinical Features of Hymenopteran Hypersensitivity

Some patients develop purely local symptom each time they are stung. Painful, tender, inflammatory swelling progressing from the site of the sting and may involve the whole limb and persist for up to a week. However, there is a low risk of such people developing systemic (anaphylactic) reactions to subsequent stings. In a separate group of patients, a sting precipitates anaphylaxis: premonitory itching or tingling of scalp, axillae, or groins; flushing; dizziness; syncope; wheezing; abdominal colic (uterine colic in women), diarrhea, incontinence of urine and feces; and tachycardia and visual disturbances that may evolve rapidly within minutes of the sting. Signs include urticaria; angioedema of lips, gums, mouth, and tongue; generalized pruritic erythema with swelling; edema of the glottis; profound hypotension; and loss of consciousness. Deaths have occurred after only 2 minutes. Serum sickness may develop a week or more later. The risk of reactions is increased by β-blockers, ACE inhibitors, and cyclooxygenase-1 and -2 inhibitors.

Diagnosis of Anaphylaxis and Venom Hypersensitivity

Raised plasma mast-cell tryptase concentrations (peak at 0.5–1.5 h, last 6–8 h) confirm anaphylaxis. Detection of venom-specific IgE in serum (radioallergosorbent test) by skin testing or live sting challenge confirms type 1 hypersensitivity. Those who have suffered systemic anaphylaxis, have a 50% to 60% risk of a reacting to subsequent stings. Children who have generalized urticaria after a sting have only a 10% chance of reacting when stung again.

Treatment

Barbed bee stings must be removed immediately to prevent injection of more venom. Vespids can sting repeatedly. Ice packs and aspirin are effective in relieving pain. Wasp stings may become infected because some species feed on rotting meat. Massive local reactions may require histamine H_1 blocker, aspirin, nonsteroidal anti-inflammatory agents, and even corticosteroids.

Systemic anaphylaxis demands urgent epinephrine (adrenaline: adults, 0.5–1 mL; children, 0.01 mg/kg of 0.1% [1:1000]) intramuscularly into the anterolateral thigh. Adrenergic β_2 receptor agonists (eg, salbutamol) are given for bronchoconstriction. The roles of histamine H_1 blockers, such as chlorphenamine maleate (adults, 10 mg;

children, 0.2 mg/kg) and corticosteroids is uncertain. People with identified hypersensitivity should wear an identifying tag and must be trained to self-administer 0.1% epinephrine (adrenaline).

SCORPIONS (SCORPIONES: BUTHIDAE, HEMISCORPIIDAE)
Epidemiology

In Brazil in 2016, a total of 91,000 scorpion stings were reported, more than three times the number of snakebites, with 121 deaths, 12 more than from snakebite. Arizona reports 15,000 (mainly *Centruroides exilicauda/sculpturatus*) stings per year, with no fatalities since 1968. Among an estimated 250,000 stings per year by *Centruroides* sp in Mexico, deaths have decreased to 50 per year. In Tunisia, there are about 40,000 stings per year, 1000 hospital admissions, and 100 deaths from *Androctonus*, *Buthus*, and *Leiurus* sp stings. In Iran, *Androctonus* and *Buthus* sp, and especially *Hemiscorpius lepturus*, cause fatalities. In Maharashtra, India, stings by Konkan red scorpions (*Hottentota tamulus*) are common and may prove fatal in adults and children.

Prevention

Exclude scorpions from houses with a row of ceramic tiles at the base of outside walls, making the doorsteps at least 20 cm high, and by using residual insecticides (1% lindane or dieldrin) indoors.

Clinical Features

Many stings are excruciatingly painful. The exception is *H lepturus*, whose stings may be painless. Scorpion venom ion channel toxins release endogenous acetylcholine and catecholamines, producing early cholinergic and later adrenergic effects. Vomiting, profuse sweating, piloerection, alternating bradycardia and tachycardia, abdominal colic, diarrhea, incontinence, and priapism are followed by hypertension, shock, tachyarrhythmia and bradyarrhythmia, EKG evidence of myocarditis, and pulmonary edema. Neurotoxic effects (*Centruroides* sp) include erratic eye movements, fasciculations, muscle spasms that may be misinterpreted as tonic-clonic convulsions, and respiratory embarrassment. Ptosis and dysphagia are reported from *Parabuthus* envenoming (South and East Africa) (**Fig. 12**), thrombotic strokes from *Nebo hierichonticus* stings in the Middle East, acute pancreatitis from *Tityus trinitatis* in Trinidad, and local necrosis, hemolysis and AKI from *H lepturus*.

Treatment

The most effective analgesia is local anesthetic, administered by digital block in stings on fingers and toes. Antivenom has proved effective in Arizona and India.[42,43] Cardiovascular symptoms may respond to ancillary vasodilator treatment with prazosin (α_1-blocker).[44] Dobutamine is effective for left ventricular failure that evolves despite early prazosin therapy.[45]

SPIDERS (ARANEAE)

The danger of spider bites has been grossly exaggerated. Few species have proved to be of genuine medical importance.[46]

Epidemiology

In Brazil, there were 29,000 spider bites in 2016 with 22 deaths. *Loxosceles* sp (recluse spiders) (**Fig. 13**) cause frequent bites in Central and Southern America. In the south-central United States, brown recluse spider (*Loxosceles reclusa*) bites caused at least

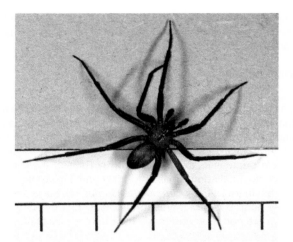

Fig. 12. Chilean recluse spider (*Loxosceles laeta*) from Brazil. This is the most dangerous species. (© 2018 David A. Warrell.)

six deaths during the last century. Most bites occur in bedrooms while people are asleep or dressing. Black and brown widow spiders (*Latrodectus* sp) are cosmopolitan in distribution. Rare fatalities have been reported in Australia (*Loxosceles hasselti*) and in the United States (*Loxosceles mactans*). Latin American banana spiders (*Phoneutria* sp) cause bites there and in temperate countries in imported bunches of bananas, causing a few bites and deaths. The Sydney funnel web spider (*Atrax robustus*), the most dangerous of all, is restricted to south-eastern Australia and Tasmania an area around Sydney.

Clinical Features

Necrotic araneism
Only *Loxosceles* sp have caused "necrotic araneism."[46] Bites are usually painless and pass unnoticed but, over several hours, burning pain evolves at the bite site, with swelling and appearance of the characteristic "red-white-and-blue sign," with a

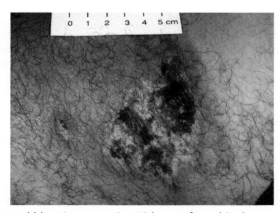

Fig. 13. Red-white-and-blue sign appearing 12 hours after a bite by a recluse spider (*Loxosceles gaucho*) in Brazil. (© 2018 David A. Warrell.)

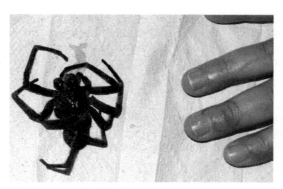

Fig. 14. Armed or wandering spider (*Phoneutria nigriventer*) from Brazil that bit a patient on her middle finger causing severe pain but no systemic symptoms. (© 2018 David A. Warrell.)

penumbra of red vasodilatation, an inner annulus of white vasoconstriction, and a cyanotic, prenecrotic center (**Fig. 14**). A blackened eschar develops, which sloughs in a few weeks, leaving a full thickness necrotic ulcer that may involve an entire limb or area of the face.

Visceral loxosclism affects
In 10% of cases there is fever, headache, scarlatiniform rash, jaundice, hemoglobinemia, and hemoglobinuria and AKI resulting from intravascular hemolysis and disseminated intravascular coagulation with a case fatality of about 5%.

Neurotoxic araneism
Bites by *Latrodectus*, *Phoneutria* (**Fig. 15**), and *Atrax* sp cause immediate pain with development of local sweating and piloerection (goose bumps). Painful regional

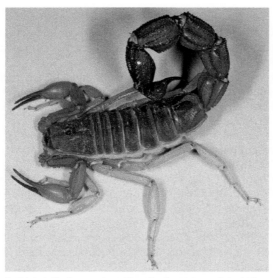

Fig. 15. Granulated thick-tailed scorpion (*Parabuthus granulatus*) from Southern Africa. (© 2018 David A. Warrell.)

lymphadenopathy, headache, nausea, vomiting, profuse generalized sweating, fever, tachycardia, hypertension, restlessness, irritability, psychosis, priapism, rhabdomyolysis, and diffuse rash may develop. Painful muscle spasms, tremors, and rigidity may affect the face and jaws (producing trismus) and abdominal muscles (simulating acute abdomen).

Treatment

First aid with pressure-immobilization (discussed previously) is recommended for rapidly developing funnel-web spider envenoming. Antivenoms against venoms of *Latrodectus* sp, *Atrax* sp, and *Phoneutria* sp are available.

SUMMARY

This article discusses the epidemiology, prevention, clinical features, and treatment of venomous bites by snakes, lizards, and spiders; stings by fish, jellyfish, echinoderms, insects, and scorpions; and poisoning by ingestion of fish, turtles, and shellfish.

WEB SITES

http://www.toxinology.com/. Accessed November 15, 2018.
http://globalcrisis.info/latestantivenom.htm. Accessed November 15, 2018.
http://www.toxinfo.org/antivenoms/. Accessed November 15, 2018.
http://www.who.int/bloodproducts/AntivenomGLrevWHO_TRS_1004_web_Annex_5.pdf?ua=1. Accessed November 15, 2018.
http://www.who.int/snakebites/resources/9789290231684/en/. Accessed November 15, 2018. African snakebite guidelines
http://apps.who.int/iris/handle/10665/249547. Accessed November 15, 2018. SE Asian Region snakebite guidelines
http://www.vapaguide.info/. Accessed November 15, 2018. VAPAGuide General advice

REFERENCES

1. Weinstein SA, Warrell DA, White J, et al. "Venomous" bites from non-venomous snakes: a critical analysis of risk and management of "colubrid" snake bites. Waltham Mass (MA): Elsevier; 2011.
2. Mohapatra B, Warrell DA, Suraweera W, et al. Snakebite mortality in India: a nationally representative mortality survey. PLoS Negl Trop Dis 2011;5(4):e1018.
3. Rahman R, Faiz MA, Selim S, et al. Annual incidence of snake bite in rural Bangladesh. PLoS Negl Trop Dis 2010;4(10):e860.
4. Ediriweera DS, Kasturiratne A, Pathmeswaran A, et al. Mapping the risk of snakebite in Sri Lanka: a national survey with geospatial analysis. PLoS Negl Trop Dis 2016;10(7):e0004813.
5. Sharma SK, Chappuis F, Jha N, et al. Impact of snake bites and determinants of fatal outcomes in southeastern Nepal. Am J Trop Med Hyg 2004;71(2):234–8.
6. Gutiérrez JM, Calvete JJ, Habib AG, et al. Snakebite envenoming. Nat Rev Dis Primers 2017;3:17063.
7. Ariaratnam CA, Sheriff MH, Theakston RD, et al. Distinctive epidemiologic and clinical features of common krait (*Bungarus caeruleus*) bites in Sri Lanka. Am J Trop Med Hyg 2008;79(3):458–62.
8. Schioldann E, Mahmood MA, Kyaw MM, et al. Why snakebite patients in Myanmar seek traditional healers despite availability of biomedical care at

hospitals? Community perspectives on reasons. PLoS Negl Trop Dis 2018;12(2): e0006299.

9. Warrell DA. Commissioned article: management of exotic snakebites. QJM 2009; 102(9):593–601.

10. Chappuis F, Sharma SK, Jha N, et al. Protection against snake bites by sleeping under a bed net in southeastern Nepal. Am J Trop Med Hyg 2007;77:197–9.

11. Mackessy SP, editor. Handbook of venoms and toxins of reptiles. Boca Raton (FL): CRC Press; 2010.

12. WHO AFRO. Available at: http://apps.who.int/iris/handle/10665/249547. Accessed November 15, 2018.

13. Naik BS. "Dry bite" in venomous snakes: a review. Toxicon 2017;133:63–7.

14. Warrell DA, Greenwood BM, Davidson NM, et al. Necrosis, haemorrhage and complement depletion following bites by the spitting cobra (*Naja nigricollis*). Q J Med 1976;45(177):1–22.

15. WHO SEARO. Available at: http://apps.who.int/iris/handle/10665/249547. Accessed November 15, 2018.

16. Phillips RE, Theakston RD, Warrell DA, et al. Paralysis, rhabdomyolysis and hae-molysis caused by bites of Russell's viper (*Vipera russelli pulchella*) in Sri Lanka: failure of Indian (Haffkine) antivenom. Q J Med 1988;68(257):691–715.5.

17. Sano-Martins IS, Fan HW, Castro SC, et al. Reliability of the simple 20 minute whole blood clotting test (WBCT20) as an indicator of low plasma fibrinogen concentration in patients envenomed by Bothrops snakes. Butantan Institute Antivenom Study Group. Toxicon 1994;32(9):1045–50.

18. Tun-Pe, Aye-Aye-Myint, Khin-Aye-Han, et al. Local compression pads as a first-aid measure for victims of bites by Russell's viper (*Daboia russelii siamensis*) in Myanmar. Trans R Soc Trop Med Hyg 1995;89:293–5.

19. de Silva HA, Pathmeswaran A, Ranasinha CD, et al. Low-dose adrenaline, prom-ethazine, and hydrocortisone in the prevention of acute adverse reactions to an-tivenom following snakebite: a randomised, double-blind, placebo-controlled trial. PLoS Med 2011;8(5):e1000435.

20. Isbister GK, Shahmy S, Mohamed F, et al. A randomised controlled trial of two infusion rates to decrease reactions to antivenom. PLoS One 2012;7(6):e38739.

21. Ho M, Warrell DA, Looareesuwan S, et al. Clinical significance of venom antigen levels in patients envenomed by the Malayan pit viper (*Calloselasma rhodos-toma*). Am J Trop Med Hyg 1986;35(3):579–87.

22. Boyer LV, Seifert SA, Clark RF, et al. Recurrent and persistent coagulopathy following pit viper envenomation. Arch Intern Med 1999;159(7):706–10.

23. Faiz MA, Ahsan MF, Ghose A, et al. Bites by the Monocled Cobra, *Naja kaouthia*, in Chittagong Division, Bangladesh: epidemiology, clinical features of envenom-ing and management of 70 identified cases. Am J Trop Med Hyg 2017;96(4): 876–84.

24. Watt G, Theakston RD, Hayes CG, et al. Positive response to edrophonium in pa-tients with neurotoxic envenoming by cobras (*Naja philippinensis*). A placebo-controlled study. N Engl J Med 1986;315(23):1444–8.

25. Sethi KD, Rivner MH, Swift TR. Ice pack test for myasthenia gravis. Neurology 1987;37(8):1383–5.

26. Chu ER, Weinstein SA, White J, et al. Venom ophthalmia caused by venoms of spitting elapid and other snakes: report of ten cases with review of epidemiology, clinical features, pathophysiology and management. Toxicon 2010;56:259–72.

27. Beck DD. Biology of Gila monster and beaded lizards. Berkeley (CA): University of California Press; 2005.

28. Halstead BW. Poisonous and venomous marine animals of the world. Princeton (NJ): Darwin Press; 1988.

29. Sutherland SK, Tibballs J. Australian animal toxins. The creatures, their toxins and care of the poisoned patient. 2nd edition. Melbourne (Australia): Oxford University Press; 2001.

30. Williamson JA, Fenner PJ, Burnett JW, et al, editors. Venomous and poisonous marine animals: a medical and biological handbook. Sydney (Australia): University of New South Wales Press; 1996.

31. Casewell NR, Visser JC, Baumann K, et al. The evolution of fangs, venom, and mimicry systems in blenny fishes. Curr Biol 2017;27(8):1184–91.

32. Friedman MA, Fernandez M, Backer LC, et al. An updated review of ciguatera fish poisoning: clinical, epidemiological, environmental, and public health management. Mar Drugs 2017;15(3) [pii:E72].

33. Bagnis RA, Kuberski T, Laugier S. Clinical observations on 3009 cases of ciguatera (fish poisoning) in the Southern Pacific. Am J Trop Med Hyg 1979;28: 1067–73.

34. Fussy A, Pommier P, Lumbroso C, et al. Chelonitoxism: new case reports in French Polynesia and review of the literature. Toxicon 2007;49(6):827–32.

35. James KJ, Carey B, O'Halloran J, et al. Shellfish toxicity: human health implications of marine algal toxins. Epidemiol Infect 2010;138(7):927–40.

36. Feng C, Teuber S, Gershwin ME. Histamine (scombroid) fish poisoning: a comprehensive review. Clin Rev Allergy Immunol 2016;50(1):64–9.

37. Mullins ME, Hoffman RS. Is mannitol the treatment of choice for patients with ciguatera fish poisoning? Clin Toxicol (Phila) 2017;55(9):947–55.

38. Jouiaei M, Yanagihara AA, Madio B, et al. Ancient venom systems: a review on cnidaria toxins. Toxins (Basel) 2015;7(6):2251–71.

39. Little M, Fitzpatrick R, Seymour J. Successful use of heat as first aid for tropical Australian jellyfish stings. Toxicon 2016;122:142–4.

40. Alfaya Arias T, Soriano Gómis V, Soto Mera T, et al. Key issues in Hymenoptera venom allergy: an update. J Investig Allergol Clin Immunol 2017;27(1):19–31.

41. França FO, Benvenuti LA, Fan HW, et al. Severe and fatal mass attacks by 'killer' bees (Africanized honey bees–Apis mellifera scutellata) in Brazil: clinicopathological studies with measurement of serum venom concentrations. Q J Med 1994;87(5):269–82.

42. Boyer LV, Theodorou AA, Berg RA, et al. Antivenoms for critically ill children with neurotoxicity from scorpion slings. N Engl J Med 2009;360:2090–8.

43. Natu VS, Kamerkar SB, Geeta K, et al. Efficacy of anti-scorpion venom serum over prazosin in the management of severe scorpion envenomation. J Postgrad Med 2010;56(4):275–80.

44. Bawaskar HS, Bawaskar PH. Management of the cardiovascular manifestations of poisoning by the Indian red scorpion (Mesobuthus tamulus). Br Heart J 1992;68:478–80.

45. Patil SN. A retrospective analysis of a rural set up experience with special reference to dobutamine in prazosin-resistant scorpion sting cases. J Assoc Physicians India 2009;57:301–4.

46. Isbister GK, White J, Currie BJ, et al. Spider bites: addressing mythology and poor evidence. Am J Trop Med Hyg 2005;72:361–4.

Malaria
What's New in the Management of Malaria?

Katherine Plewes, MSc, MD, DPhil, FRCPC[a,b], Stije J. Leopold, MD, PhD[a],
Hugh W.F. Kingston, BMBCh, MRCP, PhD[c,d],
Arjen M. Dondorp, MD, PhD[c,e,*]

KEYWORDS

- Malaria • Plasmodium • Management • Antimalarials • Resistance

KEY POINTS

- Intravenous artesunate for severe malaria and oral artemisinin-based combination therapies for uncomplicated malaria are first-line treatment for all *Plasmodium* species causing disease in humans.
- Species-specific diagnosis is important to guide appropriate primaquine administration for gametocytocidal treatment of falciparum malaria to reduce transmission in endemic areas, and for radical treatment of vivax and ovale malaria to prevent relapse.
- Severe malaria management requires early renal replacement therapy for acute kidney failure and cautious fluid resuscitation to prevent lethal pulmonary edema.
- Post-artesunate delayed-onset hemolysis of once-infected red blood cells is an expected consequence of the removal of pyknotic ring form parasites through splenic pitting after artesunate treatment.
- Artemisinin and partner drug resistant falciparum malaria is spreading in the Greater Mekong Subregion, and increasingly causes treatment failure of artemisinin-based combination therapies.

Disclosure Statement: The authors declare that they have no relationship with a commercial company that has a direct financial interest in subject matter or materials discussed in article or with a company making a competing product.
[a] Malaria Department, Mahidol Oxford Research Unit, Faculty of Tropical Medicine, Mahidol University, 3/F 60th, Anniversary Chalermprakiat Building, 420/6 Rajvithi Road, Bangkok 10400, Thailand; [b] Department of Medicine, University of British Columbia, Vancouver General Hospital, 452D Heather Pavilion East, 2733 Heather Street, Vancouver, British Columbia V5Z 3J5, Canada; [c] Nuffield Department of Clinical Medicine, University of Oxford, Old Road Campus, Headington, Oxford OX3 7BN, UK; [d] Malaria Department, Mahidol Oxford Research Unit, Faculty of Tropical Medicine, Mahidol University, 3/F 60th, Anniversary Chalermprakiat Building, 420/6 Rajvithi Road, Bangkok 10400, Thailand; [e] Mahidol-Oxford Tropical Medicine Research Unit (MORU), Faculty of Tropical Medicine, Mahidol University, 3/F 60th, Anniversary Chalermprakiat Building, 420/6 Rajvithi Road, Bangkok 10400, Thailand
* Corresponding author. Mahidol-Oxford Tropical Medicine Research Unit (MORU), Faculty of Tropical Medicine, Mahidol University, 3/F 60th, Anniversary Chalermprakiat Building, 420/6 Rajvithi Road, Bangkok 10400, Thailand.
E-mail address: Arjen@tropmedres.ac

Infect Dis Clin N Am 33 (2019) 39–60
https://doi.org/10.1016/j.idc.2018.10.002
id.theclinics.com
0891-5520/19/© 2018 Elsevier Inc. This is an open access article under the CC BY-NC-ND license
(http://creativecommons.org/licenses/by-nc-nd/4.0/).

INTRODUCTION

Malaria affected an estimated 216 million people causing 445,000 deaths in 2016.[1] This reduced burden of disease and death is a result of more than a century of worldwide effort and research aimed at improving prevention, diagnosis, and management of malaria.

Since the first description of a protozoan parasite causing malaria,[2] it is now recognized that 6 *Plasmodium* species cause infection in humans living in tropical and subtropical regions. *Plasmodium falciparum* and *Plasmodium vivax* cause the most infections worldwide with differing geographic distributions. The contribution of *Plasmodium malariae,* and sympatric species *Plasmodium ovale curtisi* and *Plasmodium ovale wallikeri* to the global burden of disease is low. The zoonotic *Plasmodium knowlesi*, jumping species from Macaque monkeys, is predominantly found in Southeast Asia. Molecular diagnostics have recently identified human cases of zoonotic *Plasmodium simium* and *Plasmodium cynomolgi*; however, the prevalence and clinical impact of these species are unclear.[3,4]

Plasmodium infections result in a spectrum of clinical effects, including asymptomatic parasitemia, uncomplicated malaria, severe malaria, and death. Severe and fatal malaria are predominantly caused by *P falciparum* principally due to endothelial cytoadherence causing sequestration of mature-staged infected red blood cells in vital organs. This results in microcirculatory obstruction and end-organ dysfunction. Although *P vivax* and *P knowlesi* infection can cause severe malaria,[5,6] cytoadherence-mediated sequestration has not been clearly observed. Understanding factors related to the infecting parasite species and host immunity is critical to optimizing treatment and preventing death. This review highlights recent developments in our understanding of malaria pathophysiology and the translation to new aspects of management.

DIAGNOSIS

Appropriate species-specific management of malaria requires early confirmation of the diagnosis. All febrile travelers, particularly visiting friend and relative travelers, returning from malaria-endemic areas should be considered to have malaria until proven otherwise. Febrile patients living in or recently immigrating from endemic regions should have malaria ruled out. The clinical features of severe and uncomplicated malaria are nonspecific; therefore, a parasitologic diagnosis is required by microscopy or a rapid diagnostic test (RDT). Regardless of species, a diagnosis of severe or uncomplicated malaria can be made based on specific diagnostic criteria (**Box 1**).

Microscopic analysis of stained thick and thin blood smears is the diagnostic reference standard. Thick-smear diagnosis allows sensitive parasitemia quantification (as low as 30 parasites per microliter), and thin-smear diagnosis permits speciation and prognostic assessment via parasite staging and proportion of pigment-containing neutrophils. In severe falciparum malaria, the presence of late-stage parasites and/ or more than 5% of neutrophils containing pigment predict poor outcomes.[7,8] In unstable transmission regions, nonimmune patients with signs of severity and low parasitemia may reflect a high sequestered parasite biomass and should not falsely reassure the treating physician.[8] A high parasitemia in the absence of signs of severity is associated with increased mortality. Large differences between the number of peripheral blood infected cells and number of sequestered infected cells may exist, such that rapid increases in parasitemia can occur in synchronous infections.[9] In regions of high transmission, diagnosis is challenging because partially immune parasitemic individuals are asymptomatic. RDTs detecting *P falciparum* histidine-rich protein 2

> **Box 1**
> **Diagnostic criteria for severe malaria**
>
> I. Falciparum malaria
>   Clinical criteria
>   - Prostration
>   - Convulsions (>2 within 24 hours)
>   - Coma (Glasgow Coma Scale <11 in adults or Blantyre Coma Scale <3 in children)
>   - Respiratory distress (acidotic breathing)
>   - Shock (capillary time ≥3s, with or without systolic blood pressure <80 mm Hg [adults], less than 70 mm Hg [children])
>   - Pulmonary edema (confirmed radiologically)
>   - Abnormal bleeding
>   - Jaundice
>   - Anuria
>   - Hemoglobinuria (blackwater)
>   - Repeated vomiting
>   Laboratory criteria
>   - Anemia (hemoglobin <70 g/L in adults, <50 g/L in children)
>   - Acidosis (base deficit >8 mEq/L or bicarbonate <15 mmol/L, or venous lactate >5 mM)
>   - Hypoglycemia (blood glucose <2.2 mmol/L or <40 mg/dL)
>   - Renal impairment (creatinine >265 μmol/L [3 mg/dL] or blood urea >20 mmol/L)
>   - Jaundice (bilirubin >50 μM [3 mg/dL] and parasite count >100,000/μL)
>   - Hyperparasitemia >10%
>
> II. Knowlesi malaria
>   Clinical criteria
>   - Criteria as per falciparum malaria
>   - Inability to tolerate oral therapy
>   Laboratory criteria
>   - Criteria as per falciparum malaria with modified parasitemia cutoffs as follows
>   - Jaundice and parasitemia >20,000/μL
>   - Parasitemia >100,000/μL
>
> III. Vivax malaria
>   - Criteria as per falciparum malaria excluding parasite density thresholds
>
> *Data from* World Health Organization. Severe malaria. Trop Med Int Health 2014;19 Suppl 1:7–131.

(PfHRP2) have a detection threshold of approximately 200 parasites per microliter but new ultrasensitive PfHRP2 RDTs can detect parasitemias as low as 2 to 4 parasites per microliter.[10] However, PfHRP2-based RDTs are not quantitative, remain positive for up to 1 month, exhibit prozone effect at high parasitemias, and may be falsely negative in individuals with PfHRP2 gene deletions, which is reported mainly from South America as well as increasingly from Africa.[11–14]

In Southeast Asia, speciation may be challenging, as young ring stages of *P knowlesi*, *P falciparum*, and *P vivax* look similar, whereas mature trophozoites of *P knowlesi* and *P malariae* also may be confused. In Africa, *P vivax* is sporadically being diagnosed in Duffy-negative populations, suggesting alternative mechanisms of red blood cell invasion.[15] In absence of a peripheral blood smear, an RDT with a panspecific or species-specific lactate dehydrogenase (pLDH) or aldolase is required for diagnosing nonfalciparum infections. In high resourced regions, diagnosis by polymerase chain reaction should be pursued for accurate species-specific diagnosis and treatment of exported malaria, particularly from Africa and Southeast Asia.

CASE MANAGEMENT

Uncomplicated falciparum malaria can progress rapidly to severe disease and death, particularly in nonimmune individuals. Physicians must be alert to the fact that decreasing transmission in Africa will result in older age groups being at risk for severe malaria as premunition (protection from disease despite presence of peripheral blood parasites) is lost (**Fig. 1**). Thus, it is important that a malaria diagnosis is made soon after onset of malaria symptoms and antimalarial treatment started without delay. If severe malaria is suspected, particularly in high-risk groups, but parasitologic diagnosis is delayed antimalarial treatment should be started immediately. Treatment requires combination therapy with at least 2 effective antimalarials with different mechanisms of action to prevent drug resistance. Antimalarial dosing must be weight-based to ensure necessary drug concentrations; population specific age-based derived schedules can be more practical to implement. Goals of care are to prevent progression of disease and death by ensuring rapid clinical cure and parasite clearance. In malaria-endemic regions, treatment also aims to reduce transmission of a treated infection. In low transmission areas additional gametocytocidal therapy is added to further reduce transmission potential. In malaria caused by P vivax or P ovale, additional hypnozoitocidal therapy is indicated to prevent relapse infection.

SEVERE MALARIA

Severe malaria is mainly caused by P falciparum, but also observed in P vivax and P knowlesi infections. It is rarely seen with the other Plasmodium species. Severe malaria caused by any Plasmodium species is a medical emergency requiring prompt administration of an effective antimalarial and supportive management, ideally in an intensive care unit. In resource-limited settings, transfer to higher-level facilities should be considered if mechanical ventilation, renal replacement therapy (RRT) or hemodynamic monitoring are required. Mortality from severe malaria is still 10% to 20% despite optimal treatment and reaches 100% if left untreated.[16,17] Mortality in pregnant women is approximately 50%. Coma, kidney dysfunction and acidosis independently predict mortality in both non-pregnant adults and children with severe falciparum malaria.[18–20] Severe malaria is more likely in pregnant women in the second and third trimesters compared to other adults and is more often complicated by pulmonary edema and hypoglycemia. Severe knowlesi malaria is associated with hyperparasitemia due to its 24-h erythrocytic cycle, shock, acute kidney injury (AKI) and respiratory failure.[21,22] Severe vivax malaria is most commonly associated with respiratory failure, AKI and severe anemia.[23]

Antimalarials

Immediate antimalarial treatment

Intravenous artesunate is first-line treatment for severe malaria worldwide caused by any Plasmodium species. All adults and children with severe malaria, including infants, lactating women, and pregnant women in all trimesters should receive intravenous artesunate for at least 24 hours until oral medication is tolerated (**Box 2**).[17] Two landmark randomized controlled trials (RCTs) showed that intravenous artesunate is superior to intravenous quinine, reducing mortality by 35% (95% CI 18.5–47.6) in Southeast Asian adults and by 22% (95% CI 8.1–36.9) in African children.[24,25] Artesunate is well-tolerated and rapidly metabolized to its active metabolite dihydroartemisinin, reaching peak concentrations within 10 minutes and is rapidly eliminated (half-life 45 minutes).[26] It has broad stage specificity, killing young circulating ring-staged parasites up to late-staged sequestered parasites (**Fig. 2**).[9,27] This activity against circulating ring-

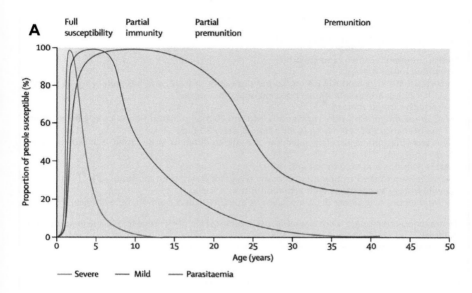

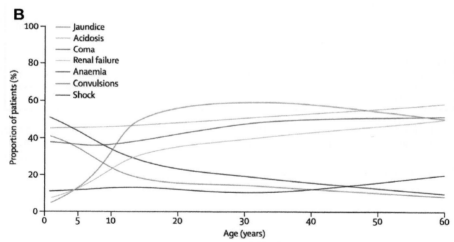

Fig. 1. Relationship between age and malaria severity in moderate transmission intensity regions. (*A*) Repeated exposures lead to acquired protection against severe malaria then against illness from malaria then in adulthood protective against microscopy-detected parasitemia.[18] With decreasing transmission intensity protection against illness and parasitemia (*blue* and *green curves*) will be lost and older age groups will be at risk of severe disease (*red curve shifting to right*). (*B*) Manifestations of severe falciparum by age in unstable transmission regions. (*From* White NJ, Pukrittayakamee S, Hien TT, Faiz MA, Mokuolu OA, Dondorp AM. Malaria. Lancet 2014; 383:723-35. *Reprinted* with permission from Elsevier (The Lancet, 2014; 383:723–35)

stage parasites is considered its critical advantage over quinine, as artesunate kills parasites before they can mature and sequester in the microvasculature.[28] Quinine has more adverse drug effects, including hypoglycemia, hyperinsulinemia, cardiotoxicity, and hypotension, particularly if given as a rapid injection rather than infusion.[23] Artemether showed a smaller survival benefit than does artesunate, likely due to its

> **Box 2**
> **Antimalarial treatment of severe malaria**
>
> Adults, pregnant women, and children
>   First-line initial therapy
>   • Artesunate intravenously 2.4 mg/kg per dose at hour 0, 12, and 24, then every 24 hours[a]
>   ○ If <20 kg: artesunate intravenous 3.0 mg/kg per dose
>   Alternative initial therapy
>   • Quinine dihydrochloride intravenous infusion 20 mg/kg loading dose (over 4 hours) then
>   maintenance dose 10 mg/kg (over 2 hours) every 8 hours[b]
>   • Artemether intramuscular[c] injection 3.2 mg/kg loading dose, then 1.6 mg/kg every
>   24 hours
>   After 24 hours and able to eat and drink[d]
>   • Artemisinin-based combination therapy orally for 3 days (not mefloquine[e])
>   Travel history to countries with artemisinin resistance
>   • Intravenous artesunate PLUS intravenous quinine (expert opinion, no evidence)
>
> If intravenous artesunate is not available, use artemether in preference to quinine in adults and
> children.
>   [a] Artesunate dose does not need to be adjusted if renal impairment or liver dysfunction
> present.
>   [b] Quinine requires dose adjustment according to renal dysfunction after 48 hours of full
> dosage. Dose adjustments are not required if receiving dialysis but quinine should be given
> post-RRT dosing if on dialysis.
>   [c] Intramuscular injections administered to anterior thigh.
>   [d] See uncomplicated malaria treatment (see **Box 3**) for oral artemisinin-based combination
> therapy options and alternatives.
>   [e] Mefloquine increases risk of postmalaria neurologic syndrome and is contraindicated in pa-
> tients with epilepsy or neuropsychiatric disorders.
>   *Data from* World Health Organization guidelines for the treatment of malaria. 3rd edition.
> 2015. Available at: http://www.who.int/malaria/publications/atoz/9789241549127/en/. Accessed
> April 24, 2017.

erratic intramuscular absorption.[29] Pre-referral rectal formulated artesunate given to severely ill children younger than 6 unable to take oral medications may reduce mortality.[30] Parasite clearance with artesunate typically occurs within 72 hours and should be documented by assessing thick and thin smears every 6 to 12 hours.

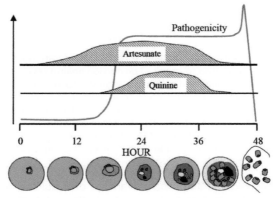

Fig. 2. Stage of parasite development and pathogenicity with rough estimates of stage specificity and "time windows" of antimalarial drug effects. (*Adapted from* White NJ, Krishna S. Treatment of malaria: some considerations and limitations of the current methods of assessment. Trans R Soc Trop Med Hyg 1989;83:767–77; with permission.)

Follow-on antimalarial treatment

After a minimum of 24 hours of intravenous antimalarial treatment and when oral medication can be tolerated, treatment must be completed with an effective, full course of an oral artemisinin-cased combination therapy (ACT) (**Box 3**). If an ACT is not available, then a non-ACT regimen can be used. Mefloquine should not be given as

---

Box 3
Antimalarial oral treatment of uncomplicated malaria

Uncomplicated *Plasmodium falciparum*, and *Plasmodium knowlesi* malaria
Artemisinin-based combination therapy (ACT): 3-day regimens
- Artemether-lumefantrine (1.4–4.4/10–16 mg/kg) by mouth (PO) twice daily x 3 days (with fat-containing food)**
- Dihydroartemisinin-piperaquine (4/18 mg/kg) PO daily for 3 days
  - If <25 kg: Dihydroartemisinin 4 (2.5–10) mg/kg and Piperaquine 24 (20–32) mg/kg PO daily for 3 days
- Artesunate (4 mg/kg) plus mefloquine (8 mg/kg) PO daily for 3 days[a]
- Artesunate (4 mg/kg) plus amodiaquine (10 mg/kg) PO daily for 3 days[a]
- Artesunate (4 mg/kg) PO daily for 3 days plus single-dose sulfadoxine-pyrimethamine (25/1.25 mg/kg)[b]

ACT: 7-day regimens
- Artesunate (2 mg/kg) PO daily plus tetracycline (4 mg/kg) PO every 6 hours for 7 days[c]
- Artesunate (2 mg/kg) PO daily plus doxycycline 100 mg PO twice daily for 7 days[c]
- Artesunate (2 mg/kg) PO daily plus clindamycin (20mg/kg) PO divided 2 times daily for 7 days[d]

Non-ACT regimens
- Atovaquone-proguanil (15/6 mg/kg) PO daily for 3 days
- Quinine (10 mg/kg) plus EITHER tetracycline OR doxycycline OR clindamycin for 7 days[c,d]

Uncomplicated *P falciparum*, and travel to countries with artemisinin resistance[f]
- Atovaquone-proguanil (15/6 mg/kg) PO daily for 3 days
- Quinine (10 mg/kg) plus EITHER tetracycline OR doxycycline OR clindamycin for 7 days[c,d]

Uncomplicated chloroquine-sensitive *Plasmodium vivax*, *Plasmodium ovale*, or *Plasmodium malariae*[e]
- Chloroquine (10 mg base/kg) per day at hour 0 and hour 24 then 5 mg base/kg at hour 48

Uncomplicated chloroquine-resistant *P. vivax*[e]
- Oral ACT (except sulfadoxine-pyrimethamine) for 3 days
- Quinine (10 mg/kg) plus EITHER tetracycline OR doxycycline OR clindamycin for 7 days[c,d]

[a] World Health Organization prequalified fixed-dose tablets preferable to loose tablets.
[b] Chloroquine-resistant *P vivax can be* treated with any oral ACT *except* artesunate plus sulfadoxine-pyrimethamine.
[c] Doxycycline preferred, as it does not accumulate in renal failure and it can be dosed daily. Contraindicated in children younger than 8 years and pregnant/lactating women (Class D).
[d] Recommended in first-trimester pregnant women.
[e] *P vivax* and *P ovale* should be followed by a course of primaquine for radical cure to prevent relapse. Contraindicated if glucose-6-phosphate-dehydrogenase deficient, pregnant or age younger than 6 months. Primaquine 0.5 mg base/kg daily for 14 days (G6PD normal; East Asia and Oceania); Primaquine 0.25 mg base/kg daily for 14 days (G6PD normal; elsewhere) or 0.75 mg base/kg weekly for 8 weeks (G6PD deficient).
[f] Admit patient, monitor clinical and parasitologic response until recovery or parasite clearance, follow-up at 4 weeks to ensure cure.
** Number of tablets per dose according to pre- defined weight bands (5–14 kg: 1 tablet; 15–24 kg: 2 tablets; 25–34 kg: 3 tablets; and > 34 kg: 4 tablets) given twice a day for 3 days.
Data from World Health Organization Guidelines for the treatment of malaria. 3rd edition. 2015. Available at: http://www.who.int/malaria/publications/atoz/9789241549127/en/. Accessed April 24, 2017.

follow-on treatment if impaired consciousness was present at diagnosis due to the increased risk of neuropsychiatric complications. In returning travelers, follow-on anti-malarial medication should be different from any prophylactic drug used during travel. In severe vivax malaria, a full course of radical treatment with primaquine should also be given after recovery.

Cerebral Malaria and Convulsions

Cerebral malaria is a clinical malaria syndrome of impaired consciousness character-ized by unrousable coma, as defined in **Box 1**, in the absence of hypoglycemia, convul-sions, sedative drugs, and nonmalarial meningoencephalitis. Generalized convulsions are observed in approximately 80% of children and 15% of adults and may progress to status epilepticus and coma.[24,25] Blood cultures should be drawn and glucose should be checked 4-hourly, especially if there is a decline in the coma score. Hypoglycemia is more frequent in children, pregnant women, and patients receiving quinine. In comatose children with suspected cerebral malaria, lumbar puncture does not increase mortality even when swelling on MRI brain or papilledema is present.[31] Funduscopic examination for malaria retinopathy is specific, but not highly sensitive, for the diagnosis of cerebral malaria and is prognostic in patients with severe malaria.[32,33] Patients should be posi-tioned in the lateral recovery position, alternating sides every 2 hours.[23] A large random-ized controlled trial is currently being conducted to assess whether recovery positioning in acutely comatose adults decreases aspiration pneumonia and improves outcomes (ClinicalTrials.gov NCT02427633). An oropharyngeal airway may be sufficient and/or bridge until endotracheal intubation is possible if the patient cannot maintain a patent airway. Nasogastric tube with suction may protect from aspiration but it should be clearly communicated to avoid early enteral feeding because feeding within 60 hours is associated with an increased risk of aspiration pneumonia.[34]

Supportive therapies include glucose and acetaminophen to maintain euglycemia and fever control. Mannitol administration to reduce intracranial pressure in patients is not recommended.[17] An RCT of a single dose of mannitol in children with cerebral malaria found no impact on clinical outcomes compared with placebo.[35] In adults with cerebral malaria and brain swelling on computed tomography imaging, mannitol pro-longed coma recovery time compared with controls not receiving mannitol.[36] RCTs of dexamethasone to reduce vasogenic edema in adults[37] and children[38] found no benefit on coma recovery or survival and is therefore not recommended. Corticoste-roids increase the risk for gastrointestinal bleeding, seizures, and prolonged coma res-olution times compared with placebo. Seizure prophylaxis with phenobarbital or fosphenytoin has not shown to be beneficial in preventing seizures, where the former was associated with increased mortality likely due to respiratory depression.[39–41] Therefore, routine seizure prophylaxis is currently not recommended in patients with seizures or cerebral malaria. Witnessed seizures should be treated with up to 2 doses of a benzodiazepine 10 minutes apart with careful respiratory monitoring. Recurrent seizures likely indicate status epilepticus and should be treated with phenytoin or phenobarbital loading, then maintenance dosing in a highly monitored setting.

Shock, Dehydration, and Acidosis

Fluid management is a critical but challenging intervention in the management of se-vere malaria. Patients present at differing times during their infections with variable de-grees of hypovolemia, acidosis, and AKI. Most adult patients have a stable blood pressure in the low-normal range. Thus, fluid therapy should be individualized, as adult patients are at risk of developing pulmonary capillary leakage and subsequent acute respiratory distress syndrome (ARDS), particularly if excess fluids are administered too rapidly. However, ARDS can develop after admission unpredictably and irrespective of fluid administration. In a study of Bangladeshi adults, 70% of patients were hypovolemic at the time ARDS developed.[42] Clinical assessment and invasive hemodynamic monitoring at admission do not necessarily reflect effective circulating blood volume nor predict fluid responsiveness or ARDS.[42–44] Further, correction of fluid deficits has not been shown to improve acidosis or AKI and increases the incidence of ARDS. This is likely due to the sequestration with subsequent microvascular obstruction and tissue hypoperfusion driving the acidosis and acute tubular injury that is not corrected by fluid loading. Aggressive fluid resuscitation in pediatric patients with compensated hemodynamic shock is also harmful. A landmark multinational study in African children with severe febrile illness and compensated shock showed a relative risk for death of 1.45 (95% CI 1.13–1.86; $P = .003$), with fluid bolus therapy (20 or 40 mL/kg of 0.9% saline or 5% albumin).[45] The case fatality rate of the 1793 children with a positive malaria slide was 9.2% with fluid bolus therapy compared with 5.8% in the control group (relative risk for death of 1.59; 95% CI 1.10–2.31). The increased mortality was suggested to be due to cardiovascular collapse rather than fluid overload in a retrospective analysis.[46]

Hemodynamic shock is not common on admission in severe malaria (approximately 16% of adults and 12% of children) and should prompt investigation for an alternative cause of the septic syndrome.[24,25] Concomitant bacteremia is observed in 6% to 13% of children and adults with malaria, and is frequently associated with increased mortality.[47–49] The incidence of bacteremia is likely underestimated due to minimal microbiological diagnostics and frequent preadmission antibiotic use in resource-limited settings. Gram-negative organisms are most commonly isolated, particularly nontyphoidal *Salmonella*, followed by *Streptococcus pneumoniae* and *Staphylococcus aureus*.[47–49] Gram-negative bacteremia complicating malaria is thought to be due to intestinal translocation from sequestration-mediated increased gut permeability, along with macrophage and neutrophil dysfunction.[47,50,51] Shock and leukocytosis are frequently associated with concomitant bacteremia in malaria; however, there is no reliable clinical or laboratory predictor. The metabolic acidosis in severe malaria is predominantly due to lactic acid from sequestration-induced tissue hypoxia. However, hydroxyphenyllactic and other gut-derived microbial acids are also elevated and predictive of mortality (ClinicalTrials.gov NCT02451904).[52] Thus, loss of gut integrity likely contributes to acidosis and gram-negative bacteremia in severe malaria; whether these gut-derived acids are predictive biomarkers of bacteremia is yet to be determined.

Given the frequently fatal outcome of ARDS even in settings with mechanical ventilation, the World Health Organization (WHO) recommends individualized restrictive fluid management, keeping the patient slightly dry (**Table 1**). Isotonic crystalloids (not colloids) are recommended because there is some evidence for harm using colloids in resuscitation.[23,53] However, fluid type has yet to be trialed in adult malaria. Dextrose-containing fluids should be used in unconscious patients to maintain glucose concentrations greater than 4 mmol/L. Transfusion is recommended for children with a hemoglobin less than 5 g/dL in areas of moderate to high transmission, and less than 7 g/dL in adults and children in low transmission regions.[23] An RCT is currently being conducted to evaluate best transfusion strategies to prevent death in severely anemic African children, as evidence for the recommended threshold is lacking (ISRCTN84086586). As anemia can develop rapidly, hematocrit should be monitored every 6 to 12 hours. Preparation for transfusion should occur at higher thresholds in patients with hyperparasitemia and/or blackwater fever because of the expected drop in hemoglobin. Recently, a more conservative weight-based fluid strategy assessed in adult patients hospitalized with malaria, found that administering

Table 1
General guidelines for fluid management in severe malaria

Clinical Status	Adults	Children
1. No severe dehydration, no anuria, no shock	Initial: 0.9% saline intravenous (IV) 2–4 mL/kg per h for 6 h[c] Maintenance: 5% dextrose/0.9% saline IV 2–3 mL/kg per h Monitoring: every 2 h for first 6 h	Initial: 0.9% saline[b] IV 3–5 mL/kg per h for 3–4 h[c] Maintenance: 5% dextrose IV 2–3 mL/kg per h Monitoring: every 2 h for first 6 h
2. Severe dehydration, urine output <0.5 mL/kg per hour[a]	Initial: 0.9% saline IV 10 mL/kg per h for 2 h[c] If no urine output (>0.5 mL/kg per h) response: Repeat: 5% dextrose/0.9% saline IV 5 mL/kg per h for 4 h Monitoring: every 2 h	—
3. Hemodynamic shock	Initial: 0.9% saline IV 20 mL/kg bolus If no blood pressure response: Repeat: 0.9% saline IV 20 mL/kg bolus Monitoring: every 30 min If no response start vasopressor	—

[a] Accurate urine output monitored with a urinary catheter is valuable to monitor fluid responsiveness to initial fluid administration; however, is an unreliable marker of kidney perfusion during acute kidney injury and may result in overresuscitation or underresuscitation if used to guide fluid therapy.
[b] Alternate resuscitation fluid in children: 0.45% saline/5% dextrose.[23]
[c] During initial fluid administration, assess for pulmonary crepitations and work of breathing every 2 h and reassess individualized fluid needs.
Data from World Health Organization. Severe malaria. Trop Med Int Health 2014;19 Suppl 1:7–131.

2.5 mg/kg per hour in the first 6 hours did not result in any adverse disease complications.[54] This is reassuring for the treatment of moderately severe patients without anuria, ARDS, or shock, but this strategy needs to be evaluated in a larger cohort with more severe disease. Empiric antibiotics should be initiated in pediatric severe malaria and in all patients with shock in severe malaria.[23] Antibiotic choice should be guided by local hospital susceptibility patterns, source of suspected sepsis, and ideally should be non-nephrotoxic. Inadequate hemodynamic response after initial fluid resuscitation is an indication for vasopressors to be started (see **Table 1**). Norepinephrine is recommended over dopamine and epinephrine, but evidence regarding optimal vasopressor therapy is limited. Epinephrine has been shown to worsen lactic acidosis in severe malaria.[55] Bicarbonate is not recommended unless blood pH is less than 7.10, based on sepsis guideline consensus and the potential harms with overuse.

Acute Kidney Injury

AKI, defined by WHO criteria, complicates up to 40% of *P falciparum*,[24] 55% of *P knowlesi*,[22] and 6% of *P vivax*[56] adult severe malaria and 10% of *P falciparum*[25] pediatric falciparum malaria. As the WHO AKI definition is not applicably defined for children, a high index of suspicion is needed because nearly 50% of children with falciparum malaria have AKI[57] as defined by current nephrology guidelines (creatinine rise ≥1.5 times baseline or 26.5 μmol/L increase within 48 hours).[58] Malaria is a risk for AKI, therefore all patients should have creatinine and urine output measured from admission. Sequestration contributes to the acute tubular necrosis in falciparum malaria.[59,60] Cell-free hemoglobin-mediated damage is a common pathophysiological pathway contributing to AKI in falciparum,[61] knowlesi malaria,[62] and potentially vivax malaria, although the latter has yet to be studied.

Fluid management and avoidance of nephrotoxic drugs are foundations of AKI management. Patients with severe malaria with volume depletion and less severe AKI (moderately elevated creatinine) at admission, show normalization of creatinine with careful volume expansion.[54] However, patients with severe AKI (creatinine >175–300 µmol/L) and/or anuria are not necessarily hypovolemic and are unlikely to respond to fluid administration.[42,43] There is no predictive model or biomarker to determine which patients will respond to fluid or not. Therefore, in patients with moderate AKI (creatinine >177 µmol/L), creatinine should be measured daily after initial cautious fluid administration. A low threshold for early RRT in malaria-associated AKI should be maintained. Early hemodialysis in acute renal failure reduces mortality from 75% to 26%.[63] Patients with anuria, rapidly rising creatinine (>220 µmol/L/d), or severe metabolic acidosis (pH <7.1) should have prompt RRT because rapid renal recovery is unlikely.[63,64] All RRT modalities are lifesaving; however, hemodialysis has been shown to be superior to peritoneal dialysis in reducing mortality.[65–67]

Furosemide has not been studied in malaria, and in nonmalaria, AKI is ineffective in preventing or treating AKI and potentially may be harmful.[68] Bicarbonate urine alkalization in blackwater fever has not been trialed and in general is not recommended.[58] Multiple studies in nonmalaria populations show that there is no benefit of low-dose dopamine in preventing or treating AKI and may cause harm.[69] In severe malaria, low-dose dopamine was shown to increase renal blood flow but did not improve oxygen consumption or reduce peak creatinine or RRT requirement.[55] Based on the mechanism of acetaminophen inhibiting hemoprotein-mediated AKI,[70] a recent RCT in adults with severe malaria found that acetaminophen improved kidney function and reduced AKI development, particularly in patients with high cell-free hemoglobin levels.[71] Larger studies of acetaminophen are being conducted to further assess this renoprotective effect in adults and children with falciparum and knowlesi malaria (ClinicalTrials.gov NCT03056391).

Other Adjunctive Therapies

Various other adjunctive treatments targeting the underlying pathophysiology of malaria have been evaluated without showing benefit, including heparin, desferrioxamine, anti–tumor necrosis factor antibody, levamisole, hyperimmune serum, N-acetylcysteine, and exchange transfusion.[17,72]

UNCOMPLICATED MALARIA
Plasmodium falciparum

Blood-stage cure

ACT is recommended first-line therapy for uncomplicated falciparum malaria in all populations except in first-trimester pregnancy; this latter exception might be lifted in the near future (see **Box 3**). ACT is also efficacious against nonfalciparum malaria and therefore recommended to treat mixed infections and unspeciated infections. ACT consists of an artemisinin component (artesunate, artemether, or dihydroartemisinin) that rapidly reduces parasitemia, and a second partner antimalarial drug that is slowly eliminated to kill the residual parasites. Oral ACT treatments are reliably effective with few adverse effects[73] and are available as fixed-dose combinations (artemether-lumefantrine, dihydroartemisinin-piperaquine, artesunate-amodiaquine, artesunate-sulfadoxine/pyrimethamine, artesunate-mefloquine, and recently added artesunate-pyronaridine). The recommended dosing of dihydroartemisinin-piperaquine was recently revised for children less than 25 kg after it was shown that children were suboptimally dosed resulting in reduced efficacy.[74,75] A recent meta-analysis and systematic review provides evidence of the low risk of cardiotoxicity of dihydroartemisinin-piperaquine.[76] Partner drugs with slow elimination (eg, mefloquine, piperaquine) provide 4 to 6 weeks' prophylaxis, whereas rapidly eliminated partner drugs (eg, lumefantrine) expose a risk to reinfection within a month. The choice of oral ACT depends on risk of drug resistance of the partner drug and potential for treatment failure, which is increased in regions of Southeast Asia (**Fig. 3**). Fake and substandard antimalarials are widespread; therefore, quality-assured drugs are required to maintain effectiveness and prevent selecting for drug resistance.[77]

Non-ACT regimens are still recommended in certain circumstances. Atovaquone-proguanil is highly effective for returned travelers without hyperparasitemia and who have not taken the drug as prophylaxis.[17] In endemic countries, it is not recommended for widespread use as high-grade atovaquone resistance emerges from a single point mutation. However, it can be given with artesunate plus primaquine in cases of standard ACT treatment failure. Quinine in combination with clindamycin or doxycycline is poorly tolerated but is recommended as second-line treatment in certain countries with ACT failure, as quinine remains efficacious. Quinine plus clindamycin 7-day treatment is the recommendation for uncomplicated falciparum malaria in first-trimester pregnancy.[17] However, this recommendation will likely be revised in the near future, as safety data of ACT in the first trimester are reassuring.[78]

Patients with uncomplicated malaria can be treated as outpatients if the patient remains clinically stable after confirming that oral therapy is tolerated and parasitemia has declined. If vomiting occurs within 1 hour of the oral antimalarial dosing, then the dose should be repeated. Mefloquine is associated with increased rates of vomiting and all quinolines (quinine, mefloquine, and chloroquine) are associated with

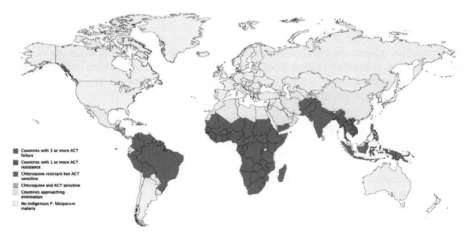

Fig. 3. Global distribution of *P falciparum* drug resistance. Countries shown by level of antimalarial resistance of local *P falciparum*. Countries approaching malaria elimination also shown (as defined in Malaria World Report 2016). (*From* Ashley EA, Phyo AP, Woodrow C. Malaria. Lancet 2018;391:1608–21. *Reprinted* with permission from Elsevier (The Lancet, 2018;391:1608–21).

orthostatic hypotension, which may result in patients not completing therapy. Higher-risk populations, including pregnant women, infants, nonimmune travelers, individuals infected with the human immunodeficiency virus, patients on tuberculosis therapy, and uncomplicated hyperparasitemic ($\geq$2% nonimmune; $\geq$4% immune) patients should be considered for admission due to increased risks of treatment failure and/or severe disease. Ideally, parasite clearance should be documented in all patients.

Gametocytocidal treatment
In low-transmission areas, primaquine should be given as a single dose (0.25 mg base/kg) with all ACT regimens for the treatment of falciparum malaria, except in pregnancy and infants.[17] This treatment serves to prevent onward transmission by killing mature stage gametocytes thereby sterilizing the infection.[79] This low dose is considered safe even in glucose-6-phosphate dehydrogenase (G6PD) deficiency, and therefore G6PD testing is not required before administration.

Plasmodium vivax, Plasmodium ovale, Plasmodium malariae, and Plasmodium knowlesi

Blood-stage cure
Unspeciated malaria and *P malariae*-like infections acquired in Southeast Asia should be treated as for uncomplicated falciparum malaria. Uncomplicated *P vivax*, *P ovale*, and *P malariae* acquired in chloroquine-sensitive regions are treated with chloroquine (see **Box 3**). While chloroquine remains efficacious against *P knowlesi*, ACT is recommended in the Malaysian malaria treatment guidelines due to the risk of misdiagnosed falciparum malaria, presence of chloroquine-resistant vivax, and trials confirming efficacy with faster parasite clearance times with ACT compared with chloroquine.[80–82] In chloroquine-resistant regions (**Fig. 4**), adults and children with uncomplicated *P vivax*, *P ovale*, *P malariae*, and *P knowlesi* should be treated with an ACT containing piperaquine, mefloquine, or lumefantrine (except first-trimester pregnancy).[17,83] Mixed infections are common in coendemic areas. Microscopy and RDT diagnostics may underestimate mixed infections. ACTs are the treatment of choice for mixed infections.

Liver-stage cure
Radical cure with primaquine is required to kill liver hypnozoites of vivax or ovale malaria to prevent relapse in all settings. Individuals with G6PD-deficiency may experience potentially dangerous dose-dependent primaquine-induced hemolysis. The severity of hemolysis also depends on the G6PD genetic variant. Testing for G6PD deficiency is required before treatment. In most trials, primaquine has been given daily for 14 days if there is no G6PD deficiency, and for 8 weeks as weekly supervised doses if G6PD deficient.[84] Adherence and hemolysis remain issues for delivery of effective radical cure. A recent trial of a 7-day course of higher-dose primaquine (1 mg base/kg) resulted in significant hemolysis in G6PD heterozygous female individuals compared with a standard 14-day course of primaquine (0.5 mg base/kg).[85] Tafenoquine is a longer-acting 8-aminoquinoline given as a single dose for radical cure that is currently under review.[86] However, this new treatment will not obviate the need for primaquine in G6PD-deficient individuals due to the risk of hemolysis.[87]

FOLLOW-ON MANAGEMENT
Post-artesunate Delayed-Onset Hemolysis

Delayed-onset hemolysis after intravenous artesunate can occur in nonimmune travelers returning from malaria-endemic regions, particularly if hyperparasitemia is

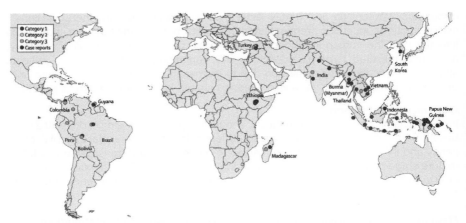

Fig. 4. Global distribution of *P vivax* chloroquine resistance. Chloroquine resistance was categorized according to the strength of evidence[99]: Category 1: greater than 10% recurrence by day, irrespective of confirmation of adequate blood chloroquine concentration; Category 2: confirmed recurrences by day 28 within reported whole-blood chloroquine concentration of greater than 100 nm; and Category 3: greater than 5% recurrences by day 28, irrespective of chloroquine concentration. Chloroquine sensitivity was confirmed if patients had enrolled after a symptomatic clinical illness, fewer than 5% recurrences had occurred by day 28, no primaquine was given before day 28, and studies had a sample size of at least 10 patients. Case reports were observations in individual patients of treatment failure during chloroquine prophylaxis, prolonged parasite clearance or *P vivax* recurrence following treatment. (*From* Price RN, von Seidlein L, Valecha N, et al. Global extent of chloroquine-resistant *Plasmodium vivax*: a systematic review and meta-analysis. Lancet Infect Dis 2014;14:982–91; and Creative Commons Attribution License (CC BY). Available at: https://doi.org/10.1016/S1473-3099(14)70855-2. Accessed September 13, 2014; with permission.)

present.[88] The mechanism of this hemolysis relates to the mechanism of clearance of young ring-stage parasites after artesunate treatment. When artesunate rapidly kills ring-stage parasites, which confers its lifesaving advantage over quinine, the dead parasites become pyknotic. These are then removed from the red cells in the spleen by a process called pitting, leaving the once-infected red cells to be recirculated.[89] The once-infected red cells retaining PfHRP2 have a shortened life span, resulting in the observed delayed hemolysis and persistently positive PfHRP2 RDT. The PfHRP2 concentration after parasite clearance predicts delayed hemolysis.[90] This phenomenon is less pronounced in African children living in high-transmission regions,[91] and post-artesunate late anemia in this setting is uncommon and not more frequent than after quinine treatment. Nonimmune patients, including travelers, should be followed up to 2 weeks after parenteral artesunate treatment to monitor hemoglobin levels, along with creatinine if hemolysis is evident.

Treatment Failures

Treatment failure is defined as the "failure to clear parasitemia or resolve clinical symptoms despite use of an antimalarial drug at correct doses," which does not equate to resistance.[17] Treatment failures can be a result of different factors, including nonadherence, inadequate drug concentrations, poor drug quality, altered pharmacokinetics, host immunity, high initial parasitemia or drug resistance. Artemether-lumefantrine (AL) treatment failures have been reported in nonimmune, returning traveling men weighing a median of 77 kg, suggesting that AL dosing may need to optimized in heavier individuals.[92] Until trials assess optimal dosing, overweight adults should be followed up to assess treatment outcomes.

Primaquine Radical Cure Failures

Failure of primaquine to prevent *P vivax* relapses has been proposed as primaquine tolerance or resistance.[93] Similar to failures in treating asexual blood parasitemia, suboptimal dosing and drug concentrations can be an alternative explanation for primaquine failures.[94] Lower primaquine efficacy and increased risk of relapse has been linked to poor or intermediate metabolism of primaquine in individuals with polymorphisms in the cytochrome P450 CYP isoform CYP2D6.[95] Tafenoquine efficacy for preventing *P vivax* relapses was not decreased in individuals with decreased CYP2D6 activity[96]; however, prospective studies are still needed to confirm this finding.

RESISTANCE
Plasmodium falciparum

P falciparum resistance to chloroquine and sulfadoxine-pyrimethamine is globally widespread. Artemisinin-resistant falciparum malaria is now prevalent in parts of Cambodia, the Lao People's Democratic Republic, Myanmar, Thailand, and Viet Nam (see **Fig. 3**).[97] Artemisinin resistance affects ring-stage parasites and is characterized by delayed parasite clearance following treatment with an artesunate monotherapy or an ACT. At the population level, artemisinin resistance is confirmed when $\geq$5% of infections carry resistance-related mutations in the Kelch13 gene in combination with a parasite clearance half-life $\geq$5 hours or persistent parasitemia $\geq$3 days after treatment assessed by light microscopy.[98] With retained full sensitivity to the ACT partner drug, ACT efficacy is largely maintained in the presence of artemisinin resistance; however, reduced efficacy of artemisinins facilitates the selection of partner drug resistance, as was observed with piperaquine and mefloquine. Once resistance to both ACT partner drugs appears, treatment failure is high, and spread of resistance accelerates quickly. Kelch13 mutations have been observed at low frequency outside Southeast Asia, including sub-Saharan Africa. However, selection for these mutations has not occurred and there is currently no confirmed artemisinin resistance in Africa.

New antimalarials are not expected within the next 5 years, and the treatment and control of falciparum malaria in the Greater Mekong Subregion (GMS) will become increasingly challenging.[97] Rotating between different ACTs, sequential treatment with 2 different ACTs or extending the current 3-day regimens have been proposed. A promising approach is deployment of triple artemisinin combinations, combining an artemisinin with 2 matching partner drugs (dihydroartemisinin–piperaquine–mefloquine and artemether–lumefantrine–amodiaquine), which are currently being trialed (ClinicalTrials.gov NCT02453308).

Plasmodium vivax

High-grade resistance to chloroquine in *P vivax* is widespread in Indonesia and Papua New Guinea and resistance has now been reported in more than 10 countries in endemic areas (see **Fig. 4**).[99] However, the geographic extent is unclear due to coadministration of primaquine, or subtherapeutic drug concentrations (inadequate dose or duration), that could mask low-level chloroquine resistance, or accentuate treatment failures, respectively.

SUMMARY

Management of malaria has changed significantly in the past 15 years, both on an individual and population level. ACTs have, together with the widespread distribution of insecticide-treated bednets, contributed to the impressive reduction in malaria transmission globally. ACTs for falciparum malaria have replaced older therapies given the undisputed survival benefit, safety, and tolerance. Further, there has been a shift toward unified ACT treatment for all human malaria infections, given the challenges in speciation and potential rise in chloroquine-vivax malaria infection. Deployment of parenteral artesunate has importantly improved case fatality. Restricted fluid management has become again the standard in severe malaria. Less progress has been made toward developing adjunctive therapies for severe malaria; however, acetaminophen is a first adjunctive treatment showing benefit by reducing AKI. Sevuparin, which inhibits sequestration, has potential to improve the compromised microcirculation in severe malaria. With malaria transmission decreasing in many parts of sub-Saharan Africa, waning immunity will shift symptomatic and severe disease to older children and adults in Africa.

At the same time, the emergence and spread of artemisinin and partner drug resistance in falciparum malaria threatens to undo the progress made in reducing malaria morbidity and mortality. Accelerated elimination of falciparum malaria in the GMS is required to contain further spread of multidrug-resistant parasite strains. This requires a well-coordinated effort to deploy malaria services to the most remote, vulnerable, and often mobile populations. In addition to conventional vector control measures and community-based facilities for early diagnosis and treatment, targeted mass drug administration of ACT and single-dose primaquine have shown potential for rapid elimination of falciparum malaria in eastern Myanmar.[100] In Africa, intermittent preventive therapy in pregnancy and infants, and seasonal childhood chemoprevention in the sub-Sahel region are being scaled up; however, increasing sulfadoxine-pyrimethamine resistance threatens its impact.[1] Enhanced deployment of long-lasting insecticide (pyrethroid)-treated bednets and indoor residual spraying with insecticide significantly reduced morbidity and mortality in high-transmission regions; however insecticide resistance may also threaten this success. Increased use of primaquine to reduce transmission of falciparum malaria may assist toward elimination, whereas increased use of primaquine to prevent relapse of vivax malaria is required for elimination of this species. Limited access to G6PD deficiency testing for safe primaquine administration is a critical issue. The emergence of zoonotic malaria infecting humans from monkey reservoirs increases the complexity of global elimination strategies. To prevent increases in malaria morbidity and mortality, WHO calls for improved access to effective interventions along with an escalation in funding for malaria control programs and research.

REFERENCES

1. World Health Organization. World malaria report 2017. Geneva (Switzerland): World Health Organization; 2017.

2. Laveran CL. Classics in infectious diseases: a newly discovered parasite in the blood of patients suffering from malaria. Parasitic etiology of attacks of malaria: Charles Louis Alphonse Laveran (1845-1922). Rev Infect Dis 1982;4:908–11.

3. Brasil P, Zalis MG, de Pina-Costa A, et al. Outbreak of human malaria caused by *Plasmodium simium* in the Atlantic Forest in Rio de Janeiro: a molecular epidemiological investigation. Lancet Glob Health 2017;5:e1038–46.

4. Ta TH, Hisam S, Lanza M, et al. First case of a naturally acquired human infection with *Plasmodium cynomolgi*. Malar J 2014;13:68–74.

5. Anstey NM, Douglas NM, Poespoprodjo JR, et al. *Plasmodium vivax*: clinical spectrum, risk factors and pathogenesis. Adv Parasitol 2012;80:151–201.

6. Barber BE, William T, Grigg MJ, et al. A prospective comparative study of knowlesi, falciparum, and vivax malaria in Sabah, Malaysia: high proportion with severe disease from *Plasmodium knowlesi* and *Plasmodium vivax* but no mortality with early referral and artesunate therapy. Clin Infect Dis 2013;56:383–97.

7. Nguyen PH, Day N, Pram TD, et al. Intraleucocytic malaria pigment and prognosis in severe malaria. Trans R Soc Trop Med Hyg 1995;89:200–4.

8. Silamut K, White NJ. Relation of the stage of parasite development in the peripheral blood to prognosis in severe falciparum malaria. Trans R Soc Trop Med Hyg 1993;87:436–43.

9. White NJ, Krishna S. Treatment of malaria: some considerations and limitations of the current methods of assessment. Trans R Soc Trop Med Hyg 1989;83:767–77.

10. Das S, Peck RB, Barney R, et al. Performance of an ultra-sensitive *Plasmodium falciparum* HRP2-based rapid diagnostic test with recombinant HRP2, culture parasites, and archived whole blood samples. Malar J 2018;17:118–24.

11. Berhane A, Anderson K, Mihreteab S, et al. Major threat to malaria control programs by *Plasmodium falciparum* lacking histidine-rich protein 2, Eritrea. Emerg Infect Dis 2018;24:462–70.

12. Beshir KB, Sepulveda N, Bharmal J, et al. *Plasmodium falciparum* parasites with histidine-rich protein 2 (pfhrp2) and pfhrp3 gene deletions in two endemic regions of Kenya. Sci Rep 2017;7:14718–27.

13. Global Malaria Programme. False-negative RDT results and implications of new reports of *P. falciparum* histidine-rich protein 2/3 gene deletions. World Health Organization; 2017. Available at: https://www.who.int/malaria/publications/atoz/information-note-hrp2-based-rdt/en/. Accessed December 7, 2017.

14. Gillet P, Scheirlinck A, Stokx J, et al. Prozone in malaria rapid diagnostics tests: how many cases are missed? Malar J 2011;10:166–76.

15. Gunalan K, Niangaly A, Thera MA, et al. *Plasmodium vivax* infections of duffy-negative erythrocytes: historically undetected or a recent adaptation? Trends Parasitol 2018;34:420–9.

16. Bruneel F, Tubach F, Corne P, et al. Severe imported falciparum malaria: a cohort study in 400 critically ill adults. PLoS One 2010;5:e13236–43.

17. World Health Organization. World Health Organization Guidelines for the treatment of malaria. Third edition. 2015. Available at: http://www.who.int/malaria/publications/atoz/9789241549127/en/. Accessed May 7, 2016.

18. Dondorp AM, Lee SJ, Faiz MA, et al. The relationship between age and the manifestations of and mortality associated with severe malaria. Clin Infect Dis 2008;47:151–7.

19. Sypniewska P, Duda JF, Locatelli I, et al. Clinical and laboratory predictors of death in African children with features of severe malaria: a systematic review and meta-analysis. BMC Med 2017;15:147–63.

20. von Seidlein L, Olaosebikan R, Hendriksen IC, et al. Predicting the clinical outcome of severe falciparum malaria in African children: findings from a large randomized trial. Clin Infect Dis 2012;54:1080–90.

21. Daneshvar C, Davis TM, Cox-Singh J, et al. Clinical and laboratory features of human *Plasmodium knowlesi* infection. Clin Infect Dis 2009;49:852–60.

22. William T, Menon J, Rajahram G, et al. Severe *Plasmodium knowlesi* malaria in a tertiary care hospital, Sabah, Malaysia. Emerg Infect Dis 2011;17:1248–55.
23. World Health Organization. Severe malaria. Trop Med Int Health 2014;19(Suppl 1): 7–131.
24. Dondorp A, Nosten F, Stepniewska K, et al. SEAQUAMAT Trial Group. Artesunate versus quinine for treatment of severe falciparum malaria: a randomised trial. Lancet 2005;366:717–25.
25. Dondorp AM, Fanello CI, Hendriksen IC, et al. Artesunate versus quinine in the treatment of severe falciparum malaria in African children (AQUAMAT): an open-label, randomised trial. Lancet 2010;376:1647–57.
26. Simpson JA, Agbenyega T, Barnes KI, et al. Population pharmacokinetics of artesunate and dihydroartemisinin following intra-rectal dosing of artesunate in malaria patients. PLoS Med 2006;3:e444–54.
27. ter Kuile F, White NJ, Holloway P, et al. *Plasmodium falciparum*: in vitro studies of the pharmacodynamic properties of drugs used for the treatment of severe malaria. Exp Parasitol 1993;76:85–95.
28. Udomsangpetch R, Pipitaporn B, Krishna S, et al. Antimalarial drugs reduce cytoadherence and rosetting *Plasmodium falciparum*. J Infect Dis 1996;173: 691–8.
29. Esu E, Effa EE, Opie ON, et al. Artemether for severe malaria. Cochrane Database Syst Rev 2014;(9):CD010678.
30. Gomes MF, Faiz MA, Gyapong JO, et al. Pre-referral rectal artesunate to prevent death and disability in severe malaria: a placebo-controlled trial. Lancet 2009; 373:557–66.
31. Moxon CA, Zhao L, Li C, et al. Safety of lumbar puncture in comatose children with clinical features of cerebral malaria. Neurology 2016;87:2355–62.
32. Beare NA, Taylor TE, Harding SP, et al. Malarial retinopathy: a newly established diagnostic sign in severe malaria. Am J Trop Med Hyg 2006;75:790–7.
33. Maude RJ, Beare NA, Abu Sayeed A, et al. The spectrum of retinopathy in adults with *Plasmodium falciparum* malaria. Trans R Soc Trop Med Hyg 2009; 103:665–71.
34. Maude RJ, Hoque G, Hasan MU, et al. Timing of enteral feeding in cerebral malaria in resource-poor settings: a randomized trial. PLoS One 2011;6:e27273–9.
35. Namutangula B, Ndeezi G, Byarugaba JS, et al. Mannitol as adjunct therapy for childhood cerebral malaria in Uganda: a randomized clinical trial. Malar J 2007; 6:138–43.
36. Mohanty S, Mishra SK, Patnaik R, et al. Brain swelling and mannitol therapy in adult cerebral malaria: a randomized trial. Clin Infect Dis 2011;53:349–55.
37. Warrell DA, Looareesuwan S, Warrell MJ, et al. Dexamethasone proves deleterious in cerebral malaria. A double-blind trial in 100 comatose patients. N Engl J Med 1982;306:313–9.
38. Hoffman SL, Rustama D, Punjabi NH, et al. High-dose dexamethasone in quinine-treated patients with cerebral malaria: a double-blind, placebo-controlled trial. J Infect Dis 1988;158:325–31.
39. Abubakar A, Van De Vijver FJ, Mithwani S, et al. Assessing developmental outcomes in children from Kilifi, Kenya, following prophylaxis for seizures in cerebral malaria. J Health Psychol 2007;12:417–30.
40. Crawley J, Waruiru C, Mithwani S, et al. Effect of phenobarbital on seizure frequency and mortality in childhood cerebral malaria: a randomised, controlled intervention study. Lancet 2000;355:701–6.

41. Gwer SA, Idro RI, Fegan G, et al. Fosphenytoin for seizure prevention in childhood coma in Africa: a randomized clinical trial. J Crit Care 2013;28:1086–92.

42. Hanson JP, Lam SW, Mohanty S, et al. Fluid resuscitation of adults with severe falciparum malaria: effects on acid-base status, renal function, and extravascular lung water. Crit Care Med 2013;41:972–81.

43. Nguyen HP, Hanson J, Bethell D, et al. A retrospective analysis of the haemodynamic and metabolic effects of fluid resuscitation in Vietnamese adults with severe falciparum malaria. PLoS One 2011;6:e25523–31.

44. Hanson J, Lam SW, Alam S, et al. The reliability of the physical examination to guide fluid therapy in adults with severe falciparum malaria: an observational study. Malar J 2013;12:348–56.

45. Maitland K, Kiguli S, Opoka RO, et al. Mortality after fluid bolus in African children with severe infection. N Engl J Med 2011;364:2483–95.

46. Maitland K, George EC, Evans JA, et al. Exploring mechanisms of excess mortality with early fluid resuscitation: insights from the FEAST trial. BMC Med 2013;11:68–82.

47. Church J, Maitland K. Invasive bacterial co-infection in African children with *Plasmodium falciparum* malaria: a systematic review. BMC Med 2014;12:31–47.

48. Nyein PP, Aung NM, Kyi TT, et al. High frequency of clinically significant bacteremia in adults hospitalized with falciparum malaria. Open Forum Infect Dis 2016;3:1–5.

49. Scott JA, Berkley JA, Mwangi I, et al. Relation between falciparum malaria and bacteraemia in Kenyan children: a population-based, case-control study and a longitudinal study. Lancet 2011;378:1316–23.

50. Cunnington AJ, Njie M, Correa S, et al. Prolonged neutrophil dysfunction after *Plasmodium falciparum* malaria is related to hemolysis and heme oxygenase-1 induction. J Immunol 2012;189:5336–46.

51. Dasari P, Reiss K, Lingelbach K, et al. Digestive vacuoles of *Plasmodium falciparum* are selectively phagocytosed by and impair killing function of polymorphonuclear leukocytes. Blood 2011;118:4946–56.

52. Herdman MT, Sriboonvorakul N, Leopold SJ, et al. The role of previously unmeasured organic acids in the pathogenesis of severe malaria. Crit Care 2015;19:317–27.

53. Perel P, Roberts I. Colloids versus crystalloids for fluid resuscitation in critically ill patients. Cochrane Database Syst Rev 2007;(4):CD000567.

54. Aung NM, Kaung M, Kyi TT, et al. The safety of a conservative fluid replacement strategy in adults hospitalised with malaria. PLoS One 2015;10:e0143062–76.

55. Day NPJ, Phu NH, Bethell DP, et al. The effects of dopamine and adrenaline infusions on acid-base balance and systemic haemodynamics in severe infection. Lancet 1996;348:219–23.

56. Rahimi BA, Thakkinstian A, White NJ, et al. Severe vivax malaria: a systematic review and meta-analysis of clinical studies since 1900. Malar J 2014;13:481–90.

57. Conroy AL, Hawkes M, Elphinstone RE, et al. Acute kidney injury is common in pediatric severe malaria and is associated with increased mortality. Open Forum Infect Dis 2016;3:1–9.

58. Kidney Disease: Improving Global Outcomes (KDIGO) Acute Kidney Injury Work Group. KDIGO clinical practice guideline for acute kidney injury. Kidney Int Suppl 2012;2:1–138.

59. Nguansangiam S, Day NP, Hien TT, et al. A quantitative ultrastructural study of renal pathology in fatal *Plasmodium falciparum* malaria. Trop Med Int Health 2007;12:1037–50.

60. Plewes K, Royakkers AA, Hanson J, et al. Correlation of biomarkers for parasite burden and immune activation with acute kidney injury in severe falciparum malaria. Malar J 2014;13:91–100.

61. Plewes K, Kingston HWF, Ghose A, et al. Cell-free hemoglobin mediated oxidative stress is associated with acute kidney injury and renal replacement therapy in severe falciparum malaria: an observational study. BMC Infect Dis 2017;17: 313–24.

62. Barber BE, Grigg MJ, Piera KA, et al. Intravascular hemolysis in severe *Plasmodium knowlesi* malaria: association with endothelial activation, microvascular dysfunction, and acute kidney injury. Emerg Microbes Infect 2018;7:106–12.

63. Tran TMT, Phu NH, Vinh H, et al. Acute renal failure in patients with severe falciparum malaria. Clin Infect Dis 1992;15:874–80.

64. Hanson J, Hasan MM, Royakkers AA, et al. Laboratory prediction of the requirement for renal replacement in acute falciparum malaria. Malar J 2011;10: 217–25.

65. Mishra OP, Gupta AK, Pooniya V, et al. Peritoneal dialysis in children with acute kidney injury: a developing country experience. Perit Dial Int 2012;32:431–6.

66. Phu NH, Hien TT, Mai NT, et al. Hemofiltration and peritoneal dialysis in infection-associated acute renal failure in Vietnam. N Engl J Med 2002;347:895–902.

67. Asinobi AO, Ademola AD, Alao MA. Haemodialysis for paediatric acute kidney injury in a low resource setting: experience from a tertiary hospital in South West Nigeria. Clin Kidney J 2016;9:63–8.

68. Ho KM, Sheridan DJ. Meta-analysis of frusemide to prevent or treat acute renal failure. Br Med J 2006;333:420–5.

69. Kellum JA, Decker JM. Use of dopamine in acute renal failure: a meta-analysis. Crit Care Med 2001;29:1526–31.

70. Boutaud O, Moore KP, Reeder BJ, et al. Acetaminophen inhibits hemoprotein-catalyzed lipid peroxidation and attenuates rhabdomyolysis-induced renal failure. Proc Natl Acad Sci U S A 2010;107:2699–704.

71. Plewes K, Kingston HWF, Ghose A, et al. Acetaminophen as a renoprotective adjunctive treatment in patients with severe and moderately severe falciparum malaria: a randomized, controlled, open-label trial. Clin Infect Dis 2018;67(7): 991–9.

72. Varo R, Crowley VM, Sitoe A, et al. Adjunctive therapy for severe malaria: a review and critical appraisal. Malar J 2018;17:47–64.

73. Adjuik M, Babiker A, Garner P, et al. Artesunate combinations for treatment of malaria: meta-analysis. Lancet 2004;363:9–17.

74. Tarning J, Rijken MJ, McGready R, et al. Population pharmacokinetics of dihydroartemisinin and piperaquine in pregnant and nonpregnant women with uncomplicated malaria. Antimicrob Agents Chemother 2012;56:1997–2007.

75. WorldWide Antimalarial Resistance Network Dihydroartemisinin-Piperaquine Study Group. The effect of dosing regimens on the antimalarial efficacy of dihydroartemisinin-piperaquine: a pooled analysis of individual patient data. PLoS Med 2013;10:e1001564–80.

76. Chan XHS, Win YN, Mawer LJ, et al. Risk of sudden unexplained death after use of dihydroartemisinin–piperaquine for malaria: a systematic review and Bayesian meta-analysis. Lancet Infect Dis 2018;18(8):913–23.

77. Nayyar GM, Breman JG, Newton PN, et al. Poor-quality antimalarial drugs in southeast Asia and sub-Saharan Africa. Lancet Infect Dis 2012;12:488–96.
78. Dellicour S, Sevene E, McGready R, et al. First-trimester artemisinin derivatives and quinine treatments and the risk of adverse pregnancy outcomes in Africa and Asia: a meta-analysis of observational studies. PLoS Med 2017;14: e1002290.
79. World Health Organization Global Malaria Programme. Single dose primaquine as a gametocytocide in *Plasmodium falciparum* malaria. Available at: http:// www.who.int/malaria/publications/atoz/who_pq_policy_recommendation/en/. Accessed December 20, 2012.
80. Barber BE, Grigg MJ, William T, et al. The treatment of *Plasmodium knowlesi* malaria. Trends Parasitol 2017;33:242–53.
81. Grigg MJ, William T, Barber BE, et al. Artemether-lumefantrine versus chloroquine for the treatment of uncomplicated *Plasmodium knowlesi* malaria: an open-label randomized controlled trial CAN KNOW. Clin Infect Dis 2018;66: 229–36.
82. Grigg MJ, William T, Menon J, et al. Artesunate-mefloquine versus chloroquine for treatment of uncomplicated *Plasmodium knowlesi* malaria in Malaysia (ACT KNOW): an open-label, randomised controlled trial. Lancet Infect Dis 2016;16: 180–8.
83. Gogtay N, Kannan S, Thatte UM, et al. Artemisinin-based combination therapy for treating uncomplicated *Plasmodium vivax* malaria. Cochrane Database Syst Rev 2013;(10):CD008492.
84. Galappaththy GN, Tharyan P, Kirubakaran R. Primaquine for preventing relapse in people with *Plasmodium vivax* malaria treated with chloroquine. Cochrane Database Syst Rev 2013;(10):CD004389.
85. Chu CS, Bancone G, Moore KA, et al. Haemolysis in G6PD heterozygous females treated with primaquine for *Plasmodium vivax* malaria: a nested cohort in a trial of radical curative regimens. PLoS Med 2017;14:e1002224–39.
86. Llanos-Cuentas A, Lacerda MV, Rueangweerayut R, et al. Tafenoquine plus chloroquine for the treatment and relapse prevention of *Plasmodium vivax* malaria (DETECTIVE): a multicentre, double-blind, randomised, phase 2b dose-selection study. Lancet 2014;383:1049–58.
87. Watson J, Taylor WRJ, Bancone G, et al. Implications of current therapeutic restrictions for primaquine and tafenoquine in the radical cure of vivax malaria. PLoS Negl Trop Dis 2018;12:e0006440–53.
88. Zoller T, Junghanss T, Kapaun A, et al. Intravenous artesunate for severe malaria in travelers, Europe. Emerg Infect Dis 2011;17:771–7.
89. Jaureguiberry S, Ndour PA, Roussel C, et al. Postartesunate delayed hemolysis is a predictable event related to the lifesaving effect of artemisinins. Blood 2014; 124:167–75.
90. Ndour PA, Larreche S, Mouri O, et al. Measuring the *Plasmodium falciparum* HRP2 protein in blood from artesunate-treated malaria patients predicts post-artesunate delayed hemolysis. Sci Transl Med 2017;9:1–11.
91. Fanello C, Onyamboko M, Lee SJ, et al. Post-treatment haemolysis in African children with hyperparasitaemic falciparum malaria; a randomized comparison of artesunate and quinine. BMC Infect Dis 2017;17:575–82.
92. Sonden K, Wyss K, Jovel I, et al. High rate of treatment failures in nonimmune travelers treated with artemether-lumefantrine for uncomplicated plasmodium falciparum malaria in Sweden: retrospective comparative analysis of effectiveness and case series. Clin Infect Dis 2017;64:199–206.

93. Spudick JM, Garcia LS, Graham DM, et al. Diagnostic and therapeutic pitfalls associated with primaquine-tolerant *Plasmodium vivax*. J Clin Microbiol 2005; 43:978–81.
94. Pedro RS, Guaraldo L, Campos DP, et al. *Plasmodium vivax* malaria relapses at a travel medicine centre in Rio de Janeiro, a non-endemic area in Brazil. Malar J 2012;11:245–51.
95. Marcsisin SR, Reichard G, Pybus BS. Primaquine pharmacology in the context of CYP 2D6 pharmacogenomics: current state of the art. Pharmacol Ther 2016; 161:1–10.
96. St Jean PL, Xue Z, Carter N, et al. Tafenoquine treatment of *Plasmodium vivax* malaria: suggestive evidence that CYP2D6 reduced metabolism is not associated with relapse in the Phase 2b DETECTIVE trial. Malar J 2016;15:97–105.
97. Dondorp AM, Smithuis FM, Woodrow C, et al. How to contain artemisinin- and multidrug-resistant falciparum malaria. Trends Parasitol 2017;33:353–63.
98. World Health Organization Global Malaria Programme. Artemisinin and artemisinin-based combination therapy resistance - Status Report. 2017. Available at: http://www.who.int/malaria/publications/atoz/artemisinin-resistance-april2017/en/. Accessed February 1, 2018.
99. Price RN, von Seidlein L, Valecha N, et al. Global extent of chloroquine-resistant *Plasmodium vivax*: a systematic review and meta-analysis. Lancet Infect Dis 2014;14:982–91.
100. Landier J, Parker DM, Thu AM, et al. Effect of generalised access to early diagnosis and treatment and targeted mass drug administration on *Plasmodium falciparum* malaria in Eastern Myanmar: an observational study of a regional elimination programme. Lancet 2018;391:1916–26.

Human African Trypanosomiasis
Progress and Stagnation

Emmanuel Bottieau, MD, PhD*, Jan Clerinx, MD

KEYWORDS

- Human African trypanosomiasis • *Trypanosoma brucei gambiense*
- *Trypanosoma brucei rhodesiense* • Clinical presentation • Diagnosis • Treatment

KEY POINTS

- Human African trypanosomiasis (HAT) is caused by 2 subspecies of the protozoon *Trypanosoma brucei, T brucei gambiense,* and *T brucei rhodesiense,* that are transmitted by tsetse flies in sub-Saharan Africa.
- The clinical course of both infections is rather different, with *T brucei gambiense* causing a chronic illness affecting predominantly the central nervous system of patients living in endemic areas, and *T brucei rhodesiense* mainly presenting as a more acute systemic febrile illness in local populations and in travelers.
- The burden of *T brucei gambiense* HAT is rapidly decreasing in Central and West Africa for 15 years, whereas *T brucei rhodesiense* infections continue to be sporadically observed in local populations as well as in travelers exposed in game reserves in East Africa.
- New antibody-based rapid diagnostic tests have the potential to simplify and accelerate the diagnosis of *T brucei gambiense* HAT in the field. Microscopy remains the main method to diagnose *T brucei rhodesiense* infection.
- Field treatment of second-stage *T brucei gambiense* HAT has evolved from highly toxic melarsoprol regimens to a safer and more convenient combination of intravenous eflornithine and oral nifurtimox, which remains, however, cumbersome for most rural settings in the tropics. Fexinidazole, a new oral treatment, has recently shown clinical noninferiority in the treatment of the second stage of the disease, and has therefore the potential to revolutionize HAT control. No progress has been achieved for the therapy of second-stage *T brucei rhodesiense* HAT, for which melarsoprol remains the only widely accepted option.

INTRODUCTION

Human African trypanosomiasis (HAT), also called sleeping sickness, is probably one of the most exemplary tropical diseases, because its vector, the blood-feeding tsetse

---

None of the authors have conflict of interest to disclose for this article.
Department of Clinical Sciences, Institute of Tropical Medicine, Nationalestraat 155, Antwerpen 2000, Belgium
* Corresponding author.
E-mail address: ebottieau@itg.be

fly (Diptera, genus *Glossina*), is exclusively distributed in intertropical Africa. It is a disease complex caused by 2 different subspecies of *Trypanosoma brucei: Trypanosoma brucei gambiense and Trypanosoma brucei rhodesiense,* which are each transmitted by different species or subspecies of *Glossina*. Despite their undistinguishable aspect under a microscope and similarities in transmission and disease evolution, both pathogens widely differ in terms of epidemiology, clinical manifestations, diagnostic approach, and response to anti-parasitic treatment. *T brucei gambiense* is by far the most prevalent subspecies and causes the anthroponotic West African HAT, which has been associated with major epidemic waves in the twentieth century. In contrast, *T brucei rhodesiense* is a zoonotic pathogen causing East African HAT that sporadically affects humans. The burden of both *T brucei gambiense* and *T brucei rhodesiense* HAT has substantially decreased for 15 years in the endemic areas, thanks to intense control efforts.[1] HAT cases are, however, occasionally seen outside Africa, where they often pose significant management challenges to physicians not familiar with tropical medicine.[2] The purpose of this review was to provide an update on the recent advances in the diagnosis and treatment of both forms of HAT, with a focus on the differing aspects and perspectives of their clinical management in the nonendemic setting.

CURRENT EPIDEMIOLOGY IN ENDEMIC COUNTRIES AND IN TRAVELERS

The distribution of HAT is highly focal, resulting in complex interactions among parasite, vector, host, and environment. Transmission occurs in rural or periurban areas when humans are exposed to the bites of forest, riverine, or savannah tsetse flies.[1] Congenital transmission is possible,[3,4] but other routes, such as laboratory accidents, blood transfusion, or organ transplantation are likely extremely rare.

There are approximately 360 historical foci of HAT distributed in 36 sub-Saharan Africa countries: 300 foci of *T brucei gambiense* HAT in 24 West and Central African countries and 60 foci of *T brucei rhodesiense* HAT in 13 East African countries; one country, Uganda, is endemic for both infections that do not regionally overlap.[5] Nowadays, approximately 70 million people live at different levels of risk for HAT infection. The Atlas of Human African Trypanosomiasis[6] provides dynamic and regularly updated information from 2000 about the number of HAT cases at the village level (accessible at http://www.who.int/trypanosomiasis_african/country/risk_AFRO/en/). *T brucei gambiense* HAT accounts for 97% of the total burden. No cases of HAT have been reported since 2010 in 15 of the countries considered as endemic.[7]

Trypanosoma brucei gambiense Human African Trypanosomiasis Is Contemplated for Elimination

Compared with the alarming levels observed in early 2000 after a long period of neglect, the total number of HAT cases has dramatically decreased to a record low number of 2164 in 2016, corresponding to a 92% reduction compared with this period (http://www.who.int/trypanosomiasis_african/news/The-world-gears-up-to-eliminate-HAT-2020/en/, accessed on June 6, 2018). This success has been made possible through major international and national reinvestments in active mass screening, vector control activities, and improved case management.[8] Currently, risk remains moderate to high (>1/10,000 inhabitants per year) for approximately 10 million people in areas where HAT is still considered a public health problem, mainly in the Democratic Republic of the Congo.[7] Recently, HAT has been included in the World Health Organization (WHO) Neglected Tropical Disease roadmap as one of the diseases targeted for elimination as a public health problem by 2020. To achieve this goal, however, the role of cryptic reservoirs such as latent human infections or possible animal reservoirs in *T brucei gambiense* HAT transmission still needs to be clarified.[9]

Trypanosoma brucei rhodesiense Human African Trypanosomiasis Remains a Persistent Threat in International Travelers

The number of *T brucei rhodesiense* HAT cases has also decreased since 2000, and moderate risk of infection is now limited to restricted areas of Uganda, Malawi, and Zambia. Progress seems to stagnate since 2011, with approximately 100 cases diagnosed per year in endemic countries.[7]

In travelers, epidemiology of HAT has evolved in the past century. In early 1900, *T brucei gambiense* HAT was predominant in the nonendemic setting and mainly seen in expatriates and soldiers.[10] For the past 25 years, the number of published cases has increased above 100, with a vast majority of *T brucei rhodesiense* infections diagnosed in all continents, including Asia recently, among short-term tourists who had visited national parks and game reserves in East Africa.[8–24] In comparison, during this period, fewer than 30 cases of *T brucei gambiense* infections have been reported outside Africa, almost exclusively in migrants or long-term expatriates, sometimes from foci considered as silent,[12] or after a very long incubation period of up to 30 years.[25] HAT accounted for 6 (0.06%) of the 10,092 international travelers presenting with systemic febrile illness in the last survey of the GeoSentinel network of travel clinics from 2007 to 2011.[26]

CLINICAL AND LABORATORY FEATURES

Both forms of HAT progress from skin infection at the site of a tsetse bite (inoculation chancre), caused by local trypanosome multiplication, to systemic symptoms following dissemination in the bloodstream and in the reticuloendothelial system (first, or early, or hemolymphatic stage). Infection gradually progresses with invasion of the central nervous system (CNS) when the parasites cross the blood-brain barrier (second, or late, or meningoencephalitic stage). The main difference, however, resides in the speed of parasite multiplication and the rapidity of symptom evolution. Systemic and neurologic symptoms may overlap, so that the distinction between first and second stage cannot rely on clinical presentation, but needs to be based on stringent laboratory criteria (**Box 1** and section on "Diagnosis").

Table 1 summarizes the approximate frequencies of the main clinical features per trypanosome subspecies and disease stage, as reported in recent series from endemic settings.[27] Most studies described, however, mixed groups of patients with first- and second-stage disease, and only a few small case series focused on first-stage only, probably because both forms of HAT are disproportionally diagnosed at the late stage in the field.

Box 1
Criteria to confirm second-stage human African trypanosomiasis

Demonstration of trypanosomes in any body fluid (blood, cervical lymph node aspirate, or cerebrospinal fluid) AND

Cerebrospinal fluid examination demonstrating:
- The presence of trypanosomes,
- And/or the presence of more than 5 white blood cells per μL

From World Health Organization. Control and surveillance of human African trypanosomiasis. World Health Organ Tech Rep Ser 2013;(984); with permission.

Table 1
Approximate frequencies (%) of clinical and laboratory features (when available) per disease stage in the main series of human African trypanosomiasis in endemic areas and in travelers

Clinical and Laboratory Features	First-Stage T.b. gambiense HAT	Second-Stage T.b. gambiense HAT	First-Stage T.b. rhodesiense HAT	First-Stage T.b. rhodesiense HAT	Second-Stage T.b. rhodesiense HAT
N evaluated	39[29] + 56[30]	2541[31]	83[38]	45[36]	138[39] +192[38]
Setting	Endemic	Endemic	Endemic	Travelers	Endemic
Non-neurological features					
Chancre	<5	0	50	85	15
Documented fever	20	15	50	100	20
Headache	80	80	70	50	95
Anorexia	—	25	—	—	85
Pruritus	45	50	—	5	20
Lymphadenopathy	60	55	50	40	30
Any edema (face,...)	15	35	25	—	40
Jaundice	—	—	—	25	—
Skin rash	—	—	—	30	—
Splenomegaly	50	15	15	25	25
Neurologic features					
Any sleeping disorder	60	75	25	10	85
Daytime sleeping	—	40	25	5	75
Insomnia	—	55	—	5	65
Behavior change	10	30	—	5	20
Motor weakness	—	35	—	—	20
Walking difficulties	—	20	—	—	50
Altered consciousness	—	15	5	<5	20
Sensory-motor deficit	—	35	—	—	20
Tremor	—	20	30	5	40
Abnormal movements	15	10	—	<5	25
Speech impairment	—	15	—	—	15
Laboratory findings					
CSF-WBC 6–19/μL	—	22	—	—	25
CSF-WBC 20–99/μL	—	32	—	—	38
CSF-WBC >100/μL	—	45	—	—	37
Trypanosomes in CSF	—	40	—	—	85
Trypanosomes in blood	30–75	30–75	95	95	95

Abbreviations: CSF, cerebrospinal fluid; HAT, human African trypanosomiasis; *T.b.*, *Trypanosoma brucei;* WBC, white blood cell.

From World Health Organization. Control and surveillance of human African trypanosomiasis. World Health Organ Tech Rep Ser 2013;(984); with permission.

Trypanosoma brucei gambiense Human African Trypanosomiasis Mainly Presents as a Slow-Progressing Neurologic Disease

The trypanosomal chancre often goes unrecognized. The first stage, which lasts for approximately 1 year on average,[28] is characterized by intermittent low-grade fever;

nonspecific symptoms, such as headache, anorexia, and asthenia; painless lymph-adenopathies with preferential cervical localization (Winterbottom sign); pruritus; and some subtle neurologic manifestations (sleep disorders, concentration disturbances).[29,30] Clinical information on the second stage is much more robust.[31] It presents with more prominent neurologic and neuropsychiatric manifestations, while most systemic symptoms tend to regress. The neurologic functions deteriorate progressively but ineluctably, causing a wide variety of symptoms and signs, which may include nocturnal insomnia, daytime hypersomnia, tremor, fasciculations, ataxia, motor weakness, archaic reflexes, abnormal behaviors, confusion, coma, or dementia.[32] If left untreated, death occurs on average from 1 to 2 years after neurologic involvement begins.[33] Subclinical myocarditis and endocrine hypothalamic-hypophyseal dysfunction are often present.[1,34,35]

In the nonendemic setting, the clinical presentation of the few reported *T brucei gambiense* HAT cases differed between Western travelers and African migrants.[36] Although the latter were almost exclusively diagnosed during the late stage of the disease,[17] with pattern and frequency of symptoms similar to those described previously, many travelers and expatriates presented with early-stage symptoms (eg, chancre, fever or rash) almost identical to those of *T brucei rhodesiense* infection (see the following section).

Trypanosoma brucei rhodesiense Human African Trypanosomiasis Is Mainly an Acute Systemic Febrile Illness

The trypanosomal inoculation chancre is often still present at the onset of systemic symptoms, such as fever, generalized tender lymphadenopathies, splenomegaly, and/or facial or generalized edema.[37,38] At that stage, parasitemia is usually high (see section of "Diagnosis"). Multiorgan failure and acute myocarditis may develop at any time during this period. Neurologic involvement may appear a few weeks later, presenting as subacute meningoencephalopathy,[39] and death usually occurs within 6 months after the initial onset of symptoms. Recent studies have shown, however, that the clinical phenotypes may dramatically differ between endemic foci, even within a single country,[38] likely due to the genetic diversity of *T brucei rhodesiense* strains. Also, the reported symptoms and signs may be biased by the high frequency of coinfections, such as malaria, helminthic diseases, or human immunodeficiency virus (HIV) in endemic areas.[37]

In the nonendemic setting, meaningful data on symptom frequencies have been collected for the early stage of *T brucei rhodesiense* HAT (see **Table 1**),[36] whereas only 10 cases with late-stage disease have been reported.[10,11,17,40] In the largest review describing 45 travelers diagnosed with first-stage *T brucei rhodesiense* HAT,[36] the trypanosomal chancre was almost always present at diagnosis, at the time of systemic symptoms that usually appear 3 to 14 days after the infective bite. Rash and jaundice were frequently observed, in 30% and 25% of the cases, respectively, whereas these features have never been reported in series from endemic countries. Symptoms of encephalopathy were present in a minority of travelers with early-stage disease. In almost all cases, thrombocytopenia, elevated levels of inflammatory parameters, liver enzymes, and bilirubin, as well as kidney dysfunction, were observed. In contrast, white blood cell count was often normal.

Of note, in travelers who have been exposed in different regions where HAT occurs, the similarities in the clinical presentation of *T brucei rhodesiense* and *T brucei gambiense* HAT could pose a serious diagnostic dilemma.[17,36]

DIAGNOSIS

Because current treatments of HAT, and in particular of its late stage, are complex and potentially toxic, all efforts should be made to first obtain a diagnosis of certainty, by demonstrating the presence of trypanosomes in any body fluid. Once the diagnosis of infection is established, the second step is to stage the disease, by looking in the cerebrospinal fluid (CSF) for trypanosomes and for indirect markers of CNS involvement.[27] The set of operational criteria that has been established by WHO to ascertain the diagnosis of second-stage HAT in endemic settings is summarized in **Box 1**. Direct identification of trypanosomes in CSF is poorly sensitive (see **Table 1**). Although the cutoff of 5 white blood cells (WBCs) per µL of CSF has often been challenged, it is the most widely accepted for clinical management, as far as the counting procedure is repeated for WBC counts between 5 and 20/µL, and that the average of both measures is taken as the final result.[41] Determination of protein levels in CSF is not systematically performed in the field and seems to have less value. Elevated concentration of immunoglobulin (Ig)M in CSF is a very sensitive marker of second-stage infection, but is not widely available.[42] Novel biomarkers are being evaluated to improve the diagnostic accuracy of second-stage HAT.[43,44]

Parasitologic Diagnosis of Trypanosoma brucei gambiense Human African Trypanosomiasis Is Notoriously Difficult

Diagnosis may be obtained by direct microscopic examination of mobile trypanosomes in blood, or after Giemsa staining (**Table 2**). Both techniques have a low diagnostic yield, even when repeated (30%). Direct examination of cervical lymph node aspirate or CSF is also poorly sensitive.[45,46] Sensitivity may be substantially improved by concentration methods that require additional laboratory infrastructure and skills not always available in endemic settings. The techniques most widely used are the microhematocrit or capillary tube centrifugation (mHTC or CTC or Woo method) and the mini-anion exchange centrifugation technique (mAECT, or "mini-column"), that increase sensitivity to 60% and 80%, respectively.[45,46] Subgenus-specific polymerase chain reaction (PCR) assays mainly targeting the 177-bp satellite DNA have been recently developed and shown high sensitivity and specificity (see **Table 2**). They are, however, for the moment available only in reference laboratories. New low-tech molecular methods such as loop-mediated isothermal amplification have been designed but are not readily available in most HAT settings.[46–48] The most interesting next-generation diagnostic for active infection by trypanosomatids is the spliced leader RNA (SL-RNA) detected by PCR.[49]

Because parasitologic diagnosis is cumbersome and poorly sensitive, antibody-based serologic assays have been developed for >50 years as screening tools. The most widely used in the field is the Card Agglutination Test for Trypanosomiasis (CATT/T b. gambiense), developed at the Institute of Tropical Medicine, Antwerp (ITMA), which has been the cornerstone of mass screening campaigns for years. Sensitivity and specificity were high enough (≥95% in most but not all HAT-endemic settings) to make it an excellent field tool to select individuals requiring additional confirmatory testing (with conventional microscopy and concentration methods).[45] Because the CATT is designed for mass screening and still requires agitator rotator, electricity, and refrigeration, there is a need for simple and individual point-of-care tests. Rapid diagnostic tests (RDTs) based on immunochromatographic lateral-flow detection of antibodies against the variant surface glycoproteins (VSGs) LiTat 1.3 and VSG LiTat 1.5 have been recently developed and evaluated.[50] The lateral-flow device HAT Sero-K-SeT test, developed by Coris BioConcept (Gembloux,

Table 2
Diagnostic accuracy of the different laboratory methods for the diagnosis of *Trypanosoma brucei gambiense* human African trypanosomiasis (HAT)

	Threshold of Detection	Sensitivity	Specificity
Microscopy-based methods			
Examination of wet blood	10,000/mL	5–55	100
Blood film (Giemsa staining)	—	25–50	100
Examination lymph node aspirate	—	20–60	100
Capillary tube centrifugation (or Woo)	500/mL	45–90	100
Mini-anion-exchange centrifugation technique	50/mL	75–90	100
Molecular methods			
Polymerase chain reaction assays	1–1000/mL	87–100	92–100
DNA-based loop-mediated isothermal amplification	100–1000/mL	75	100
Spliced leader RNA	100/mL	92	96
Antibody-based methods			
Card Agglutination Test for Trypanosomiasis	—	87–98	95
HAT Sero-*K*-SeT (Coris BioConcept, Gembloux, Belgium)	—	98–100	97–98
SD BIOLINE HAT (Standard Diagnostics, Kyonggi-do, South Korea)	—	89	95
SD BIOLINE HAT 2.0 (Standard Diagnostics, Kyonggi-do, South Korea)	—	70	98

Adapted from Chappuis F, Loutan L, Simarro P, et al. Options for field diagnosis of human African trypanosomiasis. Clin Microbiol Rev 2005;18(1):133–46; and Mitashi P, Hasker E, Lejon V, et al. Human African Trypanosomiasis diagnosis in first-line health services of endemic countries, a systematic review. PLoS Negl Trop Dis 2012;6(11); with permission.

Belgium) in collaboration with the ITMA, displayed sensitivity and specificity ≥98% in a diagnostic study on stored serum samples from *T brucei gambiense* HAT cases and healthy controls.[51] Subsequent prospective diagnostic studies in endemic foci[52] and clinical suspects[53] confirmed this excellent accuracy, with sensitivity and specificity of 98% and 98% and of 100% and 97%, respectively, comparable to those of CATT. A second HAT-RDT has been developed by Alere/Standard Diagnostics (SD; Kyonggi-do, South Korea) in partnership with the Foundation for Innovative New Diagnostics, first with native VSG antigens (SD BIOLINE HAT) and second with recombinant antigens (SD BIOLINE HAT 2.0). In large multicenter prospective studies, sensitivity of both SD HAT-RDTs was found lower than expected (71%–89%) whereas specificity was very high (98%).[54,55] However, combining any of these RDTs together or with CATT achieved a very high sensitivity. It appears therefore that both these RDTs achieve a diagnostic accuracy equivalent to that of CATT and may be used instead for both mass screening and clinical care, wherever local conditions do not favor the use of CATT.

In travelers, as in endemic settings, only a combination of microscopy-based and antibody-based methods may reach adequate sensitivity, whereas molecular assays could be of added value. This difficulty explains the diagnostic delay in patients with *T brucei gambiense* infection being explored outside Africa.[36] All methods require, however, expertise and material that is available in only a few reference laboratories, such as the ITMA in Antwerp, Belgium, or the Centers for Disease Control and Prevention, Atlanta, GA.

Diagnosis of Acute Trypanosoma brucei rhodesiense Human African Trypanosomiasis Is Straightforward

Because the parasite load in blood is usually very high at symptom onset, trypanosomes are relatively easily detected whenever a blood smear is performed, as it is common practice in a febrile traveler after a stay in Africa. In travelers, diagnosis of *T brucei rhodesiense* HAT has been almost always made by thick and thin blood film examination, often as a surprise finding.[17,36] It could, however, be missed when in such circumstances malaria diagnosis is limited to RDT. Although antibody-based assays exist for *T brucei rhodesiense* HAT, none have been developed in RDT format.

In travelers with multiple exposure to different HAT-endemic regions, species-specific diagnosis is important to select the most appropriate treatment. Molecular techniques for species differentiation are available in only a few reference settings.[47]

TREATMENT

Selection of HAT therapy still relies on the recognition of the causative trypanosome and on disease staging. To treat the hemolymphatic phase, 2 drugs have been used for decades: pentamidine and suramin. Both drugs do not penetrate the CNS. For the meningoencephalitic stage, melarsoprol, eflornithine, and the nifurtimox-eflornithine combination therapy (NECT) are the drugs currently used, but 2 new drugs, fexinidazole and acoziborole, offer promising perspectives. The current treatment recommendations for endemic and nonendemic settings and the main adverse events are presented in **Table 3**.

Trypanosoma brucei gambiense Human African Trypanosomiasis Treatment Is Being Revolutionized

Hemolymphatic stage

Pentamidine isethionate for 7 days remains the treatment of choice for first-stage infection due to *T brucei gambiense,* because it is rather well tolerated and remarkably effective (cure rate more than 93%) despite more than 50 years of widespread use throughout Africa.[56] Despite promising results in a phase 2 trial,[57] the development of panfuramide as an alternative to pentamidine was stopped in 2008 after safety concerns emerged during the phase 3 trial. Two participants developed reversible glomerulopathy.[58] Suramin has also some activity against *T brucei gambiense*, but its lower efficacy and higher toxicity preclude its use for the first-stage *T brucei gambiense* HAT. In contrast, preliminary results suggest that the new compound fexinidazole is highly effective in first-stage *T brucei gambiense* HAT (see later in this article).

Meningoencephalitic stage

Melarsoprol, an arsenical compound, has been used for more than 50 years for treatment of second-stage HAT. It has an excellent trypanocidal activity, compensating its rather low CNS penetration. However, toxicity has always been a major issue, in particular because of the encephalopathic syndrome occurring in up to 10% of the treated patients and associated with almost 50% mortality,[59] that could be only partly prevented by coadministration of prednisolone.[60] This complication seems either due

Table 3
Recommended treatment of human African trypanosomiasis in endemic settings and in travelers (and side effects per drug reported in >1% of the cases)

	First Choice	Second Choice
Trypanosoma brucei gambiense		
First-stage disease	Pentamidine 4 mg/kg per day IM or slow IV (diluted in saline in 2-h infusion) once-daily for 7 d. *Side effects: pain and swelling at the injection site, hypotension, abdominal discomfort, glucose instability and diabetes.*	Eflornithine 100 mg/kg 4 times per day (diluted in 250 mL saline for a 2-h infusion) for 14 d. NB: in children eflornithine 150 mg/kg 4 times per day (diluted in 250 mL saline for a 2-h infusion) for 14 d.
Second-stage disease	NECT: Eflornithine 200 mg/kg twice daily (diluted in 250 mL saline for a 2-h infusion) for 7 d combined with nifurtimox PO 15 mg/kg per day divided in 3 doses for 10 d. NB: in children eflornithine 300 mg/kg twice daily (diluted in 250 mL saline for a 2-h infusion) for 7 d combined with nifurtimox PO 15 mg/kg/d divided in 3 doses for 10 d. *Side effects eflornithine: headache, seizures, bone marrow toxicity. Side effects nifurtimox: headache, seizures, nausea, dizziness, tremor, skin rash.*	Eflornithine 100 mg/kg 4 times per day (diluted in 250 mL saline for a 2-h infusion) for 14 d. NB: first choice in pregnant women (nifurtimox contraindicated). NB: in children eflornithine 150 mg/kg 4 times a day (diluted in 250 mL saline for a 2-h infusion) for 14 d.
Trypanosoma brucei rhodesiense		
First-stage disease	Suramin: test dose of 100 mg IV (under monitoring) on day 1 followed by 20 mg/kg (max 1 g) on days 1, 3, 6, 14, 21 (or once a week for 5 wk). *Side effects: hypersensitivity, nephropathy, peripheral neuropathy and bone marrow toxicity.*	Pentamidine 4 mg/kg per day IM or slow IV (diluted in saline in 2-h infusion) once-daily for 7 d.
Second-stage disease	Melarsoprol: 2.2 mg/kg/d IV for 10 d (consider prednisolone 10 mg/kg preventively, or in case fever and convulsions develop after initiation of treatment). *Side effects: encephalopathic syndrome, melarsoprol reaction, hepatitis, pancreatitis, neuropathy, tremor, skin rash.*	

Abbreviations: IM, intramuscular; IV, intravenous; NECT, nifurtimox-eflornithine combination therapy; PO, by mouth.

From World Health Organization. Control and surveillance of human African trypanosomiasis. World Health Organ Tech Rep Ser 2013;(984); with permission.

to early direct cytotoxicity or late (7–10 days) antigen-mediated immune reaction related to parasite lysis. No symptoms or signs at presentation can predict the risk of developing an encephalitic syndrome, but some observations suggest that it was associated with the appearance of fever, rash, and convulsions after the start of the treatment.[59] Many other severe adverse events are possible in treated patients, such as arrhythmias, peripheral neuropathy, or hepatitis, reflecting multiorgan toxicity. In addition, treatment failure with melarsoprol was increasingly reported in many areas,[61] possibly linked with mutations in the aquaglyceroporin 2 and 3 genes.[62]

In the late 1980s, the polyamine synthesis inhibitor eflornithine (or difluoromethylornithine), emerged as an effective and much less toxic alternative drug to melarsoprol against second-stage *T brucei gambiense* HAT.[63,64] However, because of its short half-life (1.5–5.0 hours) and its low binding with proteins, adequate efficacy could be achieved only with 4 daily intravenous administrations for a 2-week period. Shorter courses of eflornithine were clearly inferior.[65]

Although manageable in well-equipped hospitals, this regimen was too cumbersome and expensive for the remote areas where the disease prevails, even with strong international support. Therefore, after pharmacologic exploration for synergism, the Drug for Neglected Diseases Initiative (DNDI) designed and conducted a pivotal randomized control trial that demonstrated that the combination of a 10-day course of oral nifurtimox with a simpler, 7-day twice-daily, intravenous course of eflornithine was not inferior to eflornithine monotherapy (cure rate more than 95%) and reduced major adverse events by half (14% vs 29%; $P = .002$).[66] Phase 4 field studies further confirmed that the NECT was safer and more convenient than, and as effective as, eflornithine monotherapy.[67,68] This treatment has been endorsed by WHO since 2012 as first-line option for second-stage *T brucei gambiense* HAT. Children require higher dosages of eflornithine because of increased renal clearance. In pregnant women, eflornithine should be administered alone because nifurtimox is mutagenic. Treatment of HAT in immunosuppressed patients has never been specifically studied, but local experience suggests that HIV coinfection does not affect treatment outcome.

Very recently, another therapeutic breakthrough has been achieved by the DNDI, with the demonstration that an oral 10-day treatment with fexinidazole, a nitroimidazole analogue, is as safe as, and not inferior to, the NECT.[69] If confirmed in additional field studies, this new drug represents the first well-tolerated single-compound oral therapy against second-stage, and possibly also first-stage, *T brucei gambiense* HAT. Another drug, acoziborole (SCYX-7158), a single-dose oral oxaborole compound,[70] has recently entered a phase 2/3 DNDI-sponsored clinical trial for the treatment of first- and second-stage *T brucei gambiense* HAT. These new treatments could become a game changer in HAT treatment and control.[71]

The need of a long-term posttreatment follow-up to ascertain definitive cure has always been a particular challenge in endemic areas. Researchers have demonstrated that the follow-up strategy of second-stage *T brucei gambiense* HAT could be shortened to 1 year maximum, instead of the previous recommendation of CSF analysis every 6 months over 2 years. Algorithms based on CSF examination have been proposed to identify definitive cure at 6 months posttreatment (no trypanosome and ≤ 5 WBC/μL), or treatment failures (presence of trypanosomes and/or more than 50 WBC/μL). Patients with 6 to 49 WBC/μL at 6 months need further follow-up at 12 months (**Fig. 1**). Treatment failure is proven when trypanosomes are seen and likely when CSF microscopy reveals more than 20 WBC/μL.[72] CSF examination 3 months after treatment does not provide reliable information. Novel biological predictors for treatment failure have been developed.[73–75] In contrast, the CATT antibody test or detection of trypanosome DNA by PCR is not appropriate for evaluation of treatment response.[76]

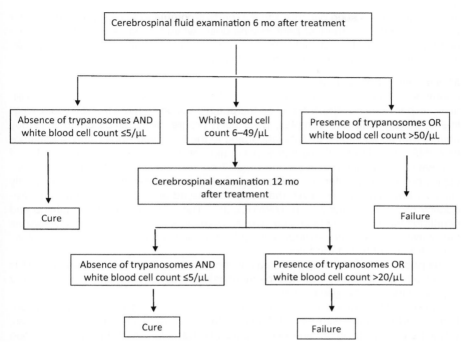

Fig. 1. Proposed algorithm for the follow-up of second-stage *T. brucei gambiense* HAT. (*Adapted from* Mumba Ngoyi D, Lejon V, Pyana P, et al. How to shorten patient follow-up after treatment for Trypanosoma brucei gambiense sleeping sickness. J Infect Dis 2010;201(3):453–63. Available at: http://www.ncbi.nlm.nih.gov/pubmed/20047500%5Cnhttp://www.ncbi.nlm.nih.gov/entrez/query.fcgi?cmd=Retrieve&db=PubMed&dopt=Citation&list_uids=20047500; with permission.)

Treatment of failure or relapse after NECT requires expert advice, because melarsoprol therapy should be considered in such cases.[27]

Trypanosoma brucei rhodesiense Human African Trypanosomiasis Treatment Did Not Progress at All

Hemolymphatic stage

Suramin is highly effective for the treatment of first-stage infection due to *T brucei rhodesiense* and has been used in the field since 1922.[56] Usually, the blood smear becomes negative within 3 days after the first dose given. Its long half-life (44–54 days) allows a once-weekly or twice-weekly administration via the intramuscular or intravenous route. A test dose of suramin needs to be administered, because of the risk of anaphylactic reaction. Nephropathy is a potential adverse event, and needs regular monitoring.

Pentamidine, which is more widely available, also has activity against *T brucei rhodesiense*, and could be considered first if the suramin therapy has to be delayed. Some cases have even been successfully treated with pentamidine only.[17,18] There is no therapeutic advantage of combining suramin and pentamidine.

In travelers who usually present very early after the onset of first-stage HAT symptoms, the systematic CSF examination is debatable because it takes several weeks before trypanosomes invade the CNS. In case the decision is taken to perform a lumbar puncture in such patients, most experts recommend to do it 2 to 3 days after the administration of the first pentamidine dose, when the parasitemia has become negative; this should avoid contaminating the CSF with blood trypanosomes and making an erroneous diagnosis of second-stage infection.

Meningoencephalitic stage

Eflornithine is not sufficiently active against *T brucei rhodesiense*,[77] and therefore melarsoprol has remained the only proven therapeutic option for more than 50 years. Regimens, initially long and complex, have been progressively simplified to a 10-day course with no additional toxicity, according to the Improved Application of Melarsoprol (IMPAMEL) III trial.[78] The same trial could not demonstrate any added value of pretreatment with suramin in second-stage *T brucei rhodesiense* HAT. It remains unclear whether concomitant administration of prednisolone can prevent, at least partly like for *T brucei gambiense* HAT, the encephalitic syndrome, but a reduction of its frequency has been suggested in IMPAMEL III.[78] The combination of eflornithine and nifurtimox has not been tried so far. There is experimental evidence that fexinidazole has activity against *T brucei rhodesiense*,[79] but no clinical trial to evaluate it as an alternative treatment has started yet.

The posttreatment follow-up strategy of second-stage *T brucei rhodesiense* HAT is not clearly established, but has been usually modeled after the classic 2-year approach for *T brucei gambiense*.

None of the HAT drugs are commercially available. For drug supply in Europe, contact should be made with Dr J.R. Franco, Control of Neglected Tropical Diseases, WHO (francoj@who.int). In the United States and Canada, HAT treatment is supplied by the Centers for Disease Control and Prevention Drug Service.

SUMMARY

Despite the rather fast-evolving HAT epidemiology, this condition will continue to be occasionally seen in the nonendemic setting, where clinical expertise for this disease is already scarce. Diagnosis and treatment of HAT in travelers have to rely on the slow but undeniable progress achieved in endemic settings, when considering the recent breakthroughs in rapid diagnostic test screening and in simplified therapeutic options. Confirmatory microscopic diagnosis and species-specific molecular identification, however, still require a level of expertise that is available in only a few reference laboratories. Effective and nontoxic drugs are still in development for use in both African populations and in travelers to treat *T brucei rhodesiense* HAT, that until now has to be managed as in the past century.

REFERENCES

1. Büscher P, Cecchi G, Jamonneau V, et al. Human African trypanosomiasis. Lancet 2017;390(10110):2397–409.
2. Lejon V, Boelaert M, Jannin J, et al. The challenge of *Trypanosoma brucei gambiense* sleeping sickness diagnosis outside Africa. Lancet Infect Dis 2003;3(12): 804–8.
3. Lestrade-Carluer de Kyvon MA, Maakaroun-Vermesse Z, Lanotte P, et al. Congenital trypanosomiasis in child born in France to African mother. Emerg Infect Dis 2016;22(5):935–7.
4. Gaillot K, Lauvin M-A, Cottier J-P. Vertical transmission of human African trypanosomiasis: clinical evolution and brain MRI of a mother and her son. PLoS Negl Trop Dis 2017;11(7):e0005642.

5. Franco JR, Simarro PP, Diarra A, et al. Epidemiology of human African trypanoso-miasis. Clin Epidemiol 2014;6(1):257–75.
6. Simarro PP, Cecchi G, Paone M, et al. The atlas of human African trypanosomi-asis: a contribution to global mapping of neglected tropical diseases. Int J Health Geogr 2010;9(1):57. Available at: http://www.ij-healthgeographics.com/content/9/1/57.
7. Franco JR, Cecchi G, Priotto G, et al. Monitoring the elimination of human African trypanosomiasis: update to 2014. PLoS Negl Trop Dis 2017;11(5):1–26.
8. Aksoy S, Buscher P, Lehane M, et al. Human African trypanosomiasis control: achievements and challenges. PLoS Negl Trop Dis 2017;11(4):1–6.
9. Büscher P, Bart JM, Boelaert M, et al. Do cryptic reservoirs threaten gambiense-sleeping sickness elimination? Trends Parasitol 2018;34(3):197–207.
10. Neuberger A, Meltzer E, Leshem E, et al. The changing epidemiology of human African trypanosomiasis among patients from nonendemic countries - 1902-2012. PLoS One 2014;9(2):1–7.
11. Migchelsen SJ, Büscher P, Hoepelman AIM, et al. Human African trypanosomi-asis: a review of non-endemic cases in the past 20 years. Int J Infect Dis 2011; 15(8):e517–24.
12. Luintel A, Lowe P, Cooper A, et al. Case of Nigeria-acquired human African trypanosomiasis in United Kingdom, 2016. Emerg Infect Dis 2017;23(7):1225–6.
13. Gómez-Junyent J, Pinazo MJ, Castro P, et al. Human African trypanosomiasis in a Spanish traveler returning from Tanzania. PLoS Negl Trop Dis 2017;11(3):1–5.
14. Streit JA, Matsumoto E. African trypanosomiasis. N Engl J Med 2016;375(24): 2380.
15. Wang X, Ruan Q, Xu B, et al. Human African trypanosomiasis in emigrant return-ing to China from Gabon, 2017. Emerg Infect Dis 2018;24(2):400–2.
16. Liu Q, Chen X-L, Chen M-X, et al. *Trypanosoma brucei rhodesiense* infection in a Chinese traveler returning from the Serengeti National Park in Tanzania. Infect Dis Poverty 2018;7(1):5–10.
17. Simarro PP, Franco JR, Cecchi G, et al. Human African trypanosomiasis in non-endemic countries (2000-2010). J Travel Med 2012;19(1):44–53.
18. Clerinx J, Vlieghe E, Asselman V, et al. Human African trypanosomiasis in a Belgian traveller returning from the Masai Mara area, Kenya, February 2012. Euro Surveill 2012;17(10):4–7.
19. Wolf T, Wichelhaus T, Göttig S, et al. *Trypanosoma brucei rhodesiense* infection in a German traveller returning from the Masai Mara area, Kenya, January 2012. Euro Surveill 2012;17(10):2–4.
20. Gobbi F, Bisoffi Z. Human African trypanosomiasis in travellers to Kenya. Euro Surveill 2012;17(10):1–3.
21. Schwartz E, Michaeli S, Steinlauf S, et al. Human African trypanosomiasis in a traveler: diagnostic pitfalls. Am J Trop Med Hyg 2012;87(2):264–6. Available at: http://www.ajtmh.org/content/journals/10.4269/ajtmh.2012.11-0512.
22. Cottle LE, Peters JR, Hall A, et al. Multiorgan dysfunction caused by travel-associated African trypanosomiasis. Emerg Infect Dis 2012;18(2):287–9.
23. Paul M, Stefaniak J, Smuszkiewicz P, et al. Outcome of acute East African trypanosomiasis in a Polish traveller treated with pentamidine. BMC Infect Dis 2014;14(1):1–8.
24. Denny MC, Lai LL, Laureno R. Human African trypanosomiasis encephalitis in the United States. Neurohospitalist 2016;6(4):170–3.
25. Sudarshi D, Lawrence S, Pickrell WO, et al. Human African trypanosomiasis pre-senting at least 29 years after infection—what can this teach us about the

pathogenesis and control of this neglected tropical disease? PLoS Negl Trop Dis 2014;8(12):8–12.

26. Leder K, Torresi J, Libman MD, et al. GeoSentinel surveillance of illness in returned travelers, 2007-2011. Ann Intern Med 2013;158(6):456–68.

27. World Health Organization. Control and surveillance of human African trypanosomiasis. World Health Organ Tech Rep Ser 2013;(984):1–237.

28. Checchi F, Filipe JAN, Haydon DT, et al. Estimates of the duration of the early and late stage of gambiense sleeping sickness. BMC Infect Dis 2008;8:1–10.

29. Boa Y, Traore M, Doua F, et al. Les différents tableaux cliniques actuels de la trypanosomiase humaine africaine à T. b. gambiense. Analyse de 300 dossiers du foyer de Daloa, Côte d'Ivoire. Bull Soc Pathol Exot Filiales 1988;81:427–44.

30. Eperon G, Schmid C, Loutan L, et al. Clinical presentation and treatment outcome of sleeping sickness in Sudanese pre-school children. Acta Trop 2007;101:31–9.

31. Blum J, Schmid C, Burri C. Clinical aspects of 2541 patients with second stage human African trypanosomiasis. Acta Trop 2006;97(1):55–64.

32. Kennedy PGE. Clinical features, diagnosis, and treatment of human African trypanosomiasis (sleeping sickness). Lancet Neurol 2013;12(2):186–94.

33. Checchi F, Funk S, Chandramohan D, et al. Updated estimate of the duration of the meningo-encephalitic stage in gambiense human African trypanosomiasis. BMC Res Notes 2015;8(1):8–10.

34. Blum JA, Burri C, Hatz C, et al. Sleeping hearts: the role of the heart in sleeping sickness (human African trypanosomiasis). Trop Med Int Health 2007;12(12):1422–32.

35. Blum JA, Schmid C, Hatz C, et al. Sleeping glands? The role of endocrine disorders in sleeping sickness (*T.b. gambiense* human African typanosomiasis). Acta Trop 2007;104(1):16–24.

36. Urech K, Neumayr A, Blum J. Sleeping sickness in travelers—do they really sleep? PLoS Negl Trop Dis 2011;5(11):e1358.

37. Kato CD, Nanteza A, Mugasa C, et al. Clinical profiles, disease outcome and co-morbidities among *T.b. rhodesiense* sleeping sickness patients in Uganda. PLoS One 2015;10(2):1–13.

38. MacLean LM, Odiit M, Chisi JE, et al. Focus-specific clinical profiles in human African trypanosomiasis caused by *Trypanosoma brucei rhodesiense*. PLoS Negl Trop Dis 2010;4(12):e906.

39. Kuepfer I, Hhary EP, Allan M, et al. Clinical presentation of *T.b. rhodesiense* sleeping sickness in second-stage patients from Tanzania and Uganda. PLoS Negl Trop Dis 2011;5(3):e968.

40. Gautret P, Clerinx J, Caumes E, et al. Imported human African trypanosomiasis in Europe, 2005-2009. Euro Surveill 2009;14(36):9–11.

41. Mumba Ngoyi D, Menten J, Pyana PP, et al. Stage determination in sleeping sickness: comparison of two cell counting and two parasite detection techniques. Trop Med Int Health 2013;18(6):778–82.

42. Lejon V, Reiber H, Legros D, et al. Intrathecal immune response pattern for improved diagnosis of central nervous system involvement in trypanosomiasis. J Infect Dis 2003;187(9):1475–83. Available at: http://www.ncbi.nlm.nih.gov/pubmed/12717630.

43. Tiberti N, Hainard A, Lejon V, et al. Cerebrospinal fluid neopterin as marker of the meningo-encephalitic stage of *Trypanosoma brucei gambiense* sleeping sickness. PLoS One 2012;7(7):e40909.

44. Tiberti N, Matovu E, Hainard A, et al. New biomarkers for stage determination in *Trypanosoma brucei rhodesiense* sleeping sickness patients. Clin Transl Med

2013;2(1):1. Available at: http://clintransmed.springeropen.com/articles/10.1186/2001-1326-2-1.

45. Chappuis F, Loutan L, Simarro P, et al. Options for field diagnosis of human African trypanosomiasis. Clin Microbiol Rev 2005;18(1):133–46.

46. Mitashi P, Hasker E, Lejon V, et al. Human African trypanosomiasis diagnosis in first-line health services of endemic countries, a systematic review. PLoS Negl Trop Dis 2012;6(11):e1919.

47. Deborggraeve S, Büscher P. Molecular diagnostics for sleeping sickness: what is the benefit for the patient? Lancet Infect Dis 2010;10(6):433–9.

48. Mumba Ngoyi D, Ali Ekangu R, Mumvemba Kodi MF, et al. Performance of parasitological and molecular techniques for the diagnosis and surveillance of gambiense sleeping sickness. PLoS Negl Trop Dis 2014;8(6):e2954.

49. González-Andrade P, Camara M, Ilboudo H, et al. Diagnosis of trypanosomatid infections: targeting the spliced leader RNA. J Mol Diagn 2014;16(4):400–4.

50. Yansouni CP, Bottieau E, Lutumba P, et al. Rapid diagnostic tests for neurological infections in central Africa. Lancet Infect Dis 2013;13(6):546–58.

51. Buscher P, Gilleman Q, Lejon V. Rapid diagnostic test for sleeping sickness. N Engl J Med 2013;368(11):1069–70.

52. Büscher P, Mertens P, Leclipteux T, et al. Sensitivity and specificity of HAT Sero-K-SeT, a rapid diagnostic test for serodiagnosis of sleeping sickness caused by *Trypanosoma brucei gambiense*: a case-control study. Lancet Glob Health 2014; 2(6):359–63.

53. Boelaert M, Mukendi D, Bottieau E, et al. A phase III diagnostic accuracy study of a rapid diagnostic test for diagnosis of second-stage human African trypanosomiasis in the Democratic Republic of the Congo. EBioMedicine 2017;27:11–7.

54. Bisser S, Lumbala C, Nguertoum E, et al. Sensitivity and specificity of a prototype rapid diagnostic test for the detection of *Trypanosoma brucei gambiense* infection: a multi-centric prospective study. PLoS Negl Trop Dis 2016;10(4):1–16.

55. Lumbala C, Biéler S, Kayembe S, et al. Prospective evaluation of a rapid diagnostic test for *Trypanosoma brucei gambiense* infection developed using recombinant antigens. PLoS Negl Trop Dis 2018;12(3):1–20.

56. Babokhov P, Sanyaolu AO, Oyibo WA, et al. A current analysis of chemotherapy strategies for the treatment of human African trypanosomiasis. Pathog Glob Health 2013;107(5):242–52.

57. Burri C, Yeramian PD, Allen JL, et al. Efficacy, safety, and dose of pafuramidine, a new oral drug for treatment of first stage sleeping sickness, in a phase 2a clinical study and phase 2b randomized clinical studies. PLoS Negl Trop Dis 2016;10(2): 1–18.

58. Pohlig G, Bernhard SC, Blum J, et al. Efficacy and safety of pafuramidine versus pentamidine maleate for treatment of first stage sleeping sickness in a randomized, comparator-controlled, international phase 3 clinical trial. PLoS Negl Trop Dis 2016;10(2):1–17.

59. Blum J, Nkunku S, Burri C. Clinical description of encephalopathic syndromes and risk factors for their occurrence and outcome during melarsoprol treatment of human African trypanosomiasis. Trop Med Int Health 2001;6(5):390–400.

60. Pepin J, Guerin C, Ethier L, et al. Trial of prednisolone for prevention of melarsoprol-induced encephalopathy in gambiense sleeping sickness. Lancet 1989;1(8649):1246–50.

61. Robays J, Nyamowala G, Sese C, et al. High failure rates of melarsoprol for sleeping sickness, Democratic Republic of Congo. Emerg Infect Dis 2008; 14(6):966–7.

62. Pyana Pati P, Van Reet N, Mumba Ngoyi D, et al. Melarsoprol sensitivity profile of *Trypanosoma brucei gambiense* isolates from cured and relapsed sleeping sickness patients from the Democratic Republic of the Congo. PLoS Negl Trop Dis 2014;8(10):5–10.

63. Milord F, Pepin J, Loko L, et al. Efficacy and toxicity of eflornithine for treatment of *Trypanosoma brucei gambiense* sleeping sickness. Lancet 1992;340:652–5.

64. Chappuis F, Udayraj N, Stietenroth K, et al. Eflornithine is safer than melarsoprol for the treatment of second-stage *Trypanosoma brucei gambiense* human African trypanosomiasis. Clin Infect Dis 2005;41(5):748–51.

65. Pépin J, Khonde N, Maiso F, et al. Short-course eflornithine in Gambian trypanosomiasis: a multicentre randomized controlled trial. Bull World Health Organ 2000;78(11):1284–95.

66. Priotto G, Kasparian S, Mutombo W, et al. Nifurtimox-eflornithine combination therapy for second-stage African *Trypanosoma brucei gambiense* trypanosomiasis: a multicentre, randomised, phase III, non-inferiority trial. Lancet 2009; 374(9683):56–64.

67. Schmid C, Kuemmerle A, Blum J, et al. In-hospital safety in field conditions of nifurtimox eflornithine combination therapy (NECT) for *T. b. gambiense* sleeping sickness. PLoS Negl Trop Dis 2012;6(11):e1920.

68. Alirol E, Schrumpf D, Amici Heradi J, et al. Nifurtimox-eflornithine combination therapy for second-stage gambiense human African trypanosomiasis: Médecins Sans Frontières experience in the Democratic Republic of the Congo. Clin Infect Dis 2013;56(2):195–203.

69. Mesu VKBK, Kalonji WM, Bardonneau C, et al. Oral fexinidazole for late-stage African *Trypanosoma brucei gambiense* trypanosomiasis: a pivotal multicentre, randomised, non-inferiority trial. Lancet 2017;391:144–54.

70. Jacobs RT, Nare B, Wring SA, et al. Scyx-7158, an orally-active benzoxaborole for the treatment of stage 2 human African trypanosomiasis. PLoS Negl Trop Dis 2011;5(6):e1151.

71. Chappuis F. Oral fexinidazole for human African trypanosomiasis. Lancet 2018; 391(10116):100–2.

72. Mumba Ngoyi D, Lejon V, Pyana P, et al. How to shorten patient follow-up after treatment for *Trypanosoma brucei gambiense* sleeping sickness. J Infect Dis 2010;201(3):453–63. Available at: http://www.ncbi.nlm.nih.gov/pubmed/ 20047500%5Cnhttp://www.ncbi.nlm.nih.gov/entrez/query.fcgi?cmd=Retrieve&db =PubMed&dopt=Citation&list_uids=20047500.

73. Lejon V, Roger I, Mumba Ngoyi D, et al. Novel markers for treatment outcome in late-stage *Trypanosoma brucei gambiense* trypanosomiasis. Clin Infect Dis 2008; 47(1):15–22.

74. Tiberti N, Lejon V, Hainard A, et al. Neopterin is a cerebrospinal fluid marker for treatment outcome evaluation in patients affected by *Trypanosoma brucei gambiense* sleeping sickness. PLoS Negl Trop Dis 2013;7(2):1–9.

75. Ilboudo H, Camara O, Ravel S, et al. *Trypanosoma brucei gambiense* spliced leader RNA is a more specific marker for cure of human African trypanosomiasis than *T. b. gambiense* DNA. J Infect Dis 2015;212(12):1996–8.

76. Deborggraeve S, Lejon V, Ekangu RA, et al. Diagnostic accuracy of PCR in gambiense sleeping sickness diagnosis, staging and post-treatment follow-up: a 2-year longitudinal study. PLoS Negl Trop Dis 2011;5(2):1–7.

77. Clerinx J, Taelman H, Bogaerts J, et al. Treatment of late stage rhodesiense trypanosomiasis using suramin and eflornithine: report of six cases. Trans R Soc Trop Med Hyg 1998;92(4):449–50.

78. Kuepfer I, Schmid C, Allan M, et al. Safety and efficacy of the 10-day melarsoprol schedule for the treatment of second stage rhodesiense sleeping sickness. PLoS Negl Trop Dis 2012;6(8):e1695.
79. Kaiser M, Bray MA, Cal M, et al. Antitrypanosomal activity of fexinidazole, a new oral nitroimidazole drug candidate for treatment of sleeping sickness. Antimicrob Agents Chemother 2011;55(12):5602–8.

Visceral Leishmaniasis
Recent Advances in Diagnostics and Treatment Regimens

Johan van Griensven, MD, MSc, PhD[a],*, Ermias Diro, MD, PhD[b]

KEYWORDS

• Visceral leishmaniasis • Diagnosis • Treatment

KEY POINTS

• Recent diagnostic advances include the development of rapid diagnostic tests.
• Molecular tests perform well, including on peripheral blood.
• Liposomal amphotericin B is safe and effective in most regions.
• Combination therapy is increasingly being explored.
• Immunosuppressed patients require adapted diagnostic and therapeutic strategies.

INTRODUCTION

Visceral leishmaniasis (VL) is a disseminated protozoan infection caused by *Leishmania donovani* and *Leishmania infantum*.[1] Exceptionally, dermatotropic species can visceralize and cause VL, particularly in immunosuppressed patients. Transmission occurs via the bite of phlebotome sand flies. Blood transfusion, intravenous drug use, organ transplantation, and congenital and laboratory accidents constitute exceptional modes of transmission. The zoonotic form, caused by *L infantum*, occurs in the Mediterranean basin, China, the Middle East, and South America, and has dogs as the main reservoir. The anthroponotic form, caused by *L donovani*, is prevalent in eastern Africa, Bangladesh, India, and Nepal.[1] Globally, an estimated 500,000 new cases occur annually. Currently, the Indian subcontinent and eastern Africa carry more than 70% of the VL burden.

The parasite exists in 2 forms. The promastigote form is found in the vector; the amastigote form is found in the host and targets the reticulo-endothelial system in various tissues, predominantly infiltrating the spleen, bone marrow, liver, and lymph nodes.[1] The spectrum of disease ranges from asymptomatic infection to

Conflict of Interest: The authors have nothing to disclose.
[a] Department of Clinical Sciences, Institute of Tropical Medicine, Nationalestraat 155, Antwerp 2000, Belgium; [b] Department of Internal Medicine, University of Gondar, Post Office Box 196, Gondar, Ethiopia
* Corresponding author.
E-mail address: jvangriensven@itg.be

Infect Dis Clin N Am 33 (2019) 79–99
https://doi.org/10.1016/j.idc.2018.10.005
id.theclinics.com
0891-5520/19/© 2018 The Author(s). Published by Elsevier Inc. This is an open access article under the CC BY-NC-ND license (http://creativecommons.org/licenses/by-nc-nd/4.0/).

life-threatening illness. Activation of macrophages and an intact T-helper cell type 1 (Th1) response contribute to immune control. Consequently, immunosuppression is a strong risk factor for VL.[2] Most commonly, the incubation period for symptomatic VL ranges from 2 to 6 months. Viable parasites may persist for decades, even after apparently successful treatment, and in the case of immunosuppression, these reactivate and cause disease.[3] Typical manifestations include chronic fever, weight loss, and hepatosplenomegaly, with pancytopenia on blood examination. Without treatment, VL is almost universally fatal. After apparently effective treatment of VL caused by L donovani, post-kala-azar dermal leishmaniasis (PKDL), a chronic skin rash, can develop. Whereas 25% to 50% of the patients in Sudan develop PKDL, it is clearly less common, and occurring longer after treatment, in the Indian subcontinent.[4]

CURRENT DIAGNOSTIC TOOLS AND STRATEGIES
Direct Parasitologic Diagnosis (Microscopy/Culture)

Traditionally, direct visualization of the parasite via microscopy (after Giemsa staining) or culture on invasive samples (spleen, bone marrow or lymph node aspirates, or liver biopsy) has been the gold standard diagnosis (**Fig. 1**).[5] Spleen aspiration is only done routinely in eastern Africa and the Indian subcontinent, while bone marrow aspiration is more commonly done in Europe, Brazil, and the United States.[1] Although specificity is high, sensitivity is not perfect, with the best performance for spleen aspirates (93%–99%), followed by bone marrow aspiration/biopsy (53%–86%). Lymph node aspiration has a fair sensitivity (53%–65%), but enlarged lymph nodes are relatively rare in VL patients, except in Sudan.[6] Correct diagnosis requires well-trained staff, which is more challenging for countries where VL is only exceptionally seen. Culture reportedly further increases sensitivity on top of microscopy, but is cumbersome and only done in selected laboratories. Although microculture gives more rapid results, this generally still leads to a diagnostic delay of several days (to weeks).[7] Microscopy or culture on noninvasive samples (peripheral blood, buffy coat, peripheral blood mononuclear cells [PBMCs]) has been evaluated also. Although microscopy on these samples tended to have a low sensitivity,[8] microculture using buffy coat and PMBCs had a sensitivity of 85% and 91%, respectively, in an Indian study, with results available within 5 to 15 days and 3 to 7 days, respectively.[7,9]

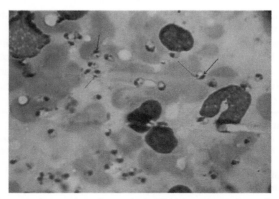

Fig. 1. Leishmania amastigotes (*small purple bodies*) in spleen tissue from a patient with visceral leishmaniasis (Gondar, Ethiopia). Red arrows show the kinetoplast, and the black arrows show the marginalized nucleus.

Serology

Historically, several serologic methods have been used, including the enzyme linked immunosorbent assay (ELISA), the indirect fluorescent antibody test (IFAT), the indirect hemagglutination assay (IHA), and immunoblotting, predominantly used in high income countries. Although performance varies across studies, methodology, and antigen used, most of these combine a fair sensitivity (80%–100%), with a fair specificity (80%–100%).[10] With the advent of new tests, some of these are currently rarely used in routine practice. Although initially crude parasite antigens were mainly used for serologic diagnosis, several recombinant proteins have been evaluated more recently. Currently, in North American reference diagnostic laboratories, the rK39 rapid diagnostic test (RDT), ELISA on crude antigen, and/or the direct agglutination test (DAT) are in use.[11] In Latin America and Spain, IFAT remains in use, but other tests such as the rK39 RDT/ELISA and DAT are increasingly being studied with promising results.[12–15]

Development of rapid diagnostic test and enzyme linked immunosorbent assay against recombinant proteins

One important step has been the development of the rK39-based RDT. The K39 protein contains 39 amino acids originating from a highly conserved kinesin region from a Brazilian *L infantum/chagasi* strain.[16] This cheap and easy to use test performs well in the Indian subcontinent and constitutes a cornerstone of the current regional VL elimination program. In a recent systematic review, sensitivity of the rK39 RDT in the Indian subcontinent was estimated at 97%, while it was only 85% in eastern Africa.[17] Intermediate values have been reported from Latin America (**Table 1**).[18] In Europe, the limited available data suggest relatively poor sensitivity (83%) in human immunodeficiency virus (HIV)-negative patients.[12] Importantly, performance of the rK39 RDT varies to some extent according to the brand used, contributing to the heterogeneity observed across studies. Only 2 rK39-based RDTs are sufficiently validated for clinical use: the Kalazar Detect (Inbios, Seattle, WA), and the IT-LEISH (BioRad, Marnes-la-Coquette, France).

The more recently developed rK28 RDT maintained high sensitivity in the Indian subcontinent, and also displayed improved sensitivity (above 95%) in east Africa.[19–22] Data from Latin America remain limited.[23] Several other recombinant proteins have been evaluated (eg, rKE16 and rK26), but these generally did not outperform rK28 or rK39 tests, at least not in all continents.[18,24]

The direct agglutination test

The DAT was developed as a serologic test that could be deployed in VL endemic areas with limited laboratory infrastructure. As most tests using whole parasite antigens, the test can be falsely positive (usually with low titers) in a number of other diseases such as Chagas disease, brucellosis, and malaria.[25]

Data suggest good sensitivity and specificity in the Indian subcontinent and Brazil (see **Table 1**).[13–15,26,27] In eastern Africa, DAT was also found substantially more sensitive than the rK39 RDT. Data from Europe are limited, but the largest and most recent study suggested only moderate diagnostic accuracy.[12] One of the disadvantages is the overnight incubation, precluding same-day results.

Serologic tests have the disadvantage in that they can be positive in patients with an asymptomatic *Leishmania* infection or those with a history of VL (precluding diagnosis of VL relapse). This has fueled interest in noninvasive tests directly detecting components of the parasite.

Table 1
Overview of key literature on the performance of the rK39 rapid diagnostic test and direct agglutination test for patients not known to have human immunodeficiency virus in different visceral leishmaniasis-endemic regions

Test	Country/Region	Sensitivity (%) (95% Confidence Interval)	Specificity (%) (95% Confidence Interval)	Comment
rK39 RDT				
Cochrane meta-analysis (2014)[17]	Indian subcontinent	97 (90–99.9)	90.2 (76.1–97.7)	Various brands
	Eastern Africa	85.3 (74.5–93.2)	91.1 (80.3–97.3)	Various brands
	Brazil	88–94	91–100	Range across three studies; no pooled estimate
WHO-TDR multicontinent study (2012)[18]	India	98.8 (96.5–99.6)	97.6 (94.8–98.9)	DiaMed IT LEISH
		99.6 (97.8–99.9)	96.0 (92.8–97.8)	Kalazar Detect
	Eastern Africa	87.2 (82.5–90.8)	96.4 (93.3–98.1)	DiaMed IT LEISH
		67.6 (61.6–73.1)	90.8 (86.6–93.8)	Kalazar Detect
	Brazil	92.0 (87.8–94.8)	95.6 (92.2–97.5)	DiaMed IT LEISH
		84.7 (79.7–88.7)	96.8 (93.9–98.4)	Kalazar Detect
Europe: largest study – Spain (2018)[12]		83.1 (75.1–91.2)	100 (99.8–100)	Kalazar Detect Case control study
DAT				
Systematic review (2006)[78]	Indian subcontinent	97.1 (94.9–98.4)	95.1 (88.1–98.5)	No pooled estimates for Brazil
	Eastern Africa	93.2 (89.1–95.8)	96.1 (89.2–98.6)	
Brazil - range across 3 studies[13–15]		90–99	88.6–98.1	—
Europe: largest study - Spain (2018)[12]		84.2 (76.3–92.1)	86.3 (81.7–90.9)	Case control study

Abbreviation: TDR, the special program for research and training in tropical diseases.

Urine Antigen Tests

There is 1 latex antigen test commercially available (KAtex, Kalon Biological, United Kingdom). Although in a Cochrane meta-analysis, specificity was high (93%), sensitivity was low (64%). Consequently, it is currently rarely used in clinical practice. Sensitivity was slightly better (84%–86%) in HIV patients.[28,29] Several new urine antigen tests have been developed in ELISA format, displaying better sensitivity.[30] Commercially available RDTs based on these antigens are not available yet. Potentially, antigen tests could be of value as a test of cure.[30]

Molecular Tests

Molecular tests are increasingly in use for VL diagnosis. A recent systematic review demonstrated high sensitivity (>95%) of polymerase chain reaction (PCR) on bone marrow, peripheral blood, or buffy coat samples, without clear differences in performance on blood between *L donovani* in Asia and east Africa and *L infantum* in the Mediterranean.[31] Data on PCR on blood from cases infected by *L infantum* in Latin America were limited but do suggest a similar performance in this continent. Similarly, the limited data on real-time PCR suggest performance comparable to conventional PCR. PCR on blood could thus be an interesting first noninvasive step in the diagnostic work-up. However, specificity was low (63%–76%) in the better designed studies (**Table 2**). On the 1 hand, this could indicate a suboptimal gold standard used (with true cases being missed); on the other hand it also indicates that in endemic areas a substantial proportion of individuals without VL are PCR positive (asymptomatic *Leishmania* infection). This indicates that a positive test should be interpreted in combination with a sound clinical case definition, and ideally other tests such as serology. High parasite loads in quantitative PCR give additional weight to VL diagnosis.

To allow implementation in field settings, loop-mediated isothermal amplification (LAMP) has been explored. As accuracy looks comparable to conventional methods, molecular tests are likely to be increasingly used in resource-constrained endemic areas also.[22,31–33] Both qualitative and quantitative tests are also being evaluated to assess cure, as they usually turn negative after treatment.[32]

Table 2
Pooled estimates from a meta-analysis of the diagnostic performance of molecular methods to diagnoses visceral leishmaniasis

Type of Study & Sample	Number of Studies	Sensitivity (95% Confidence Interval)	Specificity (95% Confidence Interval)
All studies (case control & consecutive studies combined			
PCR blood	19	93.1 (90.0–95.2)	95.6 (87.0–98.6)
PCR bone marrow	8	95.3 (91.0–97.6)	92.6 (59.3–99.1)
Consecutive studies			
PCR blood	4	92.3 (88.4–94.9)	63.3 (53.9–71.8)
PCR bone marrow	5	95.8 (80.0–98.6)	76.4 (46.3–92.4)
HIV/VL – all studies combined			
PCR buffy coat cells	4	93.1 (83.3–97.3)	96.9 (58.2–99.9)
PCR bone marrow	5	96.6 (59.2–99.8)	96.6 (80.7–99.5)

Adapted from de Ruiter CM, van der Veer C, Leeflang MM, et al. Molecular tools for diagnosis of visceral leishmaniasis: systematic review and meta-analysis of diagnostic test accuracy. J Clin Microbiol 2014;52(9):3152; with permission.

Although diagnosis and treatment vary by the geographic origin of the patient and the causative species, species identification is rarely required for patient management unless there is geographic overlap of *L infantum* and *donovani* (which is uncommon), there is doubt on the exact region of exposure (eg, exposure in different regions), or in immunosuppressed individuals in whom species not typically causing VL can visceralize (eg, *L tropica*). Species identification is typically done using enzyme electrophoresis, or increasingly by molecular methods. However, there is a range of molecular methods at hand, potentially leading to variable results between laboratories.

Diagnosis of Visceral Leishmaniasis in Immunocompromised Patients

Diagnosis of VL in immunocompromised patients (particularly HIV patients) can be challenging for several reasons. First, atypical presentations are not uncommon, whereby parasites are only found in atypical locations (eg, intestinal, oral ulcers), and bone marrow or spleen aspiration can consequently be negative.[3] Second, serologic tests tend to be less sensitive in immunocompromised patients.[34] Hence, negative results have to be interpreted carefully, and using more than 1 serologic test if available might be useful. In a meta-analysis from 2013, DAT and Western blotting were the best-performing serologic tests (**Table 3**).[35] However, the authors (Cota and colleagues[35]) acknowledged that overall evidence is still limited. For example, for DAT, there were only 4 studies in total, and no studies from the Indian subcontinent or Latin America were included. All included studies on IFAT, Western blotting, and ELISA were from Europe. Only 2 studies on the rK39 RDT were included (1 from India, 1 from Ethiopia).

Since then, several interesting studies on the rK39 RDT and DAT in HIV patients have been published. One study from Brazil reported on the rK39 RDT (sensitivity: 45.6%–46.2%; specificity: 97.0%–98.4%), DAT (sensitivity: 87.8%–89.7%; specificity: 82.3%–86.4%), and IFAT (sensitivity: 60.9%–61.5%; specificity: 87.1%–89.5%).[35] The better sensitivity of DAT compared with the rK39 RDT in HIV patients

Table 3
Diagnostic accuracy for visceral leishmaniasis of serologic and molecular tests in human immunodeficiency virus-infected patients in a systematic review

Test	Number of Studies for Sensitivity/ Specificity	Pooled Sensitivity in Random-Effects Model (%); 95% Confidence Interval	Pooled Specificity in Random-Effects Model (%); 95% Confidence Interval
Serologic			
DAT	4/3	81 (61–95)	90 (66–100)
IFAT	21/4	51 (43–58)	93 (81–99)
rK39 RDT	2	NA	NA
ELISA	5/3	66 (40–88)	90 (77–98)
Western Blotting	8/4	84 (75–91)	82 (65–94)
Molecular			
PCR whole blood	8/3	92 (83–98)	96 (80–100)
PCR bone marrow	3/0	98 (93–100)	NA

Abbreviation: NA, not available (no or too few studies available).

Data from Cota GF, de Sousa MR, de Freitas, et al. Comparison of parasitologic, serologic, and molecular tests for visceral leishmaniasis in HIV-infected patients: a cross-sectional delayed-type study. Am J Trop Med Hyg 2013;89(3):570–7.

is in line with observations in eastern Africa (DAT: 89%, rK39: 77%).[36] Similar observations were made recently in Europe evaluating DAT (sensitivity 91.3%, specificity 83.3%) and rK39 RDT (sensitivity: 67.3% specificity: 100%).[12] The fair sensitivity of DAT would thus be contributing to ruling out VL; the better specificity of the rK39 RDT would be useful to confirm VL.

In non-HIV immunosuppressive conditions, serologic tests seem to be less compromised. In a systematic review, the sensitivity of IFAT was 93% in transplant patients but only 48% in HIV patients.[37] The same review suggested a sensitivity of microscopy on bone marrow aspiration of 81% in HIV patients and 98% in transplant patients.

In the meta-analysis by Cota and colleagues,[38] molecular methods clearly outperformed serologic methods, with PCR on whole blood and bone marrow displaying high sensitivity. In a more recent meta-analysis, PCR on bone marrow and buffy coat had a high sensitivity in HIV patients (see **Table 2**). Because of the paucity of (quality) studies, no pooled estimate on peripheral blood was provided in this review. As to peripheral blood microscopy, using buffy coat or PBMCs was found to be relatively sensitive in HIV patients; sensitivity reached 56% with PBMCs, compared with 29% in HIV-negative patients.[8]

PCR has also been proposed to assess treatment response and for prediction or early detection of relapse.[39,40] Importantly, leishmanial DNA can be detected in HIV patients after treatment, without clinical significance, indicating care should be taken to diagnose VL relapse solely on a positive PCR test.[41] For this reason, quantitative PCR thresholds of parasite load have been proposed predicting relapse. However, these are highly dependent on the specific PCR protocol used and hence might not be easily generalizable.[39] Nevertheless, progressively increasing PCR levels after successful treatment should raise concern about (the risk of) VL relapse.

Diagnostic Approach

The diagnostic work-up should take into consideration the (likely) origin of the *Leishmania* infection, especially if rK39 testing is done, and the immunocompetency of the patient. If invasive samples are not to be collected for other indications (eg, to rule out hematological conditions), a step-wise approach could be taken whereby initial testing with PCR and serology (1 or 2 different tests) on peripheral blood (and possibly complemented with microscopy and/or culture) is done. Particularly in immunocompromised patients, using more than 1 serologic tests might be useful. If the diagnosis cannot be reliably ruled out or confirmed, invasive testing with PCR and microscopy (and possibly culture) is done on tissue samples (eg, bone marrow, lymph nodes). Doubtful test results like low level positive results on serology and PCR (if quantitative) would also be an indication for invasive testing. Indeed, as specificity of some tests is suboptimal, not every positive *Leishmania* test equals VL, but the pretest probabilities together with the results of various tests should be integrated to arrive to a high probability of ruling in or ruling out the disease. In case of a high clinical suspicion with negative initial *Leishmania* tests, repeating tests has been found useful also (with an initial negative bone marrow aspiration being positive when repeated).

For patients presenting with a possible VL relapse, serologic tests are of no use, as antibodies remain positive for prolonged periods after VL treatment. PCR (ideally quantitative) and direct parasitologic tests are of value here.

VISCERAL LEISHMANIASIS TREATMENT UPDATE

Untreated symptomatic VL is almost always fatal. Thus, all symptomatic patients with VL need treatment with antileishmanial drugs. Additional ancillary medications and other supportive care may also be needed. The effectiveness of antileishmanial drugs varies with the host immune status and the geographic location where the *Leishmania* infection was acquired. Thus, treatment recommendations are based on this classification. To date, liposomal amphotericin B (L-AmB) and miltefosine are the only US Food and Drug administration (FDA)-approved drugs for VL treatment (**Table 4**).

Treatment of Visceral Leishmaniasis in Immunocompetent Hosts

L-AmB is currently recommended first line antileishmanial drug based on the available efficacy data from different VL endemic regions of the world.[42] The FDA-approved dosage regimen is 3 mg/kg/d intravenously on days 1 to 5, 14, and 21 (total dose, 21 mg/kg). A large retrospective cohort study in India has shown 99% initial cure rate with 20 mg/kg of L-AmB with good safety profile and low relapse and PKDL rates.[43] The use of single-dose L-AmB (10 mg/kg) was also found effective, with a cure rate greater than 95%, and it is used in the national leishmaniasis elimination program in India.[44] Most of the experience for *L infantum* transmission regions came from the Mediterranean basin area that demonstrated good efficacy and safety.[45] Unfortunately, the efficacy of L-AmB in East Africa and Brazil was lower than expected, and higher doses may be needed (30–40 mg/kg).[42,46–48] Although the high dose has cost implications for most of the endemic regions, L-AmB remains to be the preferred choice for its safety and short regimen.

Antimonials continued to be effective in all VL endemic regions, except in the Indian subcontinent (Bihar and the neighboring regions), where parasite susceptibility to antimonials has decreased. Multicenter trials in eastern Africa have shown high efficacy and decreased hospitalization rates with combination therapy of antimonials and paromomycin.[49,50] Thus, the combination of sodium stibogluconate 20 mg/kg intravenously or intramuscularly and paromomycin 15 mg/kg intramuscularly both for 17 days is recommended as the preferred first-line regimen over 30 days of antimonial alone for VL in this region.[51] However, both of these drugs are associated with several serious adverse effects and still require prolonged hospitalization compared with the L-AmB regimen.

Other alternative antileishmanial agents are miltefosine, the only available oral antileishmanial drug in use to date, and paromomycin. Although these drugs have also been found to be highly effective in the Indian subcontinent as monotherapy, rapid emergence and spread of resistance are concerns. Use of these drugs in combination regimens has helped to overcome the challenge and maintain their effectiveness. A sequential combination therapy of liposomal amphotericin B (5 mg/kg single dose) followed by 10 days of 11 mg/kg/d paromomycin or 7 days of 50 mg/kg/d miltefosine have been found to be highly effective (98%–99%) and safe,[52,53] and are now included in World Health Organization (WHO) recommendations for the Indian subcontinent.[51] The limited experiences with these drugs in eastern Africa have shown lesser effectiveness, variable performance, and need for higher doses.[54–56] The linear dosage of miltefosine based on body weight was found to have lower steady state serum concentration and was associated with higher treatment failure among children. Allometric dosing results in optimal steady state concentration in both adults in children and is the preferred dosing algorithm for miltefosine.[57]

About 5% to 10% of primary VL cases may not show response, or may relapse after some months of the initial treatment. Nonresponding and relapsing patients can be treated by prolonging the duration of therapy, increasing dose of L-AmB, or shifting to alternative drugs.[42] The use of conventional amphotericin has decreased over time because of its high nephrotoxicity and hypokalemia. Pentamidine is also differed

Table 4
Summary of antileishmania drugs

Drugs and Mechanism of Action	Regimen	Marketing[a]	Clinical Efficacy	Toxicity	Monitoring	Cost/Course	Remark
Pentavalent antimonials • Virtually unknown mechanism; inhibition of several metabolic pathways leading to impaired macromolecule (DNA, RNA, proteins) synthesis	20 mg/kg iv or im daily for 28–30 d	GlaxoSmithKline (Pentostam) Sanofi Aventis (Glucantime) Available via CDC in USA and Special access Program in Canada	35%–95% (depending on geographic area)	Frequent, potentially severe; cardiac toxicity, pancreatitis, Nephro + hepatotoxicity	Baseline and weekly, CBC, transaminases, lipase, amylase, serum creatinine, potassium and ECG	Generic ~ $64.5 Branded ~ $85.6	Quality control issues with generic rugs Length of treatment Painful injection Toxicity Resistance in India
Amphotericin B deoxycholate • Plasma membrane inhibitor	0.75–1 mg/kg iv for 15–20 doses (daily or alternate days)	Bristol-Myers Squibb (Fungizone®)	> 97% all regions	Frequent Infusion-related reactions, nephrotoxicity, hypokalemia (in-patient care needed)	Baseline and weekly serum creatinine, BUN, potassium and urinalysis	Generic price: ~ $21	Need for slow iv infusion Dose-limiting Nephrotoxicity Potassium replacement Heat stability
Liposomal Amphotericin B • Plasma membrane inhibitor • Enhanced tissue distribution, longer half-life, less toxicity	10–30 mg/kg total dose iv; usually 3–5 mg/kg/dose Single dose (10 mg/kg) in India	Gilead via Astellas (Ambisome) FDA approved The Liposome company (Abelcet) Not FDA approved for VL	Europe and Asia: > 95%; lower in East Africa and Brazil (higher dose required)	Uncommon and mild; Nephrotoxicity	Baseline serum creatinine, blood urea nitrogen and potassium	Preferential price: $378 (21 mg/kg total dose) Commercial price: ~ 10x	Price Need for slow iv infusion Heat stability (stored <25° C)

(continued on next page)

Table 4 (continued)							
Drugs and Mechanism of Action	**Regimen**	**Marketing[a]**	**Clinical Efficacy**	**Toxicity**	**Monitoring**	**Cost/Course**	**Remark**
Miltefosine • Alkylphosphocholine drug, inhibits intracellular signalling pathways and plasma membrane	2–2.5 mg/kg/d orally daily over 28 d (India only)	Knight Therapeutics (Impavido) via Profounda in the United States, via Special Access Program in Canada FDA approved	Asia: >90% but relapse rate increasing Africa: single field study (93% in non-HIV patients	Common, usually mild and transient; gastro-intestinal (20%–55%), Nephro + hepatotoxicity Possibly teratogenic	Baseline and weekly liver and renal functions. Pregnancy test before treatment	Preferential price: approximately $80.49 Commercial price: ~ 22,000 – 34,000	Need for effective double contraception up to 3 months post treatment. Allometric dosing Easy resistance development Adverse effects affect compliance
Paromomycin Sulfate • Aminoglycoside drug, inhibits protein synthesis	15 mg/kg intramuscularly daily for 21 d (India only)	IOWH/Gland Pharma	Asia: 95% (India) Africa: 15 mg/kg: 64% (Sudan <50%) 20 mg/kg: 80% (Sudan)	Uncommon Nephrotoxicity Ototoxicity Hepatotoxicity Painful injections	Baseline and weekly renal function and audiometry	~ $23.8	Efficacy variable between and within regions Potential for easy resistance development Useful in combination therapy

Abbreviation: CBC, complete blood count.
[a] Marketing authorization holder.

from routine use in VL treatment because of its adverse effects such as diabetes mellitus (**Table 5**).

Visceral Leishmaniasis Treatment in Immunosuppressed Hosts

Visceral leishmaniasis/human immunodeficiency virus coinfection
In the presence of HIV coinfection, the existing antileishmanial drugs are associated with poor treatment responses (higher initial failure and relapse rates), more adverse events, and added toxicities and higher mortality.[34,58] A review of different regimens used for VL treatment in HIV showed higher toxicity and mortality with antimonials other than L-AmB.[59] Current guidelines recommend L-AmB at a high dose (total of 40 mg/kg).[42,51,60] One dosing regimen can be 5 mg/kg on days 1 to 5, 10, 17, and 24. However, different dosing approaches are used. Although this has good safety profile, it is less effective in eastern Africa and Latin America,[61,62] and it is associated with delayed relapses in India.[63] In an Ethiopian study, miltefosine monotherapy was found safer but less effective than antimonials.[56] A compassionate use of combination therapy of L-AmB (30 mg/kg) and miltefosine, and a recent clinical trial in Ethiopia with this combination have shown promising results, with greater than 80% initial cure rate both in primary and relapsed VL patients. A clinical trial evaluating this combination therapy or L-AmB at 40 mg/kg has been conducted, and findings are to be reported soon (https://clinicaltrials.gov/ct2/show/NCT02011958).

Antiretroviral treatment is a corner stone and should be initiated as soon as antileishmanial drugs are tolerated. The widespread use of antiretroviral treatment has resulted in dramatic reductions in the incidence of VL/HIV coinfection in southern Europe.[64] However, it appears to have only partially protective effect against relapses.[65] Repeated relapses tend be become progressively less acute, more atypical, and less responsive to treatment. Despite the use of ART, 1-year relapse rates of 30% to 60% have been reported.[34] Consequently, secondary prophylaxis is recommended after achieving parasitologic cure for patients with CD4 count level below 200 cells/μL.[60,66] These guidelines mention the limitation of data regarding when to stop secondary prophylaxis and suggest considering discontinuation of maintenance therapy when a sustained (3-6 months) CD4 level above 350 cells/μL is achieved with ART. L-AmB, antimonials, and pentamidine every 2 to 4 weeks have been used for secondary prophylaxis. Use of pentamidine infusion at a dose of 4 mg/kg every month in Ethiopia has resulted in a relapse-free survival rate of 71% 1 year after VL treatment.[67,68] Although the development of resistance is of major concern in choosing drugs for secondary prophylaxis, the mode of transmission in the region needs to be taken into consideration. In antroponothic transmission regions, HIV coinfected patients may become reservoirs of resistant strains. Thus, it is wise to preserve the first-line options from use in secondary prophylaxis.

Other immunosuppressive conditions
VL has been reported in non-HIV immunosuppressive clinical conditions such as organ transplant recipients, rheumatologic diseases, malignancies, and long-term steroid use.[2,37,69] The available data are based on case reports and case series to draw strong conclusions regarding choice of treatment. However, liposomal amphotericin B is often recommended for its good safety profile. Modifications of the immunosuppressive medications may be important during VL treatment. The treatment failure and relapse rates are less prominent when compared to patients with HIV co-infection. Thus, secondary prophylaxis is not indicated unless it was a relapsed disease.[42]

Table 5
Summary of guidelines on visceral leishmaniasis treatment recommendations

Guidelines from North America	Recommendations for Visceral Leishmaniasis Treatment
Centers for Disease Control and Prevention[42]	Immunocompetent patients • L-AmB 3 mg per kg daily, by intravenous infusion, on days 1–5, 14, and 21 (total dose of 21 mg/kg). Immunosuppressed patients • L-AmB 4 mg per kg daily on days 1–5, 10, 17, 24, 31, and 38 (total dose of 40 mg/kg). Alternatives • Amphotericin B deoxycholate 0.5–1 mg/kg either daily or every other day for a total of 15–20 mg/kg • Pentavalent antimonial (SbV) 20 mg/kg/d intravenously or intramuscularly for 28 d
AIDS*info* Guidelines for Prevention and Treatment of Opportunistic Infections in HIV-Infected Adults and Adolescents[60]	Preferred Therapy: • L-AmB 2–4 mg/kg intravenously daily (AII), or interrupted schedule (eg, 4 mg/kg on days 1–5, 10, 17, 24, 31, 38) (AII) a total dose of 20–60 mg/kg (AII) Alternative therapy: • Other amphotericin B lipid complex dosed previously described, or Amphotericin B deoxycholate 0.5–1.0 mg/kg intravenously daily for total dose of 1.5–2.0 g (BII) • Pentavalent antimony (sodium stibogluconate) 20 mg/kg intravenously or intramuscularly daily for 28 d (BII). • Miltefosine (CIII) for patients who weigh 30–44 kg: 50 mg orally bid for 28 d; for patients who weigh ≥45 kg: 50 mg orally 3 times daily for 28 d Chronic maintenance therapy for visceral leishmaniasis • Indication: for patients with visceral leishmaniasis and CD4 count <200 cells/mm³ (AII) Preferred therapy: • Liposomal amphotericin B 4 mg/kg every 2–4 wk (AII) • Amphotericin B lipid complex 3 mg/kg every 21 d (AII) Alternative therapy: • Pentavalent antimony (sodium stibogluconate) 20 mg/kg intravenously or intramuscularly every 4 weeks (BII) Discontinuation of chronic maintenance therapy • Some investigators suggest that therapy can be discontinued after a sustained (>3–6 months) increase in CD4 count to >200–350 cells/mm³ in response to ART, but others suggest that therapy should be continued indefinitely. Therefore, no recommendation can be made regarding discontinuation of chronic maintenance therapy

| Infectious Diseases Society of America (IDSA) and American Society of Tropical Medicine and Hygiene (ASTMH)[1] | **Immunocompetent**
• Ambisome 3 mg/kg/d intravenously on days 1–5, 14, and 21 (total dose, 21 mg/kg); 40 mg/kg for eastern Africa.
• Miltefosine 2.5 mg/kg/d (max 150 mg) for 28 d for VL acquired in Indian subcontinent (for age ≥12, weight ≥30, nonpregnant or breast feeding)
Alternatives:
• Pentavalent antimonial 20 mg/kg/d intravenously or intramuscularly for 28 d (where resistance is low)
• Amphotericine B (for persons with liposome-induced complement activation-related psuedoallergy)
Nonresponding or relapsing patients
• Failure with L-AmB – higher dose L-AmB, prolonged L-AmB or alternatives
• Failure with miltefosine or antimonials – L-AmB or alternative
Immunocompromised host (HIV)
• AmBisome 4 mg/kg/d intravenously, on days 1–5, 10, 17, 24, 31, and 38 (10 doses over a 38-day period), for a total dose of 40 mg/kg.
• Ambisome + miltefosine combination
• Secondary prophylaxis for CD4 <200
Other immunocompromised host (postorgan transplant)
• AmBisome 4 mg/kg/d intravenously, on days 1–5, 10, 17, 24, 31, and 38 (10 doses over a 38-day period), for a total dose of 40 mg/kg.
Special population (too young, elderly, renal or hepatic failure, pregnant, lactating)
• All need treatment; otherwise VL is fatal
• Care should be given on selection of drug, dosage, and monitoring approach |

(continued on next page)

Table 5
(continued)

Guidelines from North America	Recommendations for Visceral Leishmaniasis Treatment
WHO recommendations per region[10]	
L donovani - Indian subcontinent	• Liposomal amphotericin B: 3–5 mg/kg/d intravenously over 3–5 d for total dose of 15 mg/kg or 10 mg/kg intravenously sd
	• Combination regimens (sequential coadministration)
	• Liposomal amphotericin B (5 mg/kg intravenously sd) + miltefosine for 7 d
	• Liposomal amphotericin B (5 mg/kg intravenously sd) + paromomycin for 10 d
	• Paromomycin + miltefosine for 10 d
	• Amphotericin B deoxycholate 0.75–1 mg/kg/d intravenously, daily or on alternate days, for 15–20 doses
	• Miltefosine: children 2–11 y: 2.5 mg/kg/d; ≥12 y and < 25 kg body weight: 50 mg/d; 25–50 kg: 100 mg/d; > 50 kg: 150 mg/d; orally for 28 d
	• Paromomycin 15 mg (11 mg base)/kg/d intramuscularly for 21 d
	• Pentavalent antimonials: 20 mg Sb^{5+}/kg/d intramuscularly or intravenously for 30 in areas where they remain effective (including Nepal, Bangladesh, and certain areas in India)
	• Rescue treatment in case of nonresponse: conventional amphotericin B deoxycholate or liposomal amphotericin B at higher doses
L donovani - eastern Africa	• Combination therapy: pentavalent antimonials + paromomycin for 17 d
	• Pentavalent antimonials monotherapy
	• Liposomal amphotericin B 3–5 mg/kg/d intravenously over 6–10 d for total dose of 30 mg/kg
	• Amphotericin B deoxycholate
	• Miltefosine
L infantum regions	• Liposomal amphotericin B 3–6 mg/kg/d intravenously in 3–6 doses for a total dose of 18–21 mg/kg
	• Pentavalent antimonials 20 mg/kg Sb^{5+}/kg/d intramuscularly or intravenously for 28 d
	• Amphotericin B deoxycholate 0.75–1 mg/kg/d intravenously, daily or on alternate days for 20–30 doses, total dose of 2–3 g

For sodium stibogluconate contact the CDC Drug Service at 404-639-3670 or drugservice@cdc.gov; for emergencies, call 770-488-7100.
For miltefosine available in the United States via www.Profounda.com.

Post kala-azar dermal leishmaniasis

PKDL is a chronic skin rash that starts as erythematous macules and papules around the perioral area and progresses with nodular rash spreading all over the body. It usually comes after effective treatment of VL in *L donovani* transmission regions. Geographic variation is observed in the nature of PKDL. Although it occurs in 50% to 60% of patients in Sudan within the first 6 months of VL treatment, it is less prevalent (5%–10%) and is occurring 1 to 2 years later in the Indian subcontinent. Spontaneous recovery occurs in the majority of cases in Sudan, whereas most of the patients with PKDL in India require pharmacologic treatment. PKDL may indicate an immune reconstitution syndrome. Although the circulating parasites are cleared from the reticuloendothelial system, the skin lesions are fully parasitized and may play role in disease transmission.[4]

Depending on the extent of body involvement, PKDL is classified into 3 grades. Grade 1 is rash on the face. This is usually self-limiting and needs simple observation. Grade 2 is when the trunk is involved, with the lesions spreading down from the face. Sometimes, there may be associated mucosal involvement. Grade 3 is when it involves the extremities in addition to the face and the trunk.

Patients who show grade 2 PKDL with mucosal involvement and grade 3 PKDL need pharmacotherapy.[4] Limited data are available to guide treatment of PKDL. In eastern Africa, prolonged administration of antimonials (20 mg Sb^{5+}/kg/d for 30–60 days) with or without paromomycin, or liposomal amphotericin B (2.5 mg/kg/d for 20 days) has been recommended.[70] For the Indian subcontinent, conventional amphotericin B (1 mg/kg/d for 20 days, to be repeated up to 3–4 times at 20-day intervals) or miltefosine for 12 weeks is currently recommended by WHO.[51] L-AmB, at a total dose of 15 mg/kg divided in 5 doses, was also found effective in this region.[71] Promising findings were reported with therapeutic vaccination in Sudan.[72]

Complications and special situations

VL causes bone marrow suppression resulting in pancytopenia. VL patients are often prone to other infections because of leukopenia/neutropenia. Meticulous work-up for possible additional (predominantly bacterial) infections and timely management are critical for better outcome. They also have thrombocytopenia and anemia. Blood transfusion is another important aspect of the management.

VL may occur in individuals with different kinds of condition such as pregnancy or lactating mothers, or individuals with different organ dysfunctions such as renal failure or hepatic failure. As untreated VL can rapidly lead to deterioration and has fatal outcome, treatment should not be delayed. L-AmB is a safe option to use in these conditions. The conventional amphotericine B can be used for people with liposome-induced complement activation-related pseudo-allergy. Drug dose adjustments should also be done depending on creatinine clearance, concomitant medications. and adverse events.

Treatment monitoring

VL treatment response typically starts after 5 to 7 days of treatment initiation, with resolution of fever and improvement in appetite. This is often followed by weight gain, regression of the splenomegaly, and improvement in hematologic profiles. By the end of treatment, the spleen will become nonpalpable or tipped, and the hematology profile normalizes. However, splenomegaly might need several months to disappear completely.

In general, over 90% to 95% of immunocompetent patients demonstrate a good clinical response to treatment, with treatment unresponsiveness, death or severe toxicity seen in less than 5% to 10%.[73,74] However, treatment outcomes vary widely between different geographic regions, severity of disease, and the presence of coinfections and comorbidities. Up to 5% to 10% of immunocompetent individuals with apparent cure develop relapse, most commonly within 6 months after treatment.

Patients with underlying immunosuppression, those with partial clinical response, and those with relapsed form of disease need parasitologic assessment at the end of treatment to decide on their next management. Close follow-up for possible relapse and PKDL is important.

SUMMARY

Significant progress has been made in VL diagnostics over the last decades. Remaining challenges include the development of RDTs performing well in all VL-endemic areas. Additionally, noninvasive tests of cure are highly needed, especially for immunosuppressed patients, as they are more likely to fail treatment. In that respect, quantitative PCR and antigen tests merit further research. The same applies for the diagnosis of VL relapse. Interestingly, an RDT testing for *L donovani* antigen-specific IgG1 levels looks promising to diagnose VL relapse in immunocompetent Indian patients, with immunoglobulin 1 (IgG1) levels at very low levels in those disease-free at 6 months but high in those presenting with VL relapse.[75]

Molecular tests are expected to be increasingly used globally. In currently available studies, different types of primers and protocols were used, with limited standardization across laboratories.[31] Although available data generally suggest a consistently high sensitivity across these differences, standardization of these tests remains important. Moreover, given the relatively low number of studies on each primer, sample, species, or geographic area, additional studies are needed to get more reliable data and to discern clinically relevant differences in diagnostic performance across samples used or parasite strains. More data on the diagnostic accuracy of PCR on peripheral blood, especially in immunocompromised patients, are needed also. Immunologic markers are likely to be increasingly used to assess treatment response or to indicate safe discontinuation of secondary prophylaxis in immunocompromised patients. Whole blood assays similar to the interferon-γ release assays (IGRAs) used for TB screening have been developed and look promising.[76,77]

Several safety and effectiveness studies were reported from major *Leishmania* endemic regions of the world, as the limited available antileishmanial medicines became more accessible. The effectiveness varies with geographic region where the infection is acquired and the presence of comorbidities, importantly HIV coinfection. L-AmB has been found to be safe and effective in most endemic regions of the world and is the preferred choice to treat VL. However, higher L-AmB doses were required to treat VL in eastern Africa, where antimonials still remain the most effective although highly toxic. Combination therapy is increasing being explored and recommended to maximize effectiveness and reduce resistance development. Although antimonial combination with paromomycin has reduced the hospital stay for the eastern Africa region, L-AmB combined with miltefosine has increased effectiveness of VL treatment in HIV coinfected patients.

ACKNOWLEDGMENTS

The authors are collaborating on research activities on visceral leishmaniasis and visceral leishmaniasis/HIV co-infection in East Africa with funding from the European Union Seventh Framework Programme (FP7/2007-2013) under grant agreement n° 305178 via AfriCoLeish project and the Belgian Directorate General for Development Cooperation under the ITM-DGDC framework agreement.

REFERENCES

1. van Griensven J, Diro E. Visceral leishmaniasis. Infect Dis Clin North Am 2012; 26(2):309–22.
2. van Griensven J, Carrillo E, Lopez-Velez R, et al. Leishmaniasis in immunosuppressed individuals. Clin Microbiol Infect 2014;20(4):286–99.
3. Diro E, van Griensven J, Mohammed R, et al. Atypical manifestations of visceral leishmaniasis in patients with HIV in north Ethiopia: a gap in guidelines for the management of opportunistic infections in resource poor settings. Lancet Infect Dis 2015;15(1):122–9.
4. Zijlstra EE, Musa AM, Khalil EA, et al. Post-kala-azar dermal leishmaniasis. Lancet Infect Dis 2003;3(2):87–98.
5. Srivastava P, Dayama A, Mehrotra S, et al. Diagnosis of visceral leishmaniasis. Trans R Soc Trop Med Hyg 2011;105(1):1–6.
6. Siddig M, Ghalib H, Shillington DC, et al. Visceral leishmaniasis in Sudan. Clinical features. Trop Geogr Med 1990;42(2):107–12.
7. Maurya R, Mehrotra S, Prajapati VK, et al. Evaluation of blood agar microtiter plates for culturing leishmania parasites to titrate parasite burden in spleen and peripheral blood of patients with visceral leishmaniasis. J Clin Microbiol 2010; 48(5):1932–4.
8. Diro E, Yansouni C, Takele Y, et al. Diagnosis of visceral leishmaniasis using peripheral blood microscopy in Ethiopia: a prospective phase-III study of the diagnostic performance of different concentration techniques compared to tissue aspiration. Am J Trop Med Hyg 2017;96(1):190–6.
9. Hide M, Singh R, Kumar B, et al. A microculture technique for isolating live Leishmania parasites from peripheral blood of visceral leishmaniasis patients. Acta Trop 2007;102(3):197–200.
10. Sundar S, Rai M. Laboratory diagnosis of visceral leishmaniasis. Clin Diagn Lab Immunol 2002;9(5):951–8.
11. Aronson N, Herwaldt BL, Libman M, et al. Diagnosis and treatment of leishmaniasis: clinical practice guidelines by the Infectious Diseases Society of America (IDSA) and the American Society of Tropical Medicine and Hygiene (ASTMH). Am J Trop Med Hyg 2017;96(1):24–45.
12. Bangert M, Flores-Chavez MD, Llanes-Acevedo IP, et al. Validation of rK39 immunochromatographic test and direct agglutination test for the diagnosis of Mediterranean visceral leishmaniasis in Spain. PLoS Negl Trop Dis 2018;12(3):e0006277.
13. de Assis TS, Braga AS, Pedras MJ, et al. Multi-centric prospective evaluation of rk39 rapid test and direct agglutination test for the diagnosis of visceral leishmaniasis in Brazil. Trans R Soc Trop Med Hyg 2011;105(2):81–5.
14. Pedras MJ, de Gouvea Viana L, de Oliveira EJ, et al. Comparative evaluation of direct agglutination test, rK39 and soluble antigen ELISA and IFAT for the diagnosis of visceral leishmaniasis. Trans R Soc Trop Med Hyg 2008;102(2):172–8.
15. Oliveira E, Oliveira D, Cardoso FA, et al. Multicentre evaluation of a direct agglutination test prototype kit (DAT-LPC) for diagnosis of visceral leishmaniasis. Parasitology 2017;144(14):1964–70.
16. Burns JM Jr, Shreffler WG, Benson DR, et al. Molecular characterization of a kinesin-related antigen of Leishmania chagasi that detects specific antibody in

African and American visceral leishmaniasis. Proc Natl Acad Sci U S A 1993; 90(2):775–9.

17. Boelaert M, Verdonck K, Menten J, et al. Rapid tests for the diagnosis of visceral leishmaniasis in patients with suspected disease. Cochrane Database Syst Rev 2014;(6):CD009135.

18. Cunningham J, Hasker E, Das P, et al. A global comparative evaluation of commercial immunochromatographic rapid diagnostic tests for visceral leishmaniasis. Clin Infect Dis 2012;55(10):1312–9.

19. Mukhtar M, Abdoun A, Ahmed AE, et al. Diagnostic accuracy of rK28-based immunochromatographic rapid diagnostic tests for visceral leishmaniasis: a prospective clinical cohort study in Sudan. Trans R Soc Trop Med Hyg 2015; 109(9):594–600.

20. Pattabhi S, Whittle J, Mohamath R, et al. Design, development and evaluation of rK28-based point-of-care tests for improving rapid diagnosis of visceral leishmaniasis. PLoS Negl Trop Dis 2010;4(9) [pii:e822].

21. Bezuneh A, Mukhtar M, Abdoun A, et al. Comparison of point-of-care tests for the rapid diagnosis of visceral leishmaniasis in East African patients. Am J Trop Med Hyg 2014;91(6):1109–15.

22. Mukhtar M, Ali SS, Boshara SA, et al. Sensitive and less invasive confirmatory diagnosis of visceral leishmaniasis in Sudan using loop-mediated isothermal amplification (LAMP). PLoS Negl Trop Dis 2018;12(2):e0006264.

23. da Silva MRB, Brandao NAA, Colovati M, et al. Performance of two immunochromatographic tests for diagnosis of visceral leishmaniasis in patients coinfected with HIV. Parasitol Res 2018;117(2):419–27.

24. Teran-Angel G, Rodriguez V, Silva R, et al. Non invasive diagnostic tools for visceral leishmaniasis: a comparison of the immunoserological tests DAT, rK26 and rK39. Biomedica 2010;30(1):39–45 [in Spanish].

25. Kohanteb J, Ardehali S. Cross-reaction of sera from patients with various infectious diseases with *Leishmania infantum*. Med Princ Pract 2005;14(2):79–82.

26. Singla N, Singh GS, Sundar S, et al. Evaluation of the direct agglutination test as an immunodiagnostic tool for kala-azar in India. Trans R Soc Trop Med Hyg 1993; 87(3):276–8.

27. Sundar S, Singh RK, Maurya R, et al. Serological diagnosis of Indian visceral leishmaniasis: direct agglutination test versus rK39 strip test. Trans R Soc Trop Med Hyg 2006;100(6):533–7.

28. Vogt F, Mengesha B, Asmamaw H, et al. Accuracy of antigen detection in urine using KATex for non-invasive visceral leishmaniasis diagnosis and treatment monitoring in HIV-coinfected patients. 2017. Available at: http://www.itg.be/ Files/ECTMIH/ECTMIH%20final_programme.pdf. Accessed June 1, 2018.

29. Riera C, Fisa R, Lopez P, et al. Evaluation of a latex agglutination test (KAtex) for detection of *Leishmania* antigen in urine of patients with HIV-Leishmania coinfection: value in diagnosis and post-treatment follow-up. Eur J Clin Microbiol Infect Dis 2004;23(12):899–904.

30. Vallur AC, Tutterrow YL, Mohamath R, et al. Development and comparative evaluation of two antigen detection tests for visceral leishmaniasis. BMC Infect Dis 2015;15:384.

31. de Ruiter CM, van der Veer C, Leeflang MM, et al. Molecular tools for diagnosis of visceral leishmaniasis: systematic review and meta-analysis of diagnostic test accuracy. J Clin Microbiol 2014;52(9):3147–55.

32. Verma S, Singh R, Sharma V, et al. Development of a rapid loop-mediated isothermal amplification assay for diagnosis and assessment of cure of Leishmania infection. BMC Infect Dis 2017;17(1):223.

33. Adams ER, Schoone G, Versteeg I, et al. Development and evaluation of a novel LAMP assay for the diagnosis of cutaneous and visceral leishmaniasis. J Clin Microbiol 2018;56(7) [pii:e00386-18].

34. Alvar J, Aparicio P, Aseffa A, et al. The relationship between leishmaniasis and AIDS: the second 10 years. Clin Microbiol Rev 2008;21(2):334–59.

35. Cota GF, de Sousa MR, de Freitas Nogueira BM, et al. Comparison of parasitological, serological, and molecular tests for visceral leishmaniasis in HIV-infected patients: a cross-sectional delayed-type study. Am J Trop Med Hyg 2013;89(3): 570–7.

36. ter Horst R, Tefera T, Assefa G, et al. Field evaluation of rK39 test and direct agglutination test for diagnosis of visceral leishmaniasis in a population with high prevalence of human immunodeficiency virus in Ethiopia. Am J Trop Med Hyg 2009;80(6):929–34.

37. Antinori S, Cascio A, Parravicini C, et al. Leishmaniasis among organ transplant recipients. Lancet Infect Dis 2008;8(3):191–9.

38. Cota GF, de Sousa MR, Demarqui FN, et al. The diagnostic accuracy of serologic and molecular methods for detecting visceral leishmaniasis in HIV infected patients: meta-analysis. PLoS Negl Trop Dis 2012;6(5):e1665.

39. Molina I, Fisa R, Riera C, et al. Ultrasensitive real-time PCR for the clinical management of visceral leishmaniasis in HIV-infected patients. Am J Trop Med Hyg 2013;89(1):105–10.

40. Cruz I, Canavate C, Rubio JM, et al. A nested polymerase chain reaction (Ln-PCR) for diagnosing and monitoring *Leishmania infantum* infection in patients co-infected with human immunodeficiency virus. Trans R Soc Trop Med Hyg 2002;96(Suppl 1):S185–9.

41. Bourgeois N, Bastien P, Reynes J, et al. 'Active chronic visceral leishmaniasis' in HIV-1-infected patients demonstrated by biological and clinical long-term follow-up of 10 patients. HIV Med 2010;11(10):670–3.

42. Aronson N, Herwaldt BL, Libman M, et al. (ASTMH) IDSoAIatASoTMaH. Diagnosis and treatment of leishmaniasis: clinical practice guidelines by the Infectious Diseases Society of America (IDSA) and the American Society of Tropical Medicine and Hygiene (ASTMH). Am J Trop Med Hyg 2017;96(1):24–45.

43. Burza S, Sinha PK, Mahajan R, et al. Five-year field results and long-term effectiveness of 20 mg/kg liposomal amphotericin B (Ambisome) for visceral leishmaniasis in Bihar, India. PLoS Negl Trop Dis 2014;8(1):e2603.

44. Sundar S, Chakravarty J, Agarwal D, et al. Single-dose liposomal amphotericin B for visceral leishmaniasis in India. N Engl J Med 2010;362(6):504–12.

45. Di Masi F, Ursini T, Iannece MD, et al. Five-year retrospective Italian multicenter study of visceral leishmaniasis treatment. Antimicrob Agents Chemother 2014; 58(1):414–8.

46. Khalil EA, Weldegebreal T, Younis BM, et al. Safety and efficacy of single dose versus multiple doses of AmBisome for treatment of visceral leishmaniasis in eastern Africa: a randomised trial. PLoS Negl Trop Dis 2014;8(1):e2613.

47. Tamiru A, Tigabu B, Yifru S, et al. Safety and efficacy of liposomal amphotericin B for treatment of complicated visceral leishmaniasis in patients without HIV, North-West Ethiopia. BMC Infect Dis 2016;16(1):548.

48. Romero GAS, Costa DL, Costa CHN, et al. Efficacy and safety of available treatments for visceral leishmaniasis in Brazil: a multicenter, randomized, open label trial. PLoS Negl Trop Dis 2017;11(6):e0005706.
49. Musa A, Khalil E, Hailu A, et al. Sodium stibogluconate (SSG) & paromomycin combination compared to SSG for visceral leishmaniasis in East Africa: a randomised controlled trial. PLoS Negl Trop Dis 2012;6(6):e1674.
50. Kimutai R, Musa AM, Njoroge S, et al. Safety and effectiveness of sodium stibogluconate and paromomycin combination for the treatment of visceral leishmaniasis in Eastern Africa: results from a pharmacovigilance programme. Clin Drug Investig 2017;37(3):259–72.
51. WHO. Control of the leishmaniasis. Report of a meeting of the WHO expert committee on the control of leishmaniases. WHO technical report series 9492010, Geneva, 22–26 March 2010.
52. Sundar S, Sinha PK, Rai M, et al. Comparison of short-course multidrug treatment with standard therapy for visceral leishmaniasis in India: an open-label, non-inferiority, randomised controlled trial. Lancet 2011;377(9764):477–86.
53. Sundar S, Rai M, Chakravarty J, et al. New treatment approach in Indian visceral leishmaniasis: single-dose liposomal amphotericin B followed by short-course oral miltefosine. Clin Infect Dis 2008;47(8):1000–6.
54. Hailu A, Musa A, Wasunna M, et al. Geographical variation in the response of visceral leishmaniasis to paromomycin in East Africa: a multicentre, open-label, randomized trial. PLoS Negl Trop Dis 2010;4(10):e709.
55. Musa AM, Younis B, Fadlalla A, et al. Paromomycin for the treatment of visceral leishmaniasis in Sudan: a randomized, open-label, dose-finding study. PLoS Negl Trop Dis 2010;4(10):e855.
56. Ritmeijer K, Dejenie A, Assefa Y, et al. A comparison of miltefosine and sodium stibogluconate for treatment of visceral leishmaniasis in an Ethiopian population with high prevalence of HIV infection. Clin Infect Dis 2006;43(3):357–64.
57. Dorlo TP, Rijal S, Ostyn B, et al. Failure of miltefosine in visceral leishmaniasis is associated with low drug exposure. J Infect Dis 2014;210(1):146–53.
58. Pintado V, Martin-Rabadan P, Rivera ML, et al. Visceral leishmaniasis in human immunodeficiency virus (HIV)-infected and non-HIV-infected patients. A comparative study. Medicine (Baltimore) 2001;80(1):54–73.
59. Cota GF, de Sousa MR, Fereguetti TO, et al. Efficacy of anti-leishmania therapy in visceral leishmaniasis among HIV infected patients: a systematic review with indirect comparison. PLoS Negl Trop Dis 2013;7(5):e2195.
60. CDC. Panel on Opportunistic Infections in HIV-Infected Adults and Adolescents. Guidelines for the prevention and treatment of opportunistic infections in HIV-infected adults and adolescents: recommendations from the Centers for Disease Control and Prevention, the National Institutes of Health, and the HIV Medicine Association of the Infectious Diseases Society of America. 2013.
61. Ritmeijer K, ter Horst R, Chane S, et al. Limited effectiveness of high-dose liposomal amphotericin B (Ambisome) for treatment of visceral leishmaniasis in an Ethiopian population with high HIV prevalence. Clin Infect Dis 2011;53(12): e152–8.
62. Cota GF, de Sousa MR, de Mendonca AL, et al. Leishmania-HIV co-infection: clinical presentation and outcomes in an urban area in Brazil. PLoS Negl Trop Dis 2014;8(4):e2816.
63. Sinha PK, van Griensven J, Pandey K, et al. Liposomal amphotericin B for visceral leishmaniasis in human immunodeficiency virus-coinfected patients: 2-year treatment outcomes in Bihar, India. Clin Infect Dis 2011;53(7):e91–8.

64. Lopez-Velez R. The impact of highly active antiretroviral therapy (HAART) on visceral leishmaniasis in Spanish patients who are co-infected with HIV. Ann Trop Med Parasitol 2003;97(Suppl 1):143–7.
65. Abongomera C, Diro E, Vogt F, et al. The risk and predictors of visceral leishmaniasis relapse in human immunodeficiency virus-coinfected patients in Ethiopia: a retrospective cohort study. Clin Infect Dis 2017;65(10):1703–10.
66. WHO. Report of the Fifth Consultative Meeting on Leishmania/HIV Coinfection, March 20-22. Addis Ababa, Ethiopia, 22 Mar 2007.
67. Diro E, Ritmeijer K, Boelaert M, et al. Use of pentamidine as secondary prophylaxis to prevent visceral leishmaniasis relapse in HIV infected patients, the first twelve months of a prospective cohort study. PLoS Negl Trop Dis 2015;9(10): e0004087.
68. Diro E, Ritmeijer K, Boelaert M, et al. Long-term clinical outcomes in visceral leishmaniasis-HIV co-infected patients during and after pentamidine secondary prophylaxis in Ethiopia: a single-arm clinical trial Authors and affiliations. Clin Infect Dis 2018;66(3):444–51.
69. Bogdan C. Leishmaniasis in rheumatology, haematology and oncology: epidemiological, immunological and clinical aspects and caveats. Ann Rheum Dis 2012; 71(Suppl 2):i60–6.
70. Abongomera C, Gatluak F, Buyze J, et al. A comparison of the effectiveness of sodium stibogluconate monotherapy to sodium stibogluconate and paromomycin combination for the treatment of severe post kala azar dermal leishmaniasis in South Sudan - a retrospective cohort study. PLoS One 2016;11(9):e0163047.
71. den Boer M, Das AK, Akhter F, et al. Safety and effectiveness of short-course Ambisome in the treatment of post-kala-azar dermal leishmaniasis (PKDL): a prospective cohort study in Bangladesh. Clin Infect Dis 2018;67(5):667–75.
72. Musa AM, Khalil EA, Mahgoub FA, et al. Immunochemotherapy of persistent post-kala-azar dermal leishmaniasis: a novel approach to treatment. Trans R Soc Trop Med Hyg 2008;102(1):58–63.
73. Murray HW, Berman JD, Davies CR, et al. Advances in leishmaniasis. Lancet 2005;366(9496):1561–77.
74. Alvar J, Croft S, Olliaro P. Chemotherapy in the treatment and control of leishmaniasis. Adv Parasitol 2006;61:223–74.
75. Bhattacharyya T, Ayandeh A, Falconar AK, et al. IgG1 as a potential biomarker of post-chemotherapeutic relapse in visceral leishmaniasis, and adaptation to a rapid diagnostic test. PLoS Negl Trop Dis 2014;8(10):e3273.
76. Ibarra-Meneses AV, Ghosh P, Hossain F, et al. IFN-gamma, IL-2, IP-10, and MIG as biomarkers of exposure to leishmania spp., and of cure in human visceral leishmaniasis. Front Cell Infect Microbiol 2017;7:200.
77. Castro A, Carrillo E, San Martin JV, et al. Lymphoproliferative response after stimulation with soluble leishmania antigen (SLA) as a predictor of visceral leishmaniasis (VL) relapse in HIV+ patients. Acta Trop 2016;164:345–51.
78. Chappuis F, Rijal S, Soto A, et al. A meta-analysis of the diagnostic performance of the direct agglutination test and rK39 dipstick for visceral leishmaniasis. BMJ 2006;333(7571):723.

Cutaneous Leishmaniasis
Updates in Diagnosis and Management

Naomi E. Aronson, MD[a],*, Christie A. Joya, DO[b,1]

KEYWORDS

- Cutaneous leishmaniasis • Antimony • Amphotericin • Miltefosine
- Leishmaniasis diagnostic testing

KEY POINTS

- Cutaneous leishmaniasis is a complex disease consisting of more than 20 *Leishmania* species that have varying pathogenicity and drug susceptibility.
- Molecular diagnostic tests are sensitive and specific; they require a small lesion specimen that permits less-invasive sampling methods.
- Several test methods should be done, using a lesion specimen, to maximize diagnostic yield.
- Systemic treatments may have significant toxicity and need to be carefully considered, taking into account *Leishmania* species, geographic region of acquisition, patient comorbid health status, extent/location of lesions, and previous treatments.

INTRODUCTION

Cutaneous leishmaniasis (CL) is a severely neglected tropical disease that has been significantly increasing in numbers affected over the past decades, with a change in global prevalence from 1990 to 2013 of +174.2%.[1] This sand fly bite–transmitted parasitic infection causes chronic skin lesions that heal with scarring, often on cosmetically obvious places, leaving those affected with some disfigurement.[2] CL is endemic in regions of most continents and recently areas in Thailand, Caribbean, and Ghana are reporting emerging foci of *L enriettii* complex causing human cutaneous and/or visceral infection.[3] Leishmaniasis acquired in parts of South America also may result, even years after the skin lesions heal, with mucosal destruction of

Disclosure Statement: N.E. Aronson and C.A. Joya have no commercial or financial disclosures.
Disclaimer: The opinions and assertions expressed herein are those of the authors and do not necessarily reflect the official policy or position of the Uniformed Services University, the Department of the Navy, or the Department of Defense.
[a] Infectious Diseases Division, Uniformed Services University of the Health Sciences, 4301 Jones Bridge Road, Bethesda, MD 20814, USA; [b] U.S. Naval Medical Research Unit Number 6, Lima, Peru
[1] Present address: 3230 Lima Place, Washington DC, 20521-3230.
* Corresponding author.
E-mail address: naomi.aronson@usuhs.edu

Infect Dis Clin N Am 33 (2019) 101–117
https://doi.org/10.1016/j.idc.2018.10.004
0891-5520/19/Published by Elsevier Inc.

id.theclinics.com

the nose and pharynx (mucosal leishmaniasis [ML]). Over recent years, advances have been made in the diagnosis and treatment of CL, which are summarized in this article, with emphasis toward management approaches in North America.

DIAGNOSIS OF CUTANEOUS LEISHMANIASIS

The widespread use of more sensitive molecular diagnostic tests (such as polymerase chain reaction [PCR]) has radically changed both sample collection and the amount of time and reference laboratory support that were typical a decade ago (to confirm a leishmaniasis diagnosis). Another major advance is new antileishmanial treatments that drive more individualized therapies, which are often benefited by *Leishmania* species identification for prognosis and to direct management choices.

The first and most critical diagnostic step is for clinicians to consider a diagnosis of CL when assessing a chronic skin lesion(s) in a person with potential exposure in an endemic region (http://www.who.int/leishmaniasis/leishmaniasis_maps/en). The lesion(s) is often painless and purulence is uncommon; the location is typically on exposed areas, such as face and extremities. Appearances include ulcer (often with eschar or exudate overlying) and nodule/plaques most commonly, but lesions may also have sporotrichoid, verrucous, zosteriform, psoriasiform, eczematous, or erysipeloid features (**Figs. 1–4**).

Currently, there is no gold-standard single diagnostic test; clinical practice guidelines recommend performing several assays using a sample from an active-appearing skin lesion.[4] The sensitivity of the diagnostic assays depends on the

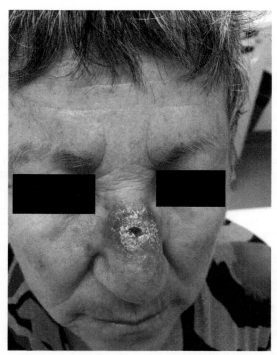

Fig. 1. Ulcerative lesion due to *L major* acquired in Morocco. (*Courtesy of* K. Billick, MD, Montreal, Canada.)

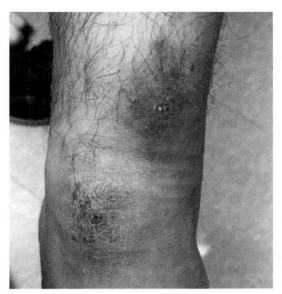

Fig. 2. Plaque-like lesions due to *L tropica* on the ankle, acquired in Syria. (*Courtesy of* S. Wood, MD, Bethesda, MD.)

number of parasites in the lesion (often equates with duration of lesion), *Leishmania* species, and type of lesion (ulcer often highest yield). There are national *Leishmania* diagnostic reference laboratories that generally provide services without charge; it is always preferable to contact them prior to obtaining samples (see **Table 3**).

Sample Collection

In CL, *Leishmania* parasites are found in the epidermis and upper levels of the dermis, so they are fairly superficial. In ulcerative lesions, the base has more parasites but also more tissue destruction; with assays, such as PCR and culture, the cleansed base is

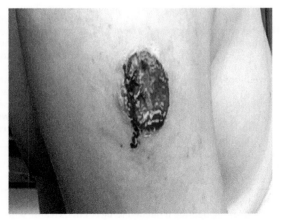

Fig. 3. Ulcerative lesion due to *L V panamensis*. (*Courtesy of* J.D. Malone, MD, San Diego, CA.)

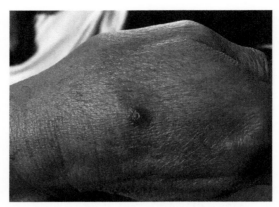

Fig. 4. Nodular lesion due to *L infantum* acquired in Sicily. (*Courtesy of* R. Maves, MD, San Diego, CA.)

the target collection site, but for histology, the less disrupted indurated border of the lesion is recommended. See **Table 1** for various sample collection techniques.

The preparation of a skin lesion for sampling is simple but key. The authors recommend the following:

- Thoroughly cleanse lesion with soap and water; rinse with water.
- Blot dry with gauze, removing any residual betadine if used.

Table 1
How to sample skin lesion for a *Leishmania* diagnosis[a]

Appearance	Methods[b]	Considerations
Ulcer	Swab using DNA collection swab, 10 times over ulcer[46]	Use for more sensitive molecular assays (eg, PCR)
	Tape strip disk, tape stripping[47]	Use for more sensitive molecular assays (eg, PCR)
	Cytology brush or dental broach[48]	For *Leishmania* culture or PCR, use for CL Detect assay
	Skin scraping with scalpel blade edge, sample about size of large rice grain[4]	Limit bleeding for best results, use local anesthesia, use 1 sampling each for smear, culture, and PCR
	Fine-needle aspirate generally from indurated border[4,48]	1-mL syringe with needle (20G–25G) with or without nonbacteriostatic saline; can be used for smear, culture, and PCR
	Shave biopsy	Use if other diagnoses under consideration as well
	4-mm punch biopsy of the indurated rim	Use if other diagnoses under consideration as well
	• Touch impression smears	Use if less-invasive testing does not
	• Press imprint smears[49]	yield diagnosis
Nodule/plaque	Skin snip (like leprosy technique)	Smear, culture, PCR
	Fine-needle aspirate	Smear, culture, PCR
	4-mm full skin thickness punch biopsy	Smear, culture, PCR

[a] Not all-inclusive of methods.
[b] Choose an active looking lesion, débride if needed to ulcer base, cleanse with detergent and water, remove any residual betadine or soap, and blot dry.

- If pertinent, débride a portion of the exudate or overlying eschar down to clean ulcer base. Generally, this is painful, and local anesthesia should be considered. Limit bleeding because it may confound the smear.
- If parasite culture is planned, sterile technique should be used.

Full-thickness skin punch biopsies should not be the first diagnostic procedure for CL, both due to a more invasive nature and because they can be lower yield.[5,6] The median number of *Leishmania* parasites found at various skin tissue levels were epidermis, 42×10^6; superior dermis, 40×10^6; inferior dermis, 26×10^6; and subcutaneous tissue, 12×10^6.[6] The primary reason to perform a punch biopsy is to evaluate other diagnostic considerations, including histopathology, fungal, or mycobacterial etiologies: in this case, only a small amount of tissue is needed for leishmaniasis culture and PCR. It is also used when noninvasive studies yield negative results.

Types of Tests for Leishmaniasis Diagnosis

Globally, tissue microscopy (a smear, tissue imprint, or drop of tissue placed on a glass slide, stained with Giemsa, and evaluated under an oil immersion lens) is the most common leishmaniasis diagnostic test. Although less sensitive than others and requiring expertise in interpretation as well as a high-power microscope lens, its advantages are mainly low cost and readily available materials. The *Leishmania* amastigote seen in human tissues is a tiny, round to oval organism approximately 3 μm to 5 μm length, with a well circumscribed nucleus and a diagnostic rod-shaped kinetoplast; it can be intracellular or extracellular (**Fig. 5**). If the kinetoplast is not seen, then *Leishmania* cannot be distinguished from *Histoplasma* or even *Sporothrix* species.

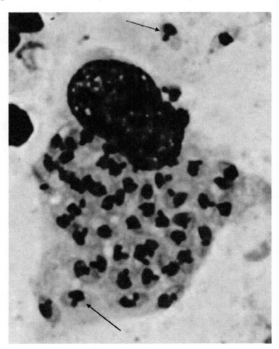

Fig. 5. Giemsa-stained skin scraping showing many intracellular amastigotes inside a mononuclear cell cytoplasm; note the rod-shaped perpendicular kinetoplast. *Arrows* indicate amastigotes. (Giemsa stain, original magnification ×250). (*Courtesy of* R. Neafie, Washington, DC.)

Histopathology is the least sensitive diagnostic method. A few practical pointers for the review of tissue histopathology for detection of *Leishmania* are to use oil immersion (100×), stain with hematoxylin-eosin but also stain sections with Brown-Hopps tissue Gram stain, resect to multiple 3-mm–thickness slices, and review areas of well-formed necrotizing and non-necrotizing granulomas carefully. Other consistent findings include an inflammatory plasma cell and lymphocyte infiltration, hypertrophied stratum corneum and necrotic ulceration, epidermal hyperplasia, parakeratosis, acanthosis, and intraepithelial abscesses.[7]

Table 2 reviews various techniques that are used for the detection of *Leishmania* parasites, concentrating on parasitologic diagnosis. The general categories of diagnostic approach are clinical, immunologic, and parasitologic. Clinical diagnosis (consistent clinical appearance and epidemiologic risk) is not considered sufficient and should always be confirmed with laboratory diagnostic testing. Immunologic diagnosis of CL is not included in **Table 2** except for the CL Detect test, because commercial serology is insufficiently sensitive to be clinically useful and the *Leishmania* skin test is not available in North America. Recent proteomic approaches may uncover more immunogenic and abundant antigens to improve serologic assays.[8] CL Detect is a Food and Drug Administration (FDA)-cleared, rapid immunochromatographic test detecting the peroxidin antigen of *Leishmania*, performed with skin lesion sampling collected with a dental broach.[9] It is particularly helpful for ulcerative lesions of recent onset (<4 months); any residual betadine interferes with assay results.

There are more than 20 *Leishmania* species associated with human infection. Unless a patient's travel history is circumscribed and there is only 1 known *Leishmania* species circulating there, species identification should be considered. Knowledge of the *Leishmania* species may allow better estimation of the risk of ML, time to healing, and response to various therapies. This is critical in immunocompromised hosts and those with medical comorbid conditions where significant risk benefit decisions must be made in treatment plans. Parasite identification has classically required parasite isolation with culture, expansion of the parasite, and then multilocus enzyme electrophoresis (so-called isoenzyme electrophoresis)[10,11] or multilocus sequence testing.[12] This testing is relegated to a few reference laboratories (**Table 3**). Because culture, albeit a definitive diagnostic test, is not highly sensitive; subject to contaminating skin flora overgrowth, nonviable organisms from transport, or finicky parasite in vitro growth; and slow (most laboratories holding cultures until 30 days before noting as no growth), this has an impact on whether species are identified (40% specimens) in a timeframe that is clinically useful.[13] Matrix-assisted laser desorption ionization (MALDI)–time of flight (TOF) mass spectrometry yields a protein spectral fingerprint of *Leishmania* species.[14–17] Although culture is required, this method has advantages of speed, and lesser cost, and, as more MALDI becomes available, this could be widely integrated into clinical laboratories. Lastly, nucleic acid amplification-based assays, such as PCR, have been developed to rapidly identify *Leishmania* species. There is great variability in gene targets, performance characteristics, methods/protocols, and a lack of commercial availability that currently limits the routine use of molecular testing for species identification. The miniexon PCR–restriction fragment length polymorphism (RFLP) genotyping has promise.[18,19]

There are 2 types of testing that are not clinically available but deserve notice: *Leishmaniavirus* coinfection and *Leishmania* drug susceptibility testing. *Leishmania* RNA viruses parasitize *Leishmania* parasites (multiple *Leishmania* species globally) and have a role in increased pathogenicity with associations with mucosal infection, lesion persistence, or increased relapse rates after treatment.[20–22] Although

Table 2
Cutaneous leishmaniasis: current diagnostic tests

Test	Considerations
Microscopy • Sample smeared on glass slide • Touch impression	• Rapid point-of-care test • Amastigote confirmed when organism with a distinct kinetoplast is seen (see **Fig. 5**) • Stain with Giemsa, Diff-Quik, Wright Giemsa, or Brown-Hopps stain • View with 100× oil immersion lens
Histopathology • Thin sections (3 mm) • Study slides for up to 1 h • 100× oil immersion	• Most organisms are superficial • Hematoxylin-eosin stain • Enhanced with Brown-Hopps tissue Gram stain • Not very sensitive
Parasite culture • Sterile collection without residual betadine on lesion • Reference laboratory, contact in advance (see **Table 3**) • Typical media is Schneider's with fetal bovine serum or NNN • Once in media, ship to laboratory at room temperature	• Prone to contamination with skin flora • Allows species identification (see narrative) ○ MLEE, MLST ○ Molecular methods, sequencing ○ PCR-RFLP ○ MALDI-TOF • Not all parasites expand well in vitro • Definitive diagnosis
Immunologic • CL Detect (InBios Seattle, WA) performed with tissue from lesion	• Point-of-care rapid test • FDA cleared • Avoid any residual betadine in sample
Recombinant polymerase amplification[50] • Lateral flow immunochromatographic strip • Targets kinetoplast DNA	• Point-of-care rapid test • Not readily available at this time
Loop-mediated isothermal amplification assay[51] • Pan–*Leishmania* spectrum • Role in resource limited settings where PCR may not be available	• Applied to boiled swabs as samples
PCR[48,52] • Multiple targets used • Multiple platforms used, real time PCR is preferred • Submit sample in high concentration ethanol (not formalin) • Can test paraffin embedded samples (lower sensitivity) • Sample can be dried onto filter paper and tested • DNA scraped off microscopy slides can provide sample • Tests vary laboratory to laboratory, comparative validation studies are needed	• Most sensitive assay • Relatively rapid • Methods allow species identification • Technique allows parasite quantitation

Abbreviations: MLEE, multilocus enzyme electrophoresis; MLST, multilocus sequence testing; NNN, Novy-MacNeal-Nicolle media.

clinical treatment failure may additionally be affected by factors other than drug susceptibility, the testing of *Leishmania* parasites for drug susceptibility remains relegated to research laboratories; although, as more therapeutic agents become available, there could be a role for testing.[23]

Table 3 Leishmaniasis diagnostic reference laboratories	
Laboratory	**Contact Information**
National Reference Centre for Parasitology, Montreal, Quebec, Canada[a]	Momar Ndao, DVM, MSc, PhD Research Institute of the McGill University Health Centre 1001 Decarie Boulevard, Room E03, 5375 Montreal, Quebec H4A 3J1, Canada Telephone +1–514–934–8347 www. mcgill.ca/tropmed/nrcp
CDC, Atlanta, GA[b]	Marcos de Almeida, PhD CDC Division of Parasitic Diseases and Malaria SMB/STAT, Unit 52 1600 Clifton Road NE Atlanta GA 30329 Telephone 404-718-4175 DPDx@cdc.gov
Walter Reed Army Institute of Research, Silver Spring, MD[c]	Sheila Peel, MSPH, PhD WRAIR Leishmania Diagnostics Laboratory 503 Robert Grant Avenue Silver Spring, MD 20910–7500 Telephone 240-595-7353 http://www.wrair.army.mil/OtherServices_LDL.aspx
WHO Collaborating Centres	http://apps.who.int/whocc/List.aspx?cc_subject= Leishmaniasis

[a] Engagement of provincial public health laboratory to forward sample is preferred.
[b] Notify state public health laboratories when submitting to CDC.
[c] Restricted to US military and Department of Defense (DoD) civilian worker samples.

TREATMENT OF CUTANEOUS LEISHMANIASIS

The primary goal of CL treatment is to reduce morbidity (ie, preventing relapse and dissemination [mucosal disease]). A majority of lesions heal slowly without specific therapy; however, therapy should be considered, especially when lesions are distressing to the patient, the lesion(s) are complex (**Fig. 6**), or if there is risk of mucosal disease. Recently, clinical practice guidelines for the diagnosis and treatment of CL were published and are available on the Infectious Diseases Society of America web site (www.idsociety.org).[4]

Although a majority of these lesions are self-healing, without significant consequences, aside from disfiguring scar, some species of the subgenus *Viannia* (ie, *L V braziliensis*, *L V guyanensis,* and *L V panamensis*) are associated with ML, which can cause significant morbidity and even mortality. Treatment of leishmaniasis may resolve lesions more quickly (potentially reducing cosmetic consequences) and decrease mucosal metastases. There is no overall drug of choice treatment of CL, because the systemic treatments available have significant toxicities and are not equally effective against all species of *Leishmania*, and healing rates among the same species differ geographically. Host cell–mediated immunity is important in control of the infection. Therefore, the treatment of CL needs to be individualized to the patient, *Leishmania* species, and the geographic region where infection was acquired.

Parallel to an assessment as to whether CL is simple or complex, treatment decisions include observation with wound care versus local therapy to the lesion versus systemic therapy (see **Fig. 6**, **Box 1a**). Drugs available for the treatment of

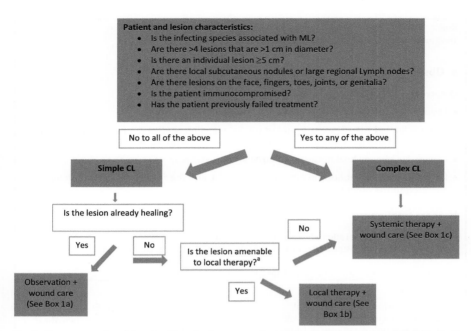

Fig. 6. Treatment algorithm for CL: a basic approach. Although CL treatment should be individualized to the patient, this is a generalized flowchart to describe a basic approach to therapy. All patients should be educated about the natural history of leishmaniasis and risks and benefits of treatment and agree to treatment plan. This does not address the treatment of pregnant patients, those with evidence of ML, or those with unusual syndromes of leishmaniasis (leishmaniasis recidivans, diffuse CL, or disseminated leishmaniasis). [a] Few lesions (<5), small lesions (<4 cm in diameter), lesions are not in a cosmetically important areas (ie, face), and not in functionally important areas.

CL are of limited availability and restricted in choices, and some have significant side effects. Historically, pentavalent antimonials (SbV) have been used for the treatment of CL; however, this treatment is not FDA approved, has some toxicity, cannot currently be given intralesionally in the United States, and there are concerns for resistance with increasing clinical failures.[23] Sodium stibogluconate (SbV) can be obtained through a Centers for Disease Control and Prevention (CDC)-sponsored investigational new drug (IND) protocol for intravenous (IV) use. Miltefosine is the only FDA-approved drug for the treatment of CL caused by *L V braziliensis*, *L V guyanensis*, and *L V panamensis*. Drugs that are used off-label in the United States are the azoles, liposomal amphotericin B (L-amB), and pentamidine; 15% topical paromomycin formulations can be compounded by individual pharmacies.

Local Therapy

For lesions that are simple and amenable to local therapy, and when a decision is made to treat, a local modality should be considered (**Box 1b**). Local therapy is generally first-line therapy for Old World cutaneous leishmaniasis (OWCL) and commonly used for New World cutaneous leishmaniasis (NWCL) that is not associated with ML (such as *LL Mexicana*). Local modalities include cryotherapy, thermotherapy, topical creams/ointments, and intralesional (IL) medications. The physical modalities

Box 1
Treatment dosing and indications for cutaneous leishmaniasis

a. Observation

Observation is reasonable in cases where all of the following apply:

- Lesions are consistent with simple CL (see **Fig. 6**).
- There is limited risk of mucosal metastasis (ie, infecting species is *L L mexicana,* an OWCL species, or, if species is unknown, the NWCL lesion was acquired north of Costa Rica).
- Lesions are already healing spontaneously at time of diagnosis.
- Patient is educated about the natural history of CL and the risks/benefits of treatment and agrees with the observation plan.

b. Local treatment

Local treatment is generally indicated for simple lesions (see **Fig. 6**)—there are a few, small lesions that are not in cosmetically or functionally important areas of the body.

Types and Administration of Local Therapy	Considerations
Cryotherapy	• Appropriate for
• Usually performed by dermatologists • Liquid nitrogen applied for 15–20 s to lesion extending 1–2 mm outside of lesion, then allowed to thaw • Repeated 3 times per session • Treatment repeated every 3 wk until healing of lesion • Success dependent on skill of operator	○ Simple lesions (see **Fig. 6**) ○ There is no risk of mucosal metastasis ○ Early lesions • Can be used in combination with SbV intralesional therapy • May consider in pregnant patients or others with contraindications to systemic therapy • Can cause permanent hypopigmentation at site
Thermotherapy	• Appropriate for
• ThermoMed device (FDA cleared) • Local anesthesia is required • Heat of 50°C is applied for 30 s to lesion extending 1–2 mm outside of lesion. • Produces second-degree burn • Success dependent on skill of operator	○ Simple small lesions (see **Fig. 6**) ○ *L L major, L L tropica, L L mexicana,* and *L V panamensis* species • Not for use over superficial nerves, cartilage, eyelids, nose, or lips • Can be used in combination with systemic therapy • May consider in pregnant patients or others with contraindications to systemic therapy
Topical paromomycin	• Appropriate for

• 15% paromomycin + 12% MBCL ointment
  ○ Trade name: Leshcutan, Israel
• 15% paromomycin cream is being developed by DoD
  ○ May be approximated by compounding pharmacies
  ○ Replaces WR 279,396
  ○ Apply to lesion bid for 20 d
  ○ Currently IND only
	○ Simple lesions (see **Fig. 6**)
	○ Ulcerative lesions
	○ *L L major* and *L V panamensis*
	• Poor response rates in *L L tropica* and *L L aethiopica* infections
	• Not recommended if there is lymphocutaneous involvement
	• Can cause significant inflammation

Intralesional therapy

- Sodium stibogluconate

  - Trade name: Pentostam
  - Not currently covered in CDC IND for parenteral therapy
  - Intradermal injection
  - 5 sites per lesion
  - 0.2–5 mL every 3–7 d until healing
  - Local anesthetic needed
- Meglumine antimoniate
  - Trade name: Glucantime
  - Not available in the United States

- Appropriate for
  - Simple lesions (see **Fig. 6**)
  - OWCL, *L V panamensis*, *L L mexicana*
- Improved efficacy when used in combination with cryotherapy

c. Systemic treatment

Systemic therapy can be used for all types of CL; however, treatment has toxicity and it should be carefully individualized based on patient characteristics. Systemic therapy can be used for simple lesions that are not amenable to local therapy, when there is risk of mucosal disease, when rapid healing is desired, and when lesion is in cosmetically or functionally important areas. It is generally the first choice for complex CL and for relapsed CL.

Types and Administration of Systemic Therapy	Considerations
Azoles	• Appropriate for
• Fluconazole	○ Lymphocutaneous CL, simple CL, and some complex CL
○ Trade name: Diflucan	○ *L L infantum*, *L L donovani*, and *L L mexicana* showed cure rates of 80%–89%.[33]
○ 200 mg po daily for 6 wk or	
○ 400 mg po daily for 6 wk	○ May be used for *L L major*; however, higher doses may be needed if infection was acquired in Iraq or North Africa.
○ Off-label use	
• Ketoconazole	
○ Trade name: Nizoral	○ Ketoconazole has reported good cure rates for *L L mexicana*, *L L major* (from Iran), and *L V panamensis*.
○ 600 mg po daily for 28 d	
○ Off-label use	• Should not be used for *L V braziliensis*
• Itraconazole	
○ Trade name: Sporanox	
○ 100 mg po bid for 42–56 d	
○ Off-label use	
Miltefosine	• Appropriate for
• Trade name: Impavido	○ Simple and complex lesions
• FDA approved for CL caused by *Viannia* species	○ *L L major*, *L L tropica*, *L V panamensis*, *L V guyanensis*, and *L V braziliensis* (not acquired in Guatemala)
• Weight-based dosing	• Expensive
• ≥45 kg body weight, 50 mg po tid for 28 d	
• Target dose is 2.5 mg/kg/d; however, limited by side effects when >150 mg/kg/d is taken	
• May be under-dosed in larger individuals	
Pentamidine isethionate	• Exclusively used for *L V guyanensis*; however, generally second line due to adverse effects
• Trade name: Pentam 300	
• Off-label use	
• 3–4 mg/kg every other day for 3–4 doses	

SbV

- Sodium stibogluconate
  - Trade name: Pentostam
  - Available from CDC under IND
  - 20 mg SbV/kg/d IV for 20 d
- Meglumine antimoniate
  - Trade name: Glucantime
  - Not available in the United States

- Appropriate for
  - Complex lesions
- Toxicity and increasing treatment failures due to resistance have relegated SbV to second-line choice in United States, Canada, and Europe

Amphotericin

- Amphotericin deoxycholate
  - Trade name: Fungizone
  - 0.5–1.0 mg/kg IV daily or every other day for cumulative dose of 15–30 mg/kg
  - Off-label use
- Liposomal amphotericin
  - Trade name: AmBisome
  - Off-label use
  - 3 mg/kg/d IV daily for d 1–5 and then d 10 or d 1–7 for cumulative dose of 18–21 mg/kg

- Appropriate for
  - Complex lesions
- Dosing is based off treatment of visceral leishmaniasis.
- Optimal dosing for CL is not well defined.
- L-amB is preferred due to less toxicity.
- Higher doses and longer therapy are required for immunocompromised hosts.
- Saline loading prior to dosing seems to partly protect against renal toxicity.

(cryotherapy and thermotherapy) may be of special use for patients who are restricted from use of systemic treatments, such as those during pregnancy and with other comorbid conditions, as well as for drug resistance.

Cryotherapy is generally well tolerated and readily available. A meta-analysis showed that cryotherapy has similar efficacy to IL antimony, with the proportion of patients cured per intention-to-treat analysis of 54% in the cryotherapy group and 68% treated with IL SbV.[24]

Thermotherapy is another option; however, it requires specialized equipment (such as ThermoMed, Thermosurgery Technologies, Inc, Phoenix, AZ) and local anesthesia. A meta-analysis showed a 73% cure rate overall for CL; however, it was somewhat less efficacious in *L V braziliensis*.[25] Most of the studies were done treating simple OWCL, although there are current trials planed in South America combining thermotherapy with miltefosine.[26]

Topical paromomycin is another local therapy that can be used for lesions that are ulcerated and due to *L L major*. A combination of paromomycin and gentamicin (WR 279,396) cream was used in a phase II clinical trial for treatment of *L V panamensis*, which showed greater efficacy in the combination therapy (87% vs 53%); a phase 3 trial in Tunisia for treatment of *L major* CL showed 81% efficacy in the paromomycin-gentamicin arm and 82% in the paromomycin arm.[27,28] A different product, 15% paromomycin in 12% methylbenzethonium chloride ([MBCL] Leishcutan), is made by Teva Pharmaceuticals (Petah Tikva, Israel).[29]

Intralesional antimony is a mainstay in many OWCL endemic regions of the world; however, it is unavailable in the United States. A recent systematic review of IL antimonials showed an overall efficacy of 75%.[30] The combination of cryotherapy and IL antimony was evaluated on systematic review and found cure rates of 82% versus 53% in IL antimony alone.[30,31] Intralesional amphotericin may bear further research as an alternative to SbV.[32]

SYSTEMIC THERAPY

If systemic therapy is necessary, the options are limited, and several have the potential for significant adverse effects. Therefore, the decision of which drug to use needs to be individualized, based on (1) the patient (ie, comorbidities, immunologic status, and if the patient is gravid, breastfeeding, or desires pregnancy in the near future), (2) the infecting species (ie, if the species is associated with ML or, if unknown, the infection was acquired in an area where ML is of concern [Bolivia, Brazil, or Peru]), and (3) the regionally observed drug susceptibilities (see **Box 1**).

For systemic therapy, the oral options are an azole (fluconazole, itraconazole, and ketoconazole) and miltefosine. Historically the azoles have reported variable cure rates; however, recent data support that they are less effective, especially for the *Viannia* subgenus. A meta-analysis showed a pooled efficacy for the azoles of 64% for the treatment of CL, with higher healing rates in *L L mexicana*, *L L infantum*, and *L L donovani*; however, the cure rates for *L L major*, *L V braziliensis*, and *L L tropica* were low.[33] In contrast, in a Cochrane systematic review of treatment of OWCL, itraconazole, 200 mg for 6 weeks to 8 weeks, was associated with healing in 85/125 (68%) subjects versus placebo 54/119 (45%).[34] A randomized controlled trial of high-dose fluconazole for *L V braziliensis* showed only a 22% cure rate on intention to treat analysis.[35] A nonrandomized study from Brazil showed that men with *L V guyanensis* infection treated with 450 mg of fluconazole daily had a 95% failure rate.[36] Azoles can have toxicity risks, including hepatotoxicity and QTc prolongation, which also need to be considered in treatment decisions.

Miltefosine is an FDA-approved oral option for the treatment of CL due to several *Viannia* species. Clinical response to the treatment of *L V braziliensis* has varied by geographic region, with port response in Guatemala and better response rates in Bolivia, Brazil, and Colombia.[37] Recent data from Colombia show a treatment failure rate of 16%; risk factors for failure were completing less than 1 month of therapy, being a child, having regional lymphadenopathy, prior meglumine antimoniate use, and adherence of less than 90%.[38]

Parenteral therapy for CL includes SbV drugs, pentamidine, and amphotericin (see **Box 1c**). SbV have been the standard of care for complex leishmaniasis for the early 20th century. Although areas of clinical antimonial resistance have been described, such as Bihar, India; national parks in Bolivia/southern Peru; and Bahia, Brazil, in other regions efficacy persists countered by toxicity and availability issues. When comparing IV treatment to intramuscular (IM) treatment using meglumine antimoniate for the treatment of *L L tropica* in Iran, there was a 95% cure rate; all of the failures were in the IM group.[39]

L-amB is one of the newer treatments for CL, its use extrapolated from is efficacy for visceral leishmaniasis with otherwise a weak supporting evidence base for CL therapy. A literature review of L-amB treatment of OWCL showed cure rates of 85%, yet the data were of poor quality and dosing regimens were variable.[40] There are fewer data for NWCL treated with amphotericin, consisting of case reports and case series with similar response rates of approximately 84%.[41,42] A retrospective analysis of returning travelers to Europe, however, showed only a 46% cure rate.[43]

In general, parenteral pentamidine is used exclusively for secondary treatment of *L V guyanensis*. Higher efficacy (85%) was seen when pentamidine was administered IV compared with IM (51%).[44] In Peru, CL treatment with 7 doses of pentamidine was inferior to SbV treatment (78% healing vs 35% in pentamidine).[45]

In addition to these treatments, all patients should have good wound care, including daily cleansings and petrolatum-based ointment. Secondary infection can complicate management and may slow the healing process.

SUMMARY

The complex nature of CL and limited treatment options that are well tolerated and effective highlight the need for further investigation. Treatment of special populations, such as, those during pregnancy, those who are HIV-infected, other immunosuppressed patients, and the elderly, can be more complicated and may require expert consultation. Approaches to CL diagnosis are focused on newer molecular methods, and the challenge is to standardize and have validated assays commercially available in the near future. As more people are traveling to or immigrating from endemic regions, CL has become a more frequently encountered diagnosis, and this article provides current information for the diagnosis and management of this neglected tropical disease.

REFERENCES

1. Global Burden of Disease Study Collaborators. Global, regional, and national incidence, prevalence, and years lived with disability for 301 acute and chronic diseases and injuries in 188 countries, 1990-2013: a systematic analysis for the Global Burden of Disease Study 2013. Lancet 2015;386(9995):743–800.
2. Bennis I, De Brouwere V, Belrhiti Z, et al. Psychosocial burden of localised cutaneous Leishmaniasis: a scoping review. BMC Public Health 2018;18(1):358.
3. Paranaiba LF, Pinheiro LJ, Torrecilhas AC, et al. Leishmania enriettii (Muniz & Medina, 1948): a highly diverse parasite is here to stay. PLoS Pathog 2017; 13(5):e1006303.
4. Aronson N, Herwaldt BL, Libman M, et al. Diagnosis and treatment of leishmaniasis: clinical practice guidelines by the Infectious Diseases Society of America (IDSA) and the American Society of Tropical Medicine and Hygiene (ASTMH). Clin Infect Dis 2016;63(12):e202–64.
5. Saab M, El Hage H, Charafeddine K, et al. Diagnosis of cutaneous leishmaniasis: why punch when you can scrape? Am J Trop Med Hyg 2015;92(3):518–22.
6. Sevilha-Santos L, Dos Santos Junior ACM, Medeiros-Silva V, et al. Accuracy of qPCR for quantifying Leishmania kDNA in different skin layers of patients with American tegumentary leishmaniasis. Clin Microbiol Infect 2018. [Epub ahead of print].
7. Magill A, Meyers WM, Neafie RC, et al. Cutaneous leishmaniasis. 2011. Available at: http://www.dtic.mil/dtic/tr/fulltext/u2/a547683.pdf. Accessed November 16, 2018.
8. Lima BS, Pires SF, Fialho LC Jr, et al. A proteomic road to acquire an accurate serological diagnosis for human tegumentary leishmaniasis. J Proteomics 2017; 151:174–81.
9. In Bios PI. CL detect™ rapid test for cutaneous leishmaniasis. 2014. Available at: http://www.inbios.com/wp-content/uploads/2016/06/900159-00-IVD-CL-Detect-Rapid-Test-Package-Insert.pdf. Accessed December 1, 2014. Update to Accessed on 16 November 2018.
10. Kreutzer RD, Christensen HA. Characterization of Leishmania spp. by isozyme electrophoresis. Am J Trop Med Hyg 1980;29(2):199–208.
11. Rioux JA, Lanotte G, Serres E, et al. Taxonomy of Leishmania. Use of isoenzymes. Suggestions for a new classification. Ann Parasitol Hum Comp 1990;65(3): 111–25.
12. El Baidouri F, Diancourt L, Berry V, et al. Genetic structure and evolution of the Leishmania genus in Africa and Eurasia: what does MLSA tell us. PLoS Negl Trop Dis 2013;7(6):e2255.

13. Weina PJ, Neafie RC, Wortmann G, et al. Old world leishmaniasis: an emerging infection among deployed US military and civilian workers. Clin Infect Dis 2004;39(11):1674–80.
14. Mouri O, Morizot G, Van der Auwera G, et al. Easy identification of leishmania species by mass spectrometry. PLoS Negl Trop Dis 2014;8(6):e2841.
15. Cassagne C, Pratlong F, Jeddi F, et al. Identification of Leishmania at the species level with matrix-assisted laser desorption ionization time-of-flight mass spectrometry. Clin Microbiol Infect 2014;20(6):551–7.
16. Lachaud L, Fernandez-Arevalo A, Normand AC, et al. Identification of leishmania by matrix-assisted laser desorption ionization-time of flight (MALDI-TOF) mass spectrometry using a free web-based application and a dedicated mass-spectral library. J Clin Microbiol 2017;55(10):2924–33.
17. Evers DL, Frye FA, Weina PJ. A simple empirical algorithm to distinguish among Leishmania braziliensis, major, and tropica species by MALDI-TOF mass spectrometry. J Microbiol Methods 2018;148:46–8.
18. Marfurt J, Nasereddin A, Niederwieser I, et al. Identification and differentiation of Leishmania species in clinical samples by PCR amplification of the miniexon sequence and subsequent restriction fragment length polymorphism analysis. J Clin Microbiol 2003;41(7):3147–53.
19. Marfurt J, Niederwieser I, Makia ND, et al. Diagnostic genotyping of old and new world leishmania species by PCR-RFLP. Diagn Microbiol Infect Dis 2003;46(2):115–24.
20. Ives A, Ronet C, Prevel F, et al. Leishmania RNA virus controls the severity of mucocutaneous leishmaniasis. Science 2011;331(6018):775–8.
21. Adaui V, Lye LF, Akopyants NS, et al. Association of the endobiont double-stranded RNA virus LRV1 with treatment failure for human leishmaniasis caused by leishmania braziliensis in Peru and Bolivia. J Infect Dis 2016;213(1):112–21.
22. Bourreau E, Ginouves M, Prevot G, et al. Presence of leishmania RNA virus 1 in leishmania guyanensis increases the risk of first-line treatment failure and symptomatic relapse. J Infect Dis 2016;213(1):105–11.
23. Ponte-Sucre A, Gamarro F, Dujardin JC, et al. Drug resistance and treatment failure in leishmaniasis: a 21st century challenge. PLoS Negl Trop Dis 2017;11(12):e0006052.
24. Lopez-Carvajal L, Cardona-Arias JA, Zapata-Cardona MI, et al. Efficacy of cryotherapy for the treatment of cutaneous leishmaniasis: meta-analyses of clinical trials. BMC Infect Dis 2016;16:360.
25. Cardona-Arias JA, Velez ID, Lopez-Carvajal L. Efficacy of thermotherapy to treat cutaneous leishmaniasis: a meta-analysis of controlled clinical trials. PLoS One 2015;10(5):e0122569.
26. Drugs for neglected diseases initiative. New hope for novel drugs for leishmaniasis. R&D Pipeline 2017. Available at: https://www.dndi.org/wp-content/uploads/2017/05/DNDi_LeishmaniasisPipeline_2017.pdf. Accessed November 16, 2018.
27. Sosa N, Capitan Z, Nieto J, et al. Randomized, double-blinded, phase 2 trial of WR 279,396 (paromomycin and gentamicin) for cutaneous leishmaniasis in Panama. Am J Trop Med Hyg 2013;89(3):557–63.
28. Ben Salah A, Ben Messaoud N, Guedri E, et al. Topical paromomycin with or without gentamicin for cutaneous leishmaniasis. N Engl J Med 2013;368(6):524–32.
29. el-On J, Halevy S, Grunwald MH, et al. Topical treatment of Old World cutaneous leishmaniasis caused by Leishmania major: a double-blind control study. J Am Acad Dermatol 1992;27(2 Pt 1):227–31.

30. Brito NC, Rabello A, Cota GF. Efficacy of pentavalent antimoniate intralesional infiltration therapy for cutaneous leishmaniasis: a systematic review. PLoS One 2017;12(9):e0184777.

31. Asilian A, Sadeghinia A, Faghihi G, et al. The efficacy of treatment with intralesional meglumine antimoniate alone, compared with that of cryotherapy combined with the meglumine antimoniate or intralesional sodium stibogluconate, in the treatment of cutaneous leishmaniasis. Ann Trop Med Parasitol 2003;97(5): 493–8.

32. Goyonlo VM, Vosoughi E, Kiafar B, et al. Efficacy of intralesional amphotericin B for the treatment of cutaneous leishmaniasis. Indian J Dermatol 2014;59(6):631.

33. Galvao EL, Rabello A, Cota GF. Efficacy of azole therapy for tegumentary leishmaniasis: a systematic review and meta-analysis. PLoS One 2017;12(10): e0186117.

34. Heras-Mosteiro J, Monge-Maillo B, Pinart M, et al. Interventions for Old World cutaneous leishmaniasis. Cochrane Database Syst Rev 2017;(12):CD005067.

35. Prates FV, Dourado ME, Silva SC, et al. Fluconazole in the treatment of cutaneous leishmaniasis caused by leishmania braziliensis: a randomized controlled trial. Clin Infect Dis 2017;64(1):67–71.

36. Francesconi VA, Francesconi F, Ramasawmy R, et al. Failure of fluconazole in treating cutaneous leishmaniasis caused by Leishmania guyanensis in the Brazilian Amazon: an open, nonrandomized phase 2 trial. PLoS Negl Trop Dis 2018;12(2):e0006225.

37. Soto J, Arana BA, Toledo J, et al. Miltefosine for new world cutaneous leishmaniasis. Clin Infect Dis 2004;38(9):1266–72.

38. Castro MDM, Cossio A, Velasco C, et al. Risk factors for therapeutic failure to meglumine antimoniate and miltefosine in adults and children with cutaneous leishmaniasis in Colombia: a cohort study. PLoS Negl Trop Dis 2017;11(4):e0005515.

39. Karamian M, Bojd MS, Salehabadi A, et al. Effectiveness of meglumine antimoniate against L. tropica in a recently emerged focus of cutaneous leishmaniasis in Birjand, eastern Islamic Republic of Iran. East Mediterr Health J 2015;21(4): 280–6.

40. Mosimann V, Neumayr A, Paris DH, et al. Liposomal amphotericin B treatment of Old World cutaneous and mucosal leishmaniasis: a literature review. Acta Trop 2018;182:246–50.

41. Wortmann G, Zapor M, Ressner R, et al. Lipsosomal amphotericin B for treatment of cutaneous leishmaniasis. Am J Trop Med Hyg 2010;83(5):1028–33.

42. Solomon M, Pavlotzky F, Barzilai A, et al. Liposomal amphotericin B in comparison to sodium stibogluconate for Leishmania braziliensis cutaneous leishmaniasis in travelers. J Am Acad Dermatol 2013;68(2):284–9.

43. Guery R, Henry B, Martin-Blondel G, et al. Liposomal amphotericin B in travelers with cutaneous and muco-cutaneous leishmaniasis: Not a panacea. PLoS Negl Trop Dis 2017;11(11):e0006094.

44. Christen JR, Bourreau E, Demar M, et al. Use of the intramuscular route to administer pentamidine isethionate in Leishmania guyanensis cutaneous leishmaniasis increases the risk of treatment failure. Travel Med Infect Dis 2018;24:31–6.

45. Andersen EM, Cruz-Saldarriaga M, Llanos-Cuentas A, et al. Comparison of meglumine antimoniate and pentamidine for peruvian cutaneous leishmaniasis. Am J Trop Med Hyg 2005;72(2):133–7.

46. Adams ER, Gomez MA, Scheske L, et al. Sensitive diagnosis of cutaneous leishmaniasis by lesion swab sampling coupled to qPCR. Parasitology 2014; 141(14):1891–7.

47. Taslimi Y, Sadeghipour P, Habibzadeh S, et al. A novel non-invasive diagnostic sampling technique for cutaneous leishmaniasis. PLoS Negl Trop Dis 2017; 11(7):e0005750.
48. Boggild AK, Valencia BM, Veland N, et al. Non-invasive cytology brush PCR diagnostic testing in mucosal leishmaniasis: superior performance to conventional biopsy with histopathology. PLoS One 2011;6(10):e26395.
49. Sousa AQ, Pompeu MM, Frutuoso MS, et al. Press imprint smear: a rapid, simple, and cheap method for the diagnosis of cutaneous leishmaniasis caused by Leishmania (Viannia) braziliensis. Am J Trop Med Hyg 2014;91(5):905–7.
50. Saldarriaga OA, Castellanos-Gonzalez A, Porrozzi R, et al. An innovative field-applicable molecular test to diagnose cutaneous leishmania viannia spp. infections. PLoS Negl Trop Dis 2016;10(4):e0004638.
51. Adams ER, Schoone G, Versteeg I, et al. Development and evaluation of a novel loop-mediated isothermal amplification assay for diagnosis of cutaneous and visceral leishmaniasis. J Clin Microbiol 2018;56(7) [pii:e00386-18].
52. Galluzzi L, Ceccarelli M, Diotallevi A, et al. Real-time PCR applications for diagnosis of leishmaniasis. Parasit Vectors 2018;11(1):273.

American Trypanosomiasis (Chagas Disease)

Luis E. Echeverria, MD[a], Carlos A. Morillo, MD, FRCPC, FESC, FHRS[b],*

KEYWORDS

- Chagas disease • Cardiomyopathy • Heart failure • Trypanosomiasis • Parasitology

KEY POINTS

- Chagas disease affects almost 8 million people, and migration from endemic to nonendemic regions has globalized the disease with approximately 350,000 infected carriers living in North America.
- The acute stage is usually asymptomatic, and less than 5% may manifest acute myocarditis.
- Of those infected with *Trypanosoma cruzi*, 20% to 40% will evolve to the cardiomyopathic stage. Predicting progression to cardiomyopathy remains a challenge.
- Etiologic treatment is highly effective, and treatment should be given to all acute infections, mothers of childbearing age, congenital infections, *T cruzi* reactivation, children less than 18 years of age, and selected cases with early cardiomyopathy.
- Chagas cardiomyopathy has an ominous course with rapidly progressing heart failure and high prevalence of sudden cardiac death.

OVERVIEW

Chagas disease (CD), also known as American trypanosomiasis, is a multisystemic disorder that can affect the cardiovascular, digestive, and central nervous systems.[1] CD is caused by *Trypanosoma cruzi*, a hemoflagellate parasite that is transmitted through various species of hematophagous reduviid insects (kissing bugs) mainly in endemic areas.[2]

CD, its vector, clinical course, and etiologic agent were first described in Brazil in 1909 by Carlos Chagas. However, there is DNA evidence that CD might be an ancient

Disclosure Statement: Dr L.E. Echevarria has no disclosures. Dr C.A. Morillo has received grant funding from the Canadian Institutes of Health Research (CIHR), Tropical Disease Research-WHO (World Health Organization) and merck for the benefit and stop-chagas respectively.
a Grupo de Estudios Epidemiológicos y Salud Pública, Heart Failure and Heart Transplant Clinic, Fundacion Cardiovascular de Colombia, Calle 155 A No. 23-58, Urbanizacion El Bosque, Floridablanca, Santander, Colombia; b Division of Cardiology, Department of Cardiac Sciences, Libin Cardiovascular Institute of Alberta, University of Calgary, Foothills Medical Centre, Room C823, 1403 29th Street Northwest, Calgary, Alberta T2N 2T9, Canada
* Corresponding author.
E-mail address: carlos.morillo@ucalgary.ca

disease because various studies have isolated *T cruzi* in tissue specimens of pre-Colombian Andean mummies dated from 7050 BC.[3] CD is an important public health problem, targets multiple systems, including the central nervous system (CNS), digestive track, immune system, and primarily, the heart. In Latin America, CD is among the most frequent causes of heart failure (HF) and reportedly responsible for up to 41% of cases in endemic areas.[4] This review discusses the mechanisms of transmission, especially sexual and oral ingestion, its worldwide epidemiology, pathogenesis, clinical manifestations, diagnosis, and current treatment.

TRANSMISSION MECHANISMS

The main transmission mechanism for CD in endemic areas is mediated by triatomine vectors. Other mechanisms of infection that are important, especially in nonendemic areas, include blood transfusion, organ transplantation, oral ingestion, laboratory accidents, vertically from mother to child, or shared intravenous needles.[5] Sexual transmission has been reported by in vivo experiments with mice; however, no reports in humans are currently available.

VECTOR TRANSMISSION

In the transmission mediated by triatomine bugs, the metacyclic trypomastigotes (infective form *T cruzi*) enters humans via triatomine excretion: triatomines have a habit of defecating while feeding on blood, and the parasite enters the host via the mucous membranes or breaks in the skin triggered by scratching while being bitten.[6] Once the parasite reaches the human host, it invades the local tissue, especially the liver, gut, spleen, lymphatic ganglia, CNS, and skeletal and cardiac muscles,[7] where it differentiates into the amastigote form and multiplies within the tissue. Once the tissue is full with amastigotes, they transform back into their flagellate infective form and lyse the cells, invading the adjacent tissues and spreading via the lymphatic system and bloodstream. When the trypomastigotes are on the peripheral circulation (**Fig. 1**), they are taken up by the triatomines during feeding.[8] It is important to note that more than 120 species of mammals, both domestic and savage, like dogs, cats, rodents, and armadillos, can be *T cruzi* hosts.[9]

In the digestive tract of the bugs, the trypomastigotes differentiate into epimastigotes (multiplicative form). After multiplication, epimastigotes differentiate again into the infective form at the final third of the digestive track, exiting through the triatomines' feces, thereby completing the life cycle. Although *T cruzi* is not pathogenic for this vector, the success in this part of *T cruzi* life cycle depends on several molecules and factors, especially the insect's intestinal microbiota, which may experience changes because of infection that include decreased fitness.[6]

ORAL TRANSMISSION

In the last years, environmental changes, especially deforestation, have affected the behavior of both the vectors and the reservoirs of *T cruzi*.[10] Vectors have migrated to new areas, generating a new form of oral transmission due to their proximity to food-handling places, leading to contamination. Oral transmission can be associated mainly with the consumption of beverages made from fruits, water, or vegetables contaminated with the feces of triatomines, or even with the complete parasite or secretions of infected mammals. Oral transmission can also be associated with the consumption of meat from undercooked infected animals, or blood from some reservoirs of the parasite, such as the armadillo (*Dasypus* spp).[11]

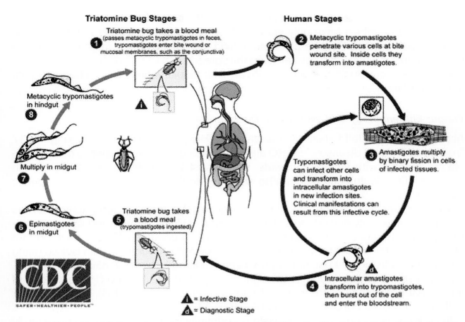

Triatomine Bug Stages

Human Stages

Fig. 1. Life cycle of American trypanosomiasis infection in humans is depicted in this cartoon. (*From* The Center for Disease Control and Prevention. Available at: www.cdc.gov/parasites/. Accessed November 1, 2018.)

After the ingestion, the invasion of the gastric epithelium by *T cruzi* involves the resistance of the trypomastigotes form to proteolytic lysis in the stomach, which is mediated by the presence of proteins in the *T cruzi* form the infective state, like gp82 and gp30.[12] These proteins allow the parasite to adhere and penetrate the cells of the gastric mucosa, enter the circulation, and then subsequently, allow the proliferation of the parasite in its amastigote state.[13]

Some reports also have considered the possibility of venereal transmission of CD. Even though this possibility has been suggested from the first reports of the disease, there are few studies on the subject.[14] It has been reported that the parasite can be found in testes, and amastigotes have been described in seminiferous tubes and ovarian thecal cells in patients with acute CD.[15] Furthermore, confirmation of *T cruzi* in menstrual blood and presence of *T cruzi* nuclear DNA in the semen of infected individuals have also been reported.[15,16]

Although there is no direct report of sexually transmitted CD in humans, animal studies provide robust evidence for venereal transmission. Inoculation of semen from CD-infected mice into the peritoneal cavity of healthy animals generates amastigote nests.[17] Furthermore, crossbreeding studies with mice have documented that sexual transmission is indeed possible in both male-female[18] and female-male transmission even in the chronic stage of the disease.[11,14] Further studies are needed to evaluate this possibility in humans, especially as a mechanism of CD spreading in nonendemic countries.

OTHER FORMS OF TRANSMISSION

CD can also be transmitted through blood transfusions, where the infective form enters freely into the bloodstream of the new host. Although most Latin American countries have taken a course of action to screen their blood banks for *T cruzi*,[19] many nonendemic countries have only started blood screenings regularly in the past few years, in risk donors. Routine blood screening, combined with a migration increase from endemic regions, may have allowed the spreading of CD in nonendemic regions.[5] The same epidemiologic risk occurs with organ transplantation, vertical transmission, and shared intravenous needles.

Chagas Epidemiology and Worldwide Distribution

According to the World Health Organization (WHO),[5] CD is classified among the 17 "neglected tropical diseases"[5]; WHO also estimates that approximately 8 million people are infected with *T cruzi* worldwide, with almost 100 million at risk of infection; in addition, 2000 deaths per year can be attributed to CD, making CD a serious public health issue.[20]

The Pan American Health Association described the endemic geography of CD as the area located between 40° north latitude (south of United States) and 45° south latitude (south of Argentina and Chile), which includes 21 countries.[9] There are important differences between CD prevalence among the endemic countries, with Bolivia being the country with highest estimated prevalence ranging between 6.8% and 18% of *T cruzi* sero-positive population.[5] Although Brazil (1.0%) and Mexico (1%) have one of the lowest prevalence of the region, together with Argentina (4.1%), they host over half of the infected population in Latin America.[3]

In endemic countries, CD transmission is primarily vector mediated, predominantly in rural areas, as rudimental infrastructure provides the environment for the development and reproduction of the vector. However, the migratory trends from rural to urban areas have put the spotlight on other forms of transmission and changed the epidemiology of CD currently affecting periurban and urban areas alike.[21]

Despite CD being endemic in Latin America, migration patterns have globalized CD, and cases have been reported in Europe, the United States, Japan, and Australia.[2] In the United States, it is estimated that around 300,000 individuals are infected,[22] although some studies report more than 250,000 cases in Texas alone and one million or more cases nationwide.[23] In Europe, it is estimated that around 45,000 to 67,000 cases of CD are present in Spain[24] with more than 100,000 cases in the entire continent[25] (**Fig. 2**). These calculations are based mainly on the number of Latin American immigrants, separated into different countries of origin and destinations, and the prevalence in the country of origin, because there is currently no epidemiologic vigilance for CD.[25] It is thought that the true prevalence may be underestimated, considering that most *T cruzi* carriers are asymptomatic. The main mechanisms of transmission are vertical from mother to child and blood transfusions, because only United States, Spain, Italy, Canada, France, and the United Kingdom perform some blood screening to detect infected patients or upfront exclude natives from endemic countries from donating.[25]

Pathophysiology and Myocardial Damage

Clinically, CD displays 2 phases. The initial, acute phase is characterized by high parasitemia, where the parasite assumes a trypomastigote form and invades the liver, gut, spleen, lymphatic ganglia, CNS, and skeletal and cardiac muscles.[3] In the acute phase, patients can either present a mild febrile disease or be asymptomatic. After the acute phase, *T cruzi* assumes the dividing form (amastigote), unleashing a local inflammatory reaction[3] (**Fig. 3**). The acute phase typically lasts 1 to 2 months and is followed by an asymptomatic indeterminate phase, without clinical manifestations.

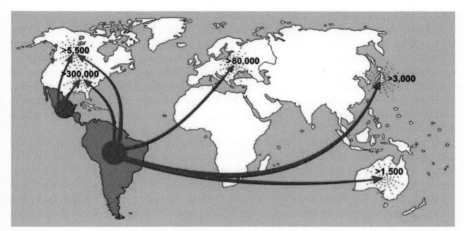

Fig. 2. Global incidence of *T cruzi*–infected carriers. (*From* Coura-Rodrigues J, Albajar-Vinas P. Chagas disease: a new worldwide challenge. Nature 2010;465:S7; with permission.)

About 30% of infected patients develop chronic CD, in which the parasites cause damage to target organs.[2]

During the first phase of the disease, myocardial involvement is caused mainly by cardiac tissue parasite invasion, consequently triggering a severe immune and inflammatory response.[3] It is theorized that the inflammatory response associated with the persistence of low-level parasitemia leads to an autoimmune response to the cardiac tissue by setting a continuous antigenic stimulation (bystander) or by mimicking the cardiac host proteins.[19]

Cardiac invasion by the amastigote form is also associated with coagulation necrosis of cardiomyocytes and hyaline degeneration of muscle fibers.[19] This coagulation necrosis can lead to microischemic areas in the border zones between the coronary arteries, without alteration of the coronary arteries themselves,[25] mainly due to diffuse collapse of intramyocardial arterioles. Experimental models of CD have shown that the microvasculature changes may appear due to a combination of occlusive platelet

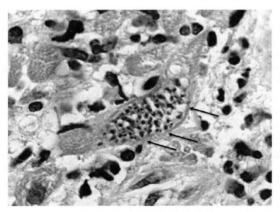

Fig. 3. Endocardial biopsy of a patient with acute infection and myocarditis. Mild interstitial edema with marked lymphocytic infiltrate and amastigote cysts of *T cruzi* (*arrows*) are shown. (Hematoxilin-Eosin, ×500).

thrombi and increased production of cytokines and immunomodulators that promote vasospasm and platelet aggregation.[19] These alterations can lead to a dilation of the left ventricle, often associated with apical and inferobasal aneurysms. Chronic heart CD is also characterized by myocytolysis, and an ongoing lymphocytic infiltration. As the adaptive immune responses elicited by the parasite eventually control the acute infection, but often fail to eliminate the parasite, variables such as parasitic load during the acute phase, the serotype of the parasite, the immune response, and the presence or absence of reinfection can influence cardiac involvement during the chronic stage of the disease.[3]

CD also causes alterations in the immune system of the host, especially during the acute phase, which extend due to the persistence of the parasite in the chronic phases. In the acute phase, polyclonal activation of B and T cells is inhibited by immunosuppression processes mediated by parasite infection.[26] It has been described that CD leads to a decreased proliferative response in lymphocytes of patients in the chronic phase, which is attributed to immunosuppressive factors capable of reducing the production of interleukin-2 (IL-2). Similarly, parasitic proteins have been described that modulate the activity of the complement system, inhibiting C3 convertase. Other hypotheses suggest that *T cruzi* infection may induce immunomodulatory molecules, such as IL-10 and transforming growth factor-β, which lead to failure in the maturation of antigen-presenting cells, a decrease in the presentation of antigens and therefore adaptive cellular responses,[21] imbalances between effector and regulatory T cells, and finally, change in the expression of stimulatory molecules and cytokines.

CLINICAL MANIFESTATIONS
Acute Chagas

After the initial infection, the incubation period varies from 7 to 15 days in the case of vector transmission and around 30 to 40 days in the transfusion transmission. Of note, the incubation period during oral transmission is significantly shorter than vector mediated.[3] The acute phase is characterized by high parasitemia, lasting around 2 months. With vector-transmitted CD, the main clinical manifestations include the presence of Romaña sign, a unilateral, painless, elastic edema of the eyelids (50%) or inoculation chagoma in the skin (25%).

Systemic symptoms of acute CD are rare and include moderate fever, malaise, headache, anorexia, diarrhea, myalgia, lymphadenopathy, hepatomegaly, splenomegaly, generalized or local edema (in limbs or face), rash, hemorrhagic manifestations, jaundice, myocarditis, tachycardia, arrhythmias, atrioventricular block, and in a small percentage, meningoencephalitis. In cases of vertical transmission, newborns can present with respiratory failure or low weight at birth or may be a premature delivery.[27]

As parasitemia is usually high in the acute phase, direct parasitologic diagnostic methods are preferred. The diagnosis is therefore made by parasite detection via microscopic examination of fresh anticoagulated blood, thin and thick blood smears, or preferably through the identification of motile trypomastigotes in samples following Strout concentration technique.[28] Polymerase chain reaction (PCR) to detect and amplify a segment of *T cruzi* genome on the host's peripheral blood or cerebrospinal fluid (CSF) is also a feasible diagnostic method. However, this method is not fully standardized, may have a high incidence of false positives, and usually requires a confirmatory test.[29]

Chronic Chagas

About 30% of infected patients enter into the chronic stage, with damage to target organs[2] (**Table 1**). Some patients, especially those infected with strains of the parasite

Table 1
Chagas disease acute and chronic phases

		CD Stages			
			Chronic Phase		
	Indeterminate Form	Chagas Cardiomyopathy		Chagas-Dilated Cardiomyopathy/HF	
Acute Phase	A	B1	B2	C	D
Patients infected by *T cruzi* with findings compatible with acute CD	Patients at risk for developing HF; positive serology, no evidence of structural cardiomyopathy or evidence of HF symptoms; normal ECG; no digestive changes	Patients with structural cardiomyopathy evidenced by ECG or echo changes, but with normal global ventricular function and neither current nor previous signs and symptoms of HF	Patients with structural cardiomyopathy characterized by global ventricular dysfunction and neither current nor previous signs and symptoms of HF	Patients with ventricular dysfunction and current or previous symptoms of HF (New York Heart Association class I, II, III, or IV)	Patients with refractory symptoms of HF at rest despite optimized clinical treatment requiring specialized interventions

that circulate in countries located in the southern cone of the continent (Brazil and Argentina), can present with exclusive or concomitant gut impairment, configuring the digestive form of the disease. These digestive alterations are caused by denervation of the autonomic plexuses of the digestive tract, which lead to disturbances in absorption, motility, and secretion, following motor coordination and dilatation, ultimately resulting in the formation of megaviscera, involving mainly the esophagus and the colon.[3]

Cardiac manifestations

The persistence of amastigotes in the myocardium often results in conduction and rhythm disturbances, sudden cardiac death, thromboembolic phenomena, and chronic systolic HF (CSHF). CSHF secondary to CD has worse prognosis compared with patients with nonchagasic HF, with about 10% of patients progressing to terminal CSHF.[3] As previously mentioned, it is thought that the interaction between chronic parasitic infection, autoimmunity, parasympathetic denervation, and anomalies in the microvasculature plays a role in the process of myocardial remodeling, the formation of scar, and, ultimately, chronic HF.[30]

Some signs and symptoms of cardiac involvement include wall-motion abnormalities, right bundle branch block and/or left anterior fascicular block, sinus bradycardia, atrial and ventricular arrhythmias, atrioventricular and intraventricular conduction disorders, such as right bundle branch block or/and left anterior fascicular block,[31] ST-T changes, thrombi, dilated cardiomyopathy with reduced left ventricular ejection fraction , and syncope[19,27,32] (Fig. 4). The presence of premature ventricular beats is also a common finding, which may identify higher-risk populations.[3] Several biomarkers, such as NT-proBNP and Hs-cTnT, have been associated with different stages and severity of Chagas cardiomyopathy.[33]

Mortality in patients with Chagas cardiomyopathy and CSHF is significantly higher than in patients with other causes. Similarly, patients with CSHF due to CD have a greater number of readmissions and complications during their hospital admissions.[27] Cardiac mortality among CD patients is split between life-threatening ventricular arrhythmias, manifesting as ventricular tachycardia/fibrillation with sudden cardiac death and progressive HF.[30]

Chronic CD is significantly associated with systemic embolism, especially cerebrovascular events. This association is particularly strong among patients with CD cardiomyopathy compared with other cardiomyopathies.[34] This differential risk might be explained by a higher incidence of atrial fibrillation around 28% and apical aneurysms compared with other cardiomyopathies.[35,36]

Central nervous system involvement

The involvement of the CNS is rare, with poor prognosis, and can result in cognitive dysfunction, including dementia, or neuritis.[1] CD with CNS involvement is defined by the finding of trypomastigotes by direct examination of CSF, amastigotes in the histopathological analysis of brain tissue, or trypomastigotes in the direct examination of blood associated with neurologic manifestations and clinical response after etiologic treatment.

CNS involvement in chronic CD is primarily related to disease reactivation, especially in immunosuppressed patients.[1] Because of the variety of etiologic agents that might cause similar clinical and imaging manifestations in immunocompromised patients, and the possibility of coinfection, it is important to perform other diagnostic tests. Clinical manifestations of neurologic CD vary in function of size, location, and number of lesions, with fever, headache, focal deficit, seizures, and sensorial loss being the most frequent findings.[37]

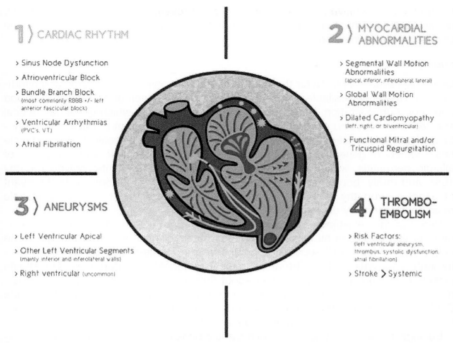

1) CARDIAC RHYTHM

> Sinus Node Dysfunction
> Atrioventricular Block
> Bundle Branch Block
  (most commonly RBBB +/- left
  anterior fascicular block)
> Ventricular Arrhythmias
  (PVC's, VT)
> Atrial Fibrillation

2) MYOCARDIAL ABNORMALITIES

> Segmental Wall Motion
  Abnormalities
  (apical, inferior, inferolateral, lateral)
> Global Wall Motion
  Abnormalities
> Dilated Cardiomyopathy
  (left, right, or biventricular)
> Functional Mitral and/or
  Tricuspid Regurgitation

3) ANEURYSMS

> Left Ventricular Apical
> Other Left Ventricular Segments
  (mainly inferior and inferolateral walls)
> Right ventricular (uncommon)

4) THROMBO-EMBOLISM

> Risk Factors:
  (left ventricular aneurysm,
  thrombus, systolic dysfunction,
  atrial fibrillation)
> Stroke > Systemic

Fig. 4. Chagas cardiomyopathy mechanical and electrical disturbances commonly observed during the evolution of cardiomyopathy. PVCs, premature ventricular contractions; RBBB, right bundle branch block; VT, ventricular tachycardia. (*From* Nunes MCP, Beaton A, Acquatella H, et al. Chagas cardiomyopathy: an update of current clinical and management. A scientific statement from the American Heart Association. Circulation 2018;138:e179; with permission.)

In the event of a suspected CD reactivation, it is important to evaluate the patient's immunologic state and look for other CD manifestations, such as pancytopenia, myocarditis, panniculitis, and bone marrow injury. Treatment must be installed as soon as possible because it generally has a low success rate.[1]

Chronic Chagas Disease Diagnosis

Because parasitic load on chronic CD is generally low, unless reactivation is demonstrated, the gold standards for diagnosis are serologic tests. The most widely used is enzyme-linked immunosorbent assay (ELISA) that detects antibodies of immunoglobulin G class against *T cruzi* on patients' serum. The WHO[20] recommends a strategy of using 2 different serologic assays, combined with epidemiologic information, because commercial ELISA-based tests present heterogenic sensitivity and specificity, and this may lead to overestimation.[29] In the case of discordant results, repeat testing is recommended. If the results persist, a third test (using PCR or western blot) is usually recommended.[38]

TREATMENT

Treatment of CD can be divided into etiologic, that is, treating directly *T cruzi* infection, or nonetiologic, treating the manifestations of the disease. The objective of etiologic treatment is to achieve parasite elimination and prevent organ damage. In contrast, nonetiologic treatment aims to prevent further morbidity and mortality related to the chronic phase of the disease.

Etiologic Treatment

Only 2 therapeutic options for the treatment of the disease: benznidazole and nifurtimox, are currently available. Benznidazole has recently been approved by the Food and Drug Administration. Benznidazole is a nitroimidazoles, which generates radical species in aerobic and anaerobic conditions,[39] and is the agent of choice for monotherapy of CD because of its extensive security and efficacy profile.[38] Benznidazole has a variety of generalized adverse effects; the most prevalent is the presence of allergic dermatitis, which affects about 20% to 30% of patients; polyneuropathy 10%, and rarely, bone marrow suppression that leads to neutropenia. In the event of either neuropathy or bone marrow suppression, treatment with benznidazole must be immediately discontinued.[3]

Benznidazole resistance has been occasionally reported, and the alternative treatment option becomes nifurtimox. Nifurtimox mechanism of action is thought to be either the production of superoxide anions or the double-strand break of the DNA through a formation of a nitro-anion radical metabolite.[40] Nifurtimox side effects include gastrointestinal symptoms in about 50% of patients (anorexia, weight loss, nausea and vomiting, abdominal discomfort). Other common side effects include CNS involvement, insomnia, irritability, and disorientation, which lead to drug discontinuation in a significant proportion of patients.[3]

Etiologic treatment is undisputed in the acute phase of CD, achieving cure rates between 65% and 80%, and even 100% in congenitally acquired disease. In general, children respond better to antiparasitic chemotherapy than adults. Antitrypanosomal treatment in the chronic stages of the disease remains controversial, because of significant toxicity profiles and the unproven role in preventing progression to cardiomyopathy. Recently, the BENEFIT (Benznidazole Evaluation for Interrupting Trypanosomiasis) trial reported nonsustained trypanocidal activity in subjects with established cardiomyopathy randomized to benznidazole evidenced by significantly reducing the detection of circulating parasites. However, these findings were not paralleled with a significant reduction in the progression of Chagas cardiomyopathy.[41] Clinical trials testing new candidate drugs and combination therapy with benznidazole in *T cruzi* carriers with no evidence of cardiac involvement, such as CHAGASAZOL (Randomized Trial of Posaconazole and Benznidazole for Chronic Chagas' Disease), STOP-CHAGAS (A Study of the Use of Oral Posaconazole in the Treatment of Asymptomatic Chronic Chagas Disease), and Treatment of adult chronic indeterminate CD with benznidazole and 3 E1224 dosing regimens: a proof-of-concept, randomized, placebo-controlled trial,[42–44] have recently been reported. Two trials demonstrated that posaconazole has trypanostatic activity during treatment; however, long-term treatment failures were greater than 90% and added no benefit when combined with benznidazole in asymptomatic *T cruzi* carriers.[42,43] Similarly, in asymptomatic *T cruzi* carriers, E1224 at different dose regimens was not superior to benznidazole at any dose regimen and failed to maintain therapeutic efficacy once treatment was finalized after 60 days.[44] These findings should not be interpreted as failure of etiologic treatment in both the indeterminate and the cardiomyopathy stages of CD. Clearly benznidazole is effective; however, better and most likely prolonged intermittent regimens should be tested before abandoning the concept of etiologic treatment. Better biomarkers that can identify subjects at risk of progression of the disease are also direly needed and should be encouraged.

In summary, treatment of *T cruzi* is indicated and recommended by guidelines in the following scenarios: acute phase, class I indication level of evidence B; chronic phase in children <18 years, class I indication level of evidence B; accidental, laboratory, and oral contamination, class I level of evidence B; asymptomatic *T cruzi* seropositive in childbearing women and neonates born from these mothers, class I level of evidence B; reactivation in chronic phase, chronic immunosuppression (ie, organ transplant in seropositive subjects), class I indication level of evidence B; trypanocidal treatment in the *T cruzi* seropositive carrier adult greater than 18 years with no evidence of cardiac or gastrointestinal impairment remains controversial because only around 20% to 30% of infected individuals will manifest cardiac CD. Nonetheless, given the efficacy in reducing or eliminating parasite load in this setting, many investigators advocate treating these individuals. Finally, trypanocidal treatment in the setting of established Chagas cardiomyopathy reduces markers of parasitemia, but these findings are not paralleled with slowing of the progression of cardiomyopathy (**Box 1, Fig. 5**).

Nonetiologic Treatment

Cardiac manifestations dominate the clinical presentation of chronic CD, and therefore, this review focuses on the treatment of HF, arrhythmias, and conduction disorders (see **Fig. 4**). Despite the fact that CD is an important cause of HF in Latin America, very few studies have included these patients in observational or randomized clinical trials. Thus, the benefits of guideline-recommended pharmacologic treatments

---

Box 1
Antitrypanosomal treatment recommendations in Chagas disease

Treatment should be considered (expert consensus)

Acute infections, regardless of the mechanism of transmission

Congenital infection

Women of childbearing age[a]

Accidental high-risk contaminations[b]

All cases of reactivation of *T cruzi* infection

Pediatric patients in chronic phase (children <18 y of age)

Treatment should be considered

Indeterminate form in patients greater than 18 y of age

Treatment should not be considered based on individual patient characteristics

Established Chagas cardiomyopathy; patients not in advanced stages may be offered treatment on the basis of a shared decision with the attending physician

Patients with established dilated cardiomyopathy

[a] After a negative pregnancy test because both drugs are contraindicated during pregnancy, and contraceptive methods should be used for women of childbearing age who will receive treatment.
[b] Contact with living parasites or cultures through skin breakage or mucosal contact, typically in a laboratory, clinical, or necroscopy setting.
Adapted from Nunes MCP, Beaton A, Acquatella H, et al. Chagas cardiomyopathy: an update of current clinical and management. A scientific statement from the American Heart Association. Circulation 2018;138:e191; with permission.

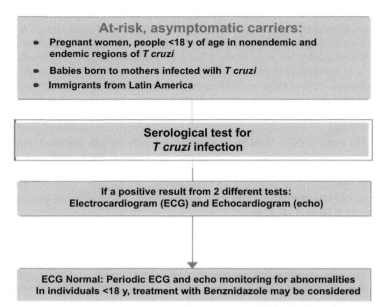

Fig. 5. Recommendations for diagnostic testing and treatment of *T cruzi* seropositive carries with and without clinical manifestations.

have not been readily established in patients with CD. In principle, the management of Chagas HF should resemble that of patients with nonischemic causes.[38] HF treatment includes as first-line therapy renin-angiotensin-aldosterone system blockade, with either an angiotensin converting enzyme inhibitor or an angiotensin receptor blocker and beta-adrenergic blockade. Not infrequently mineralocorticoid receptor antagonists with either spironolactone or eprelonone are needed to further reduce neurohumoral activation.[45]

Patients with CSHF due to CD usually have lower resting heart rates and mean arterial pressure, and reportedly a lower proportion of patients tolerate beta-blocker therapy. Beta-blockade has undoubtable benefits regarding both morbidity and mortality in nonischemic systolic HF and is the mainstay of therapy in CSHF treatment.[30] The lack of routine beta-adrenergic blockade therapy may be responsible for the worse prognosis of patients with CSHF secondary to CD compared with patients with other causes of HF; however, there is a paucity of data from randomized trials.[46]

Patients in the late stages of CHF secondary to CD usually end up with a heart transplantation, because this has become the procedure of choice for end-stage and refractory CSHF. The first heart transplant in patients with CSHF of cardiac cause was reported in Brazil in 1985 and is currently the third most common indication for heart transplantation in Latin America.[30] It is important to consider carefully monitoring the immunosuppression state and be alert to signs of CD reactivation, especially in CNS.

Atrial fibrillation and flutter are frequently observed in patients with CD, with the increased prevalence in advanced stages of the heart disease. Chronic CD is also significantly associated with systemic embolism, especially cerebrovascular events. This association is particularly strong among patients with CD-related cardiomyopathy compared with non–chagasic cardiomyopathy.[34] This differential risk might be explained by some of the CD cardiomyopathy's characteristics, such as greater incidence of atrial fibrillation and apical aneurysms compared with cardiomyopathies of other causes. Some investigators have proposed a predictive score model of ischemic stroke in CD along with prophylactic recommendations for the use of anticoagulants or ASA.[47] One of the main risks factors identified was the presence of apical aneurysm. In patients with a score of 4 to 5 points, the risk of stroke overweighed the risk of a major bleeding, thereby recommending oral anticoagulation. No data are available using direct oral anticoagulants in CD, and most experience is anecdotal.

Finally, ventricular rhythm disturbances are frequent particularly in patients with depressed ventricular systolic function. Cardiac resynchronization therapy may be an alternative in CD refractory HF; however, most CD patients have a combination of right bundle branch block and left anterior fascicular block that theoretically does not respond as well to resynchronization therapy. Despite this fact, some guidelines recommend Implantable Cardiac Defibrillator -Cardiac Resynchronization therapy for patients with sustained ventricular tachycardia, as a method to prevent sudden cardiac death.[38] Secondary prevention of sudden cardiac death with ICDs remains controversial, and benefits may be marginal as reported in a recent meta-analysis.[48]

SUMMARY

CD has been a largely neglected disease that due to changing migration patterns has trespassed endemic countries frontiers to become a global public health problem. Awareness is vital to identify global populations at risk and manage appropriately. Future research should include the inclusion of patients with Chagas cardiomyopathy and HF in large clinical trials and promote development of more efficient and safer etiologic treatment capable of eradicating *T cruzi*.

REFERENCES

1. Fernandes HJ, Barbosa LO, Machado TS, et al. Meningoencephalitis caused by reactivation of chagas disease in patient without known immunosuppression. Am J Trop Med Hyg 2017;96(2):292–4.
2. Perez CJ, Lymbery AJ, Thompson RCA. Reactivation of chagas disease: implications for global health. Trends Parasitol 2015;31(11):595–603.
3. Rassi A Jr, Rassi A, Marin-Neto JA. Chagas disease. Lancet 2010;375(9723): 1388–402.
4. Bocchi EA. Heart failure in South America. Curr Cardiol Rev 2013;9(2):147–56.
5. Angheben A, Boix L, Buonfrate D, et al. Chagas disease and transfusion medicine: a perspective from non-endemic countries. Blood Transfus 2015;13(4):540–50.
6. de Oliveira ABB, Alevi KCC, Imperador CHL, et al. Parasite-vector interaction of chagas disease: a mini-review. Am J Trop Med Hyg 2018;98(3):653–5.
7. Cordova E, Maiolo E, Corti M, et al. Neurological manifestations of Chagas' disease. Neurol Res 2010;32(3):238–44.
8. Morillo CA. Infection with Trypanosoma cruzi and progression to cardiomyopathy: what is the evidence and is the tide finally turning? Circulation 2013;127(10): 1095–7.
9. PAHO. Enfermedad de Chagas en las Américas: una revisión de la situación actual de salud pública y su visión para el futuro. 2018. Available at: https://www.paho.org/hq/index.php?option=com_content&view=article&id=14399&Itemid=72315&lang=es.

10. Abad-Franch F, Monteiro FA, Jaramillo ON, et al. Ecology, evolution, and the long-term surveillance of vector-borne Chagas disease: a multi-scale appraisal of the tribe Rhodniini (Triatominae). Acta Trop 2009;110(2–3):159–77.

11. Rueda K, Trujillo JE, Carranza JC, et al. Transmision oral de Trypanosoma cruzi: una nueva situacion epidemiologica de la enfermedad de Chagas en Colombia y otros paises suramericanos. Biomedica 2014;34(4):631–41.

12. Staquicini DI, Martins RM, Macedo S, et al. Role of GP82 in the selective binding to gastric mucin during oral infection with Trypanosoma cruzi. PLoS Negl Trop Dis 2010;4(3):e613.

13. Yoshida N, Tyler KM, Llewellyn MS. Invasion mechanisms among emerging food-borne protozoan parasites. Trends Parasitol 2011;27(10):459–66.

14. Ribeiro M, Nitz N, Santana C, et al. Sexual transmission of Trypanosoma cruzi in murine model. Exp Parasitol 2016;162:1–6.

15. Rios A, Ribeiro M, Sousa A, et al. Can sexual transmission support the enzootic cycle of Trypanosoma cruzi? Mem Inst Oswaldo Cruz 2018;113(1):3–8.

16. Hecht MM, Nitz N, Araujo PF, et al. Inheritance of DNA transferred from American trypanosomes to human hosts. PLoS One 2010;5(2):e9181.

17. Carvalho LO, Abreu-Silva AL, Hardoim Dde J, et al. Trypanosoma cruzi and myoid cells from seminiferous tubules: interaction and relation with fibrous components of extracellular matrix in experimental Chagas' disease. Int J Exp Pathol 2009;90(1):52–7.

18. Martin DL, Lowe KR, McNeill T, et al. Potential sexual transmission of Trypanosoma cruzi in mice. Acta Trop 2015;149:15–8.

19. Hidron A, Vogenthaler N, Santos-Preciado JI, et al. Cardiac involvement with parasitic infections. Clin Microbiol Rev 2010;23(2):324–49.

20. WHO. Chagas disease (American trypanosomiasis). 2014. Available at: http://www.who.int/mediacentre/factsheets/fs340/es/.

21. Ortega Zamora Y, Escamilla Rojas LJ, Villa Sandoval EM, et al. Chagas disease immunogenetics: elusive markers of disease progression. Expert Rev Cardiovasc Ther 2017;15:367–76.

22. Requena-Mendez A, Aldasoro E, de Lazzari E, et al. Prevalence of Chagas disease in Latin-American migrants living in Europe: a systematic review and meta-analysis. PLoS Negl Trop Dis 2015;9(2):e0003540.

23. Hotez PJ, Dumonteil E, Betancourt Cravioto M, et al. An unfolding tragedy of Chagas disease in North America. PLoS Negl Trop Dis 2013;7(10):e2300.

24. Neiderud CJ. How urbanization affects the epidemiology of emerging infectious diseases. Infect Ecol Epidemiol 2015;5:27060.

25. Strasen J, Williams T, Ertl G, et al. Epidemiology of Chagas disease in Europe: many calculations, little knowledge. Clin Res Cardiol 2014;103(1):1–10.

26. De Bona E, Lidani KCF, Bavia L, et al. Autoimmunity in chronic chagas disease: a road of multiple pathways to cardiomyopathy? Front Immunol 2018;9:1842.

27. Bocchi EA, Bestetti RB, Scanavacca MI, et al. Chronic chagas heart disease management: from etiology to cardiomyopathy treatment. J Am Coll Cardiol 2017;70(12):1510–24.

28. Carlier Y, Torrico F, Sosa-Estani S, et al. Congenital Chagas disease: recommendations for diagnosis, treatment and control of newborns, siblings and pregnant women. PLoS Negl Trop Dis 2011;5(10):e1250.

29. Brasil PE, Castro R, Castro L. Commercial enzyme-linked immunosorbent assay versuspolymerase chain reaction for the diagnosis of chronic Chagas disease: a systematic review and meta-analysis. Mem Inst Oswaldo Cruz 2016;111(1):1–19.

30. Benatti RD, Oliveira GH, Bacal F. Heart transplantation for chagas cardiomyopathy. J Heart Lung Transplant 2017;36(6):597–603.
31. Rojas LZ, Glisic M, Pletsch-Borba L, et al. Electrocardiographic abnormalities in Chagas disease in the general population: a systematic review and meta-analysis. PLoS Negl Trop Dis 2018;12(6):e0006567.
32. Nunes M, Beaton A, Acquatella H, et al. Chagas cardiomyopathy: an update of current clinical knowledge and management: a scientific statement from the American Heart Association. Circulation 2018;138(12):e169–209.
33. Echeverria LE, Rojas LZ, Calvo LS, et al. Profiles of cardiovascular biomarkers according to severity stages of Chagas cardiomyopathy. Int J Cardiol 2017; 227:577–82.
34. Cardoso RN, Macedo FY, Garcia MN, et al. Chagas cardiomyopathy is associated with higher incidence of stroke: a meta-analysis of observational studies. J Card Fail 2014;20(12):931–8.
35. Benchimol-Barbosa PR, Barbosa-Filho J. Atrial mechanical remodeling and new onset atrial fibrillation in chronic Chagas' heart disease. Int J Cardiol 2008;127(3): e113–5.
36. Geraldino O, Rodríguez F, Suárez M, et al. Fibrilación auricular en pacientes con diagnóstico de Chagas crónico procedentes de la zona norte del Estado Anzoátegui. Avances Cardiol 2011;31(1):10–4.
37. Rassi A Jr, Rassi A, Marcondes de Rezende J. American trypanosomiasis (Chagas disease). Infect Dis Clin North Am 2012;26(2):275–91.
38. Andrade JP, Marin Neto JA, Paola AA, et al. I Latin American Guidelines for the diagnosis and treatment of Chagas' heart disease: executive summary. Arq Bras Cardiol 2011;96(6):434–42.
39. Edwards DI. Nitroimidazole drugs–action and resistance mechanisms. I. Mechanisms of action. J Antimicrob Chemother 1993;31(1):9–20.
40. Marr JJ, Docampo R. Chemotherapy for Chagas' disease: a perspective of current therapy and considerations for future research. Rev Infect Dis 1986;8(6): 884–903.
41. Morillo CA, Marin-Neto JA, Avezum A, et al. Randomized trial of benznidazole for chronic chagas' cardiomyopathy. N Engl J Med 2015;373(14):1295–306.
42. Molina I, Gomez i Prat J, Salvador F, et al. Randomized trial of posaconazole and benznidazole for chronic Chagas' disease. N Engl J Med 2014;370(20): 1899–908.
43. Morillo CA, Waskin H, Sosa-Estani S, et al. Benznidazole and posaconazole in eliminating parasites in asymptomatic T. Cruzi carriers: the STOP-CHAGAS trial. J Am Coll Cardiol 2017;69(8):939–47.
44. Torrico F, Gascon J, Ortiz L, et al. Treatment of adult chronic indeterminate Chagas disease with benznidazole and three E1224 dosing regimens: a proof-of-concept, randomised, placebo-controlled trial. Lancet Infect Dis 2018;18(4): 419–30.
45. Yancy CW, Jessup M, Bozkurt B, et al. 2017 ACC/AHA/HFSA focused update of the 2013 ACCF/AHA guideline for the management of heart failure: a report of the American College of Cardiology/American Heart Association Task Force on Clinical Practice Guidelines and the Heart Failure Society of America. J Card Fail 2017;23(8):628–51.
46. Issa VS, Amaral AF, Cruz FD, et al. Beta-blocker therapy and mortality of patients with Chagas cardiomyopathy: a subanalysis of the REMADHE prospective trial. Circ Heart Fail 2010;3(1):82–8.

47. Sousa AS, Xavier SS, Freitas GR, et al. Prevention strategies of cardioembolic ischemic stroke in Chagas' disease. Arq Bras Cardiol 2008;91(5):306–10.
48. Carmo AAL, de Sousa MR, Agudelo JF, et al. Implantable cardioverter-defibrillator in Chagas heart disease: a systematic review and meta-analysis of observational studies. Int J Cardiol 2018;267:88–93.

Strongyloidiasis
A Neglected Tropical Disease

Alejandro Krolewiecki, MD[a], Thomas B. Nutman, MD[b],*

KEYWORDS

- Strongyloidiasis • Strongyloides • Autoinfection • Hyperinfection
- Anthelmintic therapy • Corticosteroids

KEY POINTS

- *Strongyloides stercoralis* is a unique soil transmitted helminth, which through autoinfection, can sustain chronic asymptomatic infections for decades.
- New diagnostic approaches through serology and nucleic acid amplification tests (NAATs) with superior sensitivity compared with stool microscopy are becoming more available for case management.
- In transplant candidates and subjects receiving immunosuppressive drugs (mainly corticosteroids), strongyloidiasis should be considered and treated promptly.
- Hyperinfection is a medical emergency with high mortality that requires prompt treatment initiation.
- Ivermectin is the treatment of choice for all clinical forms of strongyloidiasis, which should be treated even in asymptomatic cases.

INTRODUCTION

The *Strongyloides* group of parasites includes over 50 different species, each of them naturally infecting a limited number of mammalian species.[1] Strongyloidiasis, the human disease caused by infection with *S stercoralis*, and in rare instances in restricted geographic locations (eg, Papua New Guinea, Thailand, and Philippines) with *S fuelleborni fuelleborni* or with *S fuelleborni kelleyi*,[1–3] is a soil-transmitted helminthiasis (STH) with an global prevalence estimated to be between 30 to 100 million cases.[4,5] Infections range from asymptomatic (or subclinical) infections to symptomatic

Conflicts of Interest: Neither author has any relevant conflicts of interest to declare.

This work was supported in part by the Division of Intramural Research, National Institute of Allergy and Infectious Diseases (NIAID), National Institutes of Health (NIH).

[a] Institute for Tropical Diseases Research, Universidad Nacional de Salta/CONICET, Alvarado 751, Oran 4530, Salta, Argentina; [b] Laboratory of Parasitic Diseases, National Institute of Allergy and Infectious Diseases, National Institutes of Health, Building 4 – Room B1-03, 4 Center Drive, Bethesda, MD 20892-0425, USA

* Corresponding author.

E-mail address: tnutman@niaid.nih.gov

Infect Dis Clin N Am 33 (2019) 135–151
https://doi.org/10.1016/j.idc.2018.10.006
0891-5520/19/Published by Elsevier Inc.

id.theclinics.com

strongyloidiasis and to the potentially life-threatening hyperinfection syndrome in immunocompromised patients.[6,7] The parasite is largely confined to the tropics and subtropics, although foci of infection occur in any place where poor sanitation or other factors facilitate its transmission through fecal contamination.[5,8] The medical importance of strongyloidiasis resides in its capacity to remain clinically asymptomatic and chronically unnoticed until the host suffers alterations in its immune equilibrium that allow for accelerated larval reproduction that can lead to dissemination.[9] Infections caused by *S stercoralis* in people must be analyzed through a wide lens that incorporates all of the complexities associated with the 2-way interaction between people and helminths. Superimposed on this complex interrelationship is the chronicity of *Strongyloides* subspecies infection that can have profound parasite antigen-induced consequences to its human host that are, in turn, linked to behavioral and socioeconomic causes.

From a public health perspective, the estimated size of the population affected and at risk and its relationship to poverty and lack of adequate water and sanitation, put strongyloidiasis squarely in the neglected tropical disease (NTD) camp, although it is not currently incorporated in the World Health Organization's (WHO) strategy against STH[10] despite the growing recognition of strongyloidiasis as a disease of great public health significance.[11,12]

EPIDEMIOLOGY
Life Cycle

The unique life cycle of *S stercoralis* is a determinant for the clinical presentations in infected individuals. The alternative pathways between and within the host and the environment encompass free-living and parasitic stages. *S stercoralis* is unique among nematodes infectious for people in that larvae in the feces can give rise to a free-living generation of worms, which, in turn, give rise to infective larvae. This so-called heterogonic development process serves as an amplification mechanism that allows for increased numbers of infective larvae in the external environment. The infective larvae are active skin penetrators; oral infection, while possible, is probably of limited importance.[13] Adult female worms nested in the small intestine, most commonly in the duodenum in people, lay eggs in the mucosa that hatch into rhabditiform larvae, which are shed in the stool. Because the parasitic female's eggs hatch often within the gastrointestinal (GI) tract, the potential for autoinfection exists when precociously developing larvae attain infectivity (filariform larvae) while still in the host or through the perianal skin. When the rate of autoinfection escapes control by the host, massive repeat penetration and larval migration may result, triggering what is clinically defined as hyperinfection syndrome.

In the environment, under warm moist conditions, rhabditiform larvae can either molt into infective filariform larvae or develop through succeeding rhabditiform stages into free-living adults. Sexual reproduction occurs exclusively in the free-living stage. After dermal penetration, the filariform larvae migrate to the small intestine. The most clinically relevant, although perhaps not the predominant migration, is the classic pulmonary route, in which organisms enter the bloodstream and are carried to the lungs,[14,15] ascending the tracheobronchial tree to enter the GI tract. Only female adults are detectable in people, and subsequent reproduction occurs asexually through parthenogenesis.[16] Unique among nematodes infecting people, along with *Capillaria* subspecies, rhabditiform larvae of *S stercoralis* can transform into invasive filariform larvae before being excreted and reinfect the host by invading the intestinal wall or the perianal skin.[9] With an alteration in host immune responsiveness, even 1 adult female can multiply rapidly by parthenogenesis, leading to accelerated autoinfection or dissemination.

Transmission

The exposure of filariform larvae to the skin is the most common route of infection for *S stercoralis*.[17] The oral route is also considered as a possible route, supported by the observation of a higher prevalence of *Strongyloides* infection in patients with *Blastocystis hominis*, which is acquired by the fecal-oral route.[18] Transmission of *S stercoralis* infection after transplantation of solid organs has been suggested by several reports where only the organ donors had a history of *Strongyloides* exposure, and the disease developed in the recipient.[19,20]

As for all STH, risk factors for the acquisition of the infection are linked to exposure to a combination of 3 elements: (1) soil contamination with human feces, (2) environmental conditions that allow survival (and for the particular case of *S stercoralis*, reproduction), and (3) contact of human skin with contaminated soil. In epidemiologic studies, lack of adequate sanitation facilities within the household (but not lack of adequate water supply) was identified as a risk factor,[8] as were farming activities, walking barefoot, and living in areas with high humidity.[21,22] Latrine availability at home was found to carry a lower risk than using shared latrines.[23] The correlation between hookworms and *S stercoralis* has been examined and confirmed by 2 recent epidemiologic studies, highlighting the common infectious route of these species that access the human host through larval penetration of intact skin.[7,8]

The relationship between age and intensity of prevalence demonstrates for *S stercoralis* an age distribution similar to hookworms,[24] with prevalence rising rapidly during the first 20 years, with a slower but continued increase in prevalence through adult life.[5,25–27] Other risk factors, initially considered to be associated with an increased risk for clinically severe disease, such as human immunodeficiency virus (HIV) or human T-cell lymphotropic virus type 1 (HTLV-1) infection and alcoholism have also been found to be more frequently associated with acquisition of infection,[28,29] although in the case of alcohol abuse, the risk might be linked to malnutrition rather than pure toxicity caused by ethanol itself.[30]

The concept of strongyloidiasis as a zoonotic infection is becoming a subject of renewed interest, where evidence from DNA sequence polymorphism analysis revealed people and dogs from the same community sharing an *S stercoralis* strain that suggests a potential role for dogs in transmission.[31] This raises the possibility that dogs should also be targeted for treatment in the setting of human deworming campaigns.[32]

Global Distribution

As in most chronic infections, distribution maps highlight not just the areas where transmission occurs but also those areas where populations' movement are most significant because of the influx of immigrants and refugees.[5] Although *Strongyloides* is endemic to the tropics and subtropics, clinical suspicion should be present in all those with a present or past, even remote, exposure in endemic areas, including temperate regions such as Japan, Italy, Spain, Australia and the countries of North America.[5,33]

CLINICAL MANIFESTATIONS

In uncomplicated strongyloidiasis, many patients are asymptomatic or have mild cutaneous and/or abdominal symptoms.

Acute Strongyloidiasis

The clinical manifestations of acute strongyloidiasis are related to the path of larval migration from the site of infection to the location, most frequently the small intestine, where new adults will develop and start producing larvae. These clinical manifestations are associated with the prepatent period, defined as the time from penetration of infective larvae to production of new larvae by a mature female adult.[17] Infected individuals frequently experience irritation at the site of skin penetration that appears immediately followed occasionally by localized edema or urticaria that can last up to 3 weeks. Within a week following infection, a dry cough may occur. GI symptoms such as diarrhea, constipation, abdominal pain, or anorexia can occur following the establishment of the infection in the small intestine as early as the third week of infection.[9,17] Once larval production by the newly established adults starts (approximately 1 month following initiation of infection), new cycles of infection can be initiated through autoinfection (whether within the intestinal mucosa or in the perianal skin) that often presents as a nonspecific urticarial rash or the pathognomonic larva currens.[1,34]

Chronic Strongyloidiasis

The chronic stage of S stercoralis infections is most frequently asymptomatic or mildly symptomatic. The GI tract and skin are the main systems affected clinically. Symptomatic individuals may complain of diarrhea, constipation, intermittent vomiting or borborygmus. Because most of these symptoms are nonspecific and most frequently of mild or moderate intensity, it is difficult to suspect strongyloidiasis unless other signs or symptoms are present, despite the nonspecificity of the symptoms. Grove demonstrated in a controlled analysis with infected and uninfected individuals, among former prisoners-of-war from Australia who had been in southeast Asia, a significant increase in the presence of indigestion, diarrhea, constipation, anal pruritus, and weight loss among GI symptoms and urticaria and larva currens among dermatologic complaints.[35]

Larva currens is defined as pruritic linear streaks along the lower trunk, thighs, and buttocks resulting from migrating larvae through the subcutaneous tissues. As the larvae move, they leave behind a thin red line that gradually fades to brown and disappears within 48 hours. Compared with the cutaneous larva migrans secondary to Ancylostoma braziliensis, which is most frequently localized to the feet or ankles, larva currens caused by S stercoralis move throughout the subcutaneous tissue a speeds of 2 to 4 inches (5–10 cm) an hour.[1]

Unusual manifestations of chronic strongyloidiasis in other organs have been reported but without significantly higher prevalence in controlled studies; they include nephrotic syndrome,[36] massive upper GI bleed,[37] ascites,[38] chronic malabsorption,[39] hepatic lesions,[40] arthritis in an HLA-B27-positive individual,[41] and asthma.[42]

Severe Manifestations

In contrast to the mild clinical course of chronic strongyloidiasis that frequently goes unnoticed in the large majority of the cases, severe manifestations including the hyperinfection syndrome and disseminated strongyloidiasis occur in a minority of individuals who suffer florid clinical manifestations with potentially life-threatening consequences and a mortality rate of up to 85% to 100%.[6] Hyperinfection describes the syndrome of accelerated autoinfection caused by an alteration in the immune homestasis in the host,[9] although cases in immunocompetent individuals have been reported.[43] The concepts of autoinfection and hyperinfection are somewhat overlapping; therefore, hyperinfection syndrome denotes the presence of signs and symptoms attributable to increased larval migration caused by autoinfection with the development or exacerbation of GI and pulmonary symptoms. This is accompanied by the detection of increased numbers of larvae in stool and/or sputum and defines hyperinfection. Larvae in nondisseminated hyperinfection are increased in numbers but confined to the organs normally involved in the autoinfective cycle that occurs chronically at low scale (ie, GI tract, peritoneum, and lungs) although enteric bacteria and yeast, which can be carried by the filariform larvae or gain systemic access through intestinal ulcers, may affect any organ system.[44] Although the migratory route that allows the perpetuation of the cycle is through the GI-pulmonary-GI route, extrapulmonary migration of larvae has been shown to occur routinely during the course of chronic *S stercoralis* infections in experimentally-infected dogs.[14] Notably, many cases of hyperinfection are fatal without having larvae being detected outside the GI/pulmonary systems.

The clinical manifestations of hyperinfection vary widely, since the onset and course of the syndrome can be related to the *S stercoralis* itself, the bacteria that disseminate with the *S stercoralis* larvae or both; therefore, the presence of fever or other signs of progressive disease should trigger a search for enteric bacteria in other organ systems. The presence of eosinophilia is only seen in a minority of cases during hyperinfection; more often there is a suppression of peripheral eosinophil levels, sometimes related to corticosteroid therapy.[13,45] The presence of peripheral eosinophilia during hyperinfection appears to predict a better prognosis.[46]

GI symptoms are frequent but nonspecific and directly related to the presence of large quantities of larvae in the intestinal lumen. The symptoms relate to the invasion of the GI tract that leads to inflammation, bleeding, and ulceration. Abdominal pain (often described as crampy or bloating in nature), watery diarrhea, constipation anorexia, weight loss, difficulty swallowing, nausea, vomiting, and small bowel obstruction may result, with diffuse abdominal tenderness and hypoactive bowel sounds. Protein-losing enteropathy or ascites might appear also, as are electrolyte abnormalities that reflect these GI disturbances. Occult or gross blood is a common finding, resulting from colitis and proctitis.[1,44] Paralytic ileus with dilated and thickened loops without evidence of mechanical obstruction can be found on abdominal imaging or surgical exploration. These radiographic findings, like small bowel distension with air-fluid levels, should prompt suspicion and the search for larvae in stools when accompanied by fever, tachycardia, and hypotension.

Involvement of the respiratory system is the rule, although pulmonary symptoms occasionally are lacking. Most often symptoms related to the passage of larvae and the irritative responses are seen in disseminated infections and include dyspnea, cough, wheezing, choking, hoarseness, chest pain, hemoptysis or palpitations. Rare findings of filariform or rhabditiform larvae and even, occasionally, *S stercoralis* eggs, support the hypothesis of adult parasites actually developing in lung tissue.[47] Chest imaging most frequently shows bilateral or focal interstitial infiltrates that represent alveolar hemorrhage. Dermatologic findings include larva currens in the lower trunk, thighs, and buttocks. Petechial and purpuric rashes of these same areas, in which larvae have been demonstrated on skin biopsy, is common, including the thumbprint sign of periumbilical purpura, which radiates from the umbilical area and resembles thumbprints.[48] Vasculitis and disseminated intravascular coagulation seen associated with sepsis may also signal hyperinfection. Meningeal signs and symptoms are the most common manifestation of neurologic involvement in hyperinfection syndrome. In patients with meningitis, spinal fluid may show parameters of aseptic or alternatively demonstrate characteristics of a gram-negative bacterial infection. Bacterial meningitis unrelated to neurosurgical procedures, with spinal fluid or blood cultures identifying enteric flora, including polymicrobial infections, is a manifestation of hyper-infection. Sepsis, which is caused by gut flora that gain access to extraintestinal sites, presumably through ulcers induced by the filariform larvae or by virtue of being carried on the surface or in the intestinal tract of larvae themselves is another manifesta-tion.[44,49] Reports identifying organs to which larvae have disseminated include mesenteric lymph nodes, gallbladder, liver, diaphragm, heart, pancreas, skeletal mus-cle, kidneys, ovaries, and brain based largely on autopsy studies.[9]

Predisposing Conditions

Various drug exposures and clinical conditions that impair immune responses have been reported to predispose to hyperinfection (**Table 1**). Among the conditions asso-ciated with hyperinfection syndrome and dissemination, corticosteroids are the most

Table 1
Conditions associated with hyperinfection syndrome

Drugs/Biologics	
Immunosuppressives	Corticosteroids
	Azathioprine
	Cyclophosphamide
	Methotrexate
	Tacrolimus
Antineoplastic agents	6-mercaptopurine
	Adriamycin
	Bleomycin
	Carmustine
	Chlorambucil
	Doxorubicin
	Daunorubicin
	Ifosfamide
	Melphalan
	Mitoxantrone
	VP16
	Vinca Alkaloids
Biologics	Etanercept
	Infliximab
	Rituximab
	Antithymocyte globulin
	Muromonab-CD3 (OKT3)
	Mycophenolate mofetil
Total body irradiation	
Diseases/Syndromes	HTLV1
	Hypogammaglobulinemia (nephrotic syndrome and multiple myeloma)
	Hematologic malignancies and myelodysplastic syndromes
	Solid organ transplantation
	Hematopoietic stem cell transplantation
	HIV/immune reconstitution inflammatory syndrome (IRIS)
	Malnutrition
	Alcoholism

frequently encountered. Beyond their known immunomodulating effects, it has been postulated that corticosteroids have a direct effect on the S stercoralis parasites.[50] Hyperinfection syndrome has been described regardless of dose, duration or route of administration of corticosteroids. Even short courses (6–17 days) of corticosteroids in immunocompetent patients without underlying immunosuppressive conditions have been associated with hyperinfection syndrome and death.[51]

HTLV-1 represents a significant risk factor for the development of hyperinfection syndrome or disseminated strongyloidiasis.[52,53] The underlying mechanism appears to be associated to alterations in regulatory T-cell levels, reduced antigen driven interleukin (IL)-5 production, low total immunoglobulin E (IgE) levels.[54,55] There is also an impact of S stercoralis infection on the natural history of HTLV-1, which has been considered a cofactor in the development of HTLV-1-associated diseases.[56,57] In contrast, although stongyloidiais was once considered an AIDS-defining illness, there is no evidence of a relationship between HIV status and severe strongyloidiasis, and corticosteroids have been implicated in several cases of hyperinfection occurring in HIV-infected individuals.[9]

S stercoralis infections in the transplanted population, both in solid organ and hematologic transplants, is linked to the immunosuppression used as part of post-transplant regimens or for the treatment of conditions such as graft versus host disease (GVHD) and has been primarily linked to tacrolimus use.[58] Strongyloides infection acquisition through a cadaveric kidney has also been reported.[59]

DIAGNOSIS

The major obstacle for understanding the distribution, burden, and clinical characterization of chronic (often asymptomatic) S stercoralis infection lies in the poor sensitivity of the available diagnostic methods[11,60] and in the biology of Strongyloides, where the adult female releases eggs/larvae intermittently. Diagnosis of hyperinfection syndrome/disseminated S stercoralis infection is much less difficult given the florid clinical presentation and the large numbers of larvae often seen in the stool or other bodily fluids including cerebrospinal (CSF) and bronchoalveolar lavage fluid.

Although classic parasitologic methods looking for the identification of larvae through either culture or direct methods are still used in many laboratories; their complexity in terms of labor and their relatively low sensitivity are giving way to the incorporation of new immunological and nucleic acid amplification (NAAT)-based methods for both the clinical and public health approaches to strongyloidiasis.[60,61] Nevertheless, the lack of an acceptable gold standard for diagnosis makes it difficult to assess the accuracy of new methods.[62]

Parasitologic Methods

Definitive diagnosis relies on detection of larvae in the stool, rendering the more standard STH-egg focused techniques such as Kato-Katz, McMaster's and FLOTAC relatively useless for S stercoralis. As mentioned previously, intermittent and scanty excretion of larvae also limits the utility of standard stool studies. Among these techniques, the formalin ethyl acetate concentration technique appears as the method that is most frequently used in routine stool examination and is also a method that can be completed and yield results rapidly. Indeed, this method had a sensitivity that, in some studies, was the superior among parasitologic methods.[63] The collection of stools without preservatives improves sensitivity by maintaining larvae alive, thus allowing easier detection of moving larvae under the microscope. In the Baermann concentration method, stool is placed on coarse fabric or paper overlying a mesh screen in a funnel that is filled with warm water and connected to a clamped tube; after incubation, larvae migrate into the water and are collected by sedimentation in the water through centrifugation. This method can be further improved if the stools are previously cultured for 24 hours with charcoal. Despite its superior efficacy in diagnosing infections in different studies, this technique is cumbersome and laborious,[61,64] and other techniques such as the Harada-Mori filter paper culture or nutrient agar plate cultures are also methods with a sensitivity higher than direct smears (but require longer incubation times[65,66]). Sensitivity has improved with larger numbers of sequentially collected samples, reaching almost 100% when 7 stool samples were studied.[64,67] Invasive methods to retrieve larvae from the duodenum, where adults are most frequently found, such as duodenal aspiration and the string test, are not currently part of routine practice. Duodenal biopsy, when performed, can demonstrate parasites nested in the gastric crypts or duodenal glands, as well as eosinophil infiltration of the lamina propria,[68] although this depends on finding the correct anatomic niche.

Nucleic Acid Amplification Tests

Consistent with the trend in diagnostics, nucleic acid amplification tests (NAATs), using standard (or nested) polymerase chain reaction (PCR), qPCR, or loop mediated isothermal amplification (LAMP) assays, have been increasingly gaining traction for use in the diagnosis of S stercoralis infections.[69–73] Indeed, the improved specificity relies on the specific DNA targets used (18S rRNA, IST1, cytochrome c oxidase subunit 1 or the highly repetitive interspersed repeat sequence[74]) and improved methods for DNA extraction in stool.[70,72] As a public health tool and a multitarget clinical tool, the integration of S stercoralis qPCR in platforms that are bundled with other intestinal parasites in multiplex and multiparallel forms allows integration and screening in a standard, simplified way.[70,71,75] Although a recent systematic review warned about the limitations of these NAATs, which in this analysis were found to have an overall sensitivity of 71.8%, specificity was interpreted to be at least 93%.[76] Suboptimal sensitivity has been hypothesized to be secondary to intermittent larval production (or at least lower than the threshold of detection by the particular method) and to the presence of PCR inhibitors in stools,[77] although most of these theoretical concerns have been overcome with better technological approaches. NAAT methods have been explored in extraintestinal samples in just a few studies in urine samples in a rodent model and in a clinical study in endemic communities.[78,79]

In the setting of clinical trials to evaluate the efficacy of interventions to treat infection, proper interpretation of results also suffers from the limitations of current diagnostic methods. In a well-designed experiment, Dreyer and colleagues[67] demonstrated using the Baermann concentration technique in samples from military recruits in Brazil, that with 8 samples the cumulative sensitivity climbed from 32% with 1 sample to 67% with 8. Because of the intermittent positivity throughout the 8 separate collections from a single individual, in the setting of a clinical trial, results would be mistakenly interpreted as cure when the first but not the subsequent samples were positive. Serology offers a solution as a more reliable test of cure, as it relies on the human immune system and does not depend on intermittent larval detection in stools.[80,81]

Immunologic Methods

Several immunoassays for antibody detection, most notably enzyme-linked immunosorbent assays (ELISAs), have been increasingly used to overcome the limitations of parasitologic methods to increase diagnostic sensitivity and to simplify processing. Almost all of these tests (both in commercial and government-run laboratories) rely on measuring an IgG response to a crude soluble extract of larvae obtained from experimentally *S stercoralis*-infected animals or from related *Strongyloides* species (eg, *Strongyloides ratti*). Despite their utility, these antibody-based immunoassays have several limitations including: cross-reactivity in patients with active filarial or other STH infections, lower sensitivity in patients with hematologic malignancies or HTLV-1 infection, and the inability to distinguish between current and past infection.

To overcome some of these diagnostic obstacles, *S stercoralis*-specific recombinant antigens, such as NIE[82] and SsIR[83] have been used in several formats including ELISA,[63] luciferase immunoprecipitation systems,[63,81] and diffraction-based biosensors.[84] The use of recombinant NIE and/or SsIR has improved greatly the diagnostic accuracy and utility of these antibody-based assays.[60] The high negative predictive value of these immunoassays can be particularly useful in excluding *S stercoralis* infection as part of the differential diagnosis.[80,85]

In a blinded comparative multicenter assessment that included 399 samples, specificities above 90% were achieved, with the LIPS-NIE being the most specific[85] and most assays demonstrating sensitivities above 80% to 85%. In another trial with 101 samples, 2 commercially available ELISA kits (InBios Strongy Detects IgG ELISA - InBios International, Incorporated, Seattle, WA, and the SciMedx Strongyloides serology microwell ELISA - SciMedx Corporation, Denville, NJ), were compared with an in-house LIPS using the recombinant antigens NIE and SsIR.[86] Although there was only a 65% agreement among the 3 assays, the lack of stool microscopy (or qPCR) data makes the study uninterpretable with regards to sensitivity and specificity for *S stercoralis*.[86]

Direct antigen detection assays have been evaluated in the form of capture ELISA assays developed for *S stercoralis* coproantigen detection, but their utility awaits further testing and availability.[87]

Indirect Markers

The diagnosis of strongyloidiasis can occasionally be inferred indirectly based on elevated eosinophil or serum IgE levels in concert with appropriate clinical and epidemiologic settings. Eosinophil counts have been the most studied, as strongyloidiasis is often included in the differential diagnosis when eosinophilia is encountered either as an incidental finding or as part of the evaluation of special populations such as migrants, refugees, or returning travelers with fever.[88,89] In a recently published report in refugees from Southeast Asia to the United States, eosinophilia (>400 cells/μL) was significantly associated with a diagnosis of strongyloidiasis[90]; noteworthy, eosinophilia was not a sensitive indicator of strongyloidiasis in that study, as 27% of those positive for *S stercoralis* by qPCR were not eosinophilic. Similar findings were reached in another study with mostly African refugees; it was found that eosinophilia was absent in 33% of those definitively diagnosed with strongyloidiasis.[91] Because a significant number of individuals may have eosinophilia, strongyloidiasis should be considered in the differential diagnosis of eosinophilia in travelers or expatriates from endemic areas, particularly when accompanied by infiltrates in chest images and/or abdominal symptoms[90,92]; elevated serum IgE levels are another frequent finding in strongyloidiasis and present in 39% to 58% of the cases.[61] This association between elevated serum IgE levels and strongyloidiasis is rarely observed in HTLV-1 co-infected individuals,[54] a finding that may be linked to the inability of HTLV-I positive patients to clear *S stercoralis*.

TREATMENT

Specific antiparasitic treatment with anthelmintic drugs is indicated in all infections with *S stercoralis* regardless of the presence of symptoms or the immune status of the host.

Table 2		
Treatment for strongyloidiasis		
Clinical Syndrome	**Treatment of Choice**	**Alternative Treatment**
Asymptomatic, acute and chronic noncomplicated	Ivermectin 200 µg/kg/d orally for 2 d	Albendazole 400 mg, orally twice daily for 3–7 d Thiabendazole, 25 mg/kg orally twice daily for 3 d.
Hyperinfection	Ivermectin 200 µg/kg/d orally for at least 2 wk after stools negative for larvae	Subcutaneous ivermectin: 200 mg/kg, daily, divided doses, each arm, until negative stool examination persists for 2 wk or until patient can tolerate dosing by mouth or per rectum[a] Rectal ivermectin, 200 mg/ kg, daily, until negative stool examination persists for 2 wk[a] Albendazole 400 mg orally twice a day (in addition to ivermectin)

[a] Not FDA approved.

Treatment aims for resolution of symptoms and infection in symptomatic individuals and cure in asymptomatic individuals to prevent potential lethal complications in individuals harboring infections chronically. In contrast to the goals of drug treatments for other STH, which in the context of public health interventions target the control of these endemicities in affected communities by eliminating high and moderate intensity infections without curative goals,[93] the case of *S stercoralis* with its capacity for internal reproduction through autoinfection has a curative goal in all instances, so that the organisms are cleared completely, thereby eliminating the possibility of autoinfection.

Ivermectin is currently the drug of choice for all type of treatments. The regimen of 200 µg/kg/d for 2 days remains the treatment for uncomplicated *S stercoralis* infections as it targets both adults and larvae.[6,94] Thiabendazole (25 mg/kg/d) for 3 days is an alternative treatment, but drug availability and GI adverse effects have limited the use of this drug as ivermectin became more widely available. Albendazole at 400 mg twice a day for 3 to 7 days has been shown to be less effective than ivermectin for the treatment of uncomplicated *S stercoralis*[94,95] and is an alternative therapy (**Table 2**). A recent Cochrane Collaboration Review concluded that ivermectin has superior efficacy than albendazole and is statistically equal to thiabendazole, but the latter has more adverse events than ivermectin[94] (**Table 3**). In this review,[94] the cure rates for ivermectin, albendazole, and thiabendazole were 74% to 84%, 48%, and 69% respectively. A recent report from a nonendemic area warned of the failure of ivermectin to achieve parasitologic cure in a small group of individuals followed for up to 4 years.[96] From a public health perspective, data from different latitudes agree on the efficacy of mass drug administration with ivermectin in lowering the prevalence of *S stercoralis* infections, in some cases even years after treatment is stopped.[97–99] Hyperinfection syndrome, as a medical emergency, should prompt initiation of treatment with ivermectin immediately if this diagnosis is being considered. The regimen for severe disease is for a minimum of 2 weeks (and often until there has been evidence

Table 3
Drugs used for strongyloidiasis

Drug	Formulation	Most Relevant Adverse Events	Contraindications and Warnings
Ivermectin	3 and 6 mg tablets	Encephalopathy in those with high levels (>20,000/ml) of *Loa loa* microfilariae (mf)	Confirmed high levels of *Loa loa* mf <15 kg body weight Pregnancy Lactating women in first wk of puerperium
Albendazole	200 and 400 mg tablets	Choking in infants	First trimester pregnancy Effective contraception is recommended during therapy and for 1 mo after the last dose
Thiabendazole	Tablets, 500 mg Suspension, 500 mg/5 mL	Gastrointestinal: anorexia, nausea, vomiting, diarrhea, abdominal pain, jaundice, parenchymal liver damage. Central nervous system: dizziness, weariness, drowsiness, headache, hyperirritability, seizures, tinnitus	Activities requiring mental alertness should be avoided

of 2 full weeks of negative stool examination), although the lack of clinical trials precludes the recommendation of evidence-based guidelines. Reduction of immunosuppressive therapy should also be an important part of treatment when this is feasible.

Unorthodox methods of ivermectin administration may have to be used when patients are unable to take or absorb oral medication (even through a nasogastric tube) because of severe systemic illness or paralytic ileus. These include per rectal and parenteral formulations that come from veterinary formulations.[100]

CLOSING REMARKS

Human strongyloidiasis is a cosmopolitan public health infectious disease problem that is unique compared with other STH. These unique features must be addressed and incorporated in public health strategies for diagnosis and treatment and for individual case management. In view of growing awareness and advocacy of the importance of *S stercoralis* infection as a significant medical problem and the lack of a public health strategy,[11] new insights into the true global prevalence and the most adequate diagnostic, therapeutic, and overall public health approach for disease control are likely to change the understanding of human strongyloidiasis in the near future.

REFERENCES

1. Grove DI. Strongyloidiasis: a major roundworm infection of man. Philadelphia: Taylor & Francis; 1989.
2. Shield JM, Kow F. A comparative study of intestinal helminths in pre-school-age urban and rural children in Morobe Province, Papua New Guinea. P N G Med J 2013;56(1–2):14–31.

3. Thanchomnang T, Intapan PM, Sanpool O, et al. First molecular identification and genetic diversity of *Strongyloides stercoralis* and *Strongyloides fuelleborni* in human communities having contact with long-tailed macaques in Thailand. Parasitol Res 2017;116(7):1917–23.

4. Genta RM. Global prevalence of strongyloidiasis: critical review with epidemiologic insights into the prevention of disseminated disease. Rev Infect Dis 1989; 11(5):755–67.

5. Schär F, Trostdorf U, Giardina F, et al. *Strongyloides stercoralis*: global distribution and risk factors. PLoS Negl Trop Dis 2013;7(7):e2288.

6. Mejia R, Nutman TB. Screening, prevention, and treatment for hyperinfection syndrome and disseminated infections caused by *Strongyloides stercoralis*. Curr Opin Infect Dis 2012;25(4):458–63.

7. Becker SL, Sieto B, Silué KD, et al. Diagnosis, clinical features, and self-reported morbidity of strongyloides stercoralis and hookworm infection in a co-endemic setting. PLoS Negl Trop Dis 2011;5(8):e1292.

8. Echazú A, Bonanno D, Juarez M, et al. Effect of poor access to water and sanitation as risk factors for soil-transmitted helminth infection: selectiveness by the infective route. PLoS Negl Trop Dis 2015;9(9):e0004111.

9. Keiser PB, Nutman TB. *Strongyloides stercoralis* in the immunocompromised population. Clin Microbiol Rev 2004;17(1):208–17.

10. WHO. Preventive chemotherapy to control soil-transmitted helminth infections in at-risk population groups. Geneva (Switzerland): WHO; 2017. p. 87.

11. Krolewiecki AJ, Lammie P, Jacobson J, et al. A public health response against *Strongyloides stercoralis*: time to look at soil-transmitted helminthiasis in full. PLoS Negl Trop Dis 2013;7(5):e2165.

12. Olsen A, van Lieshout L, Marti H, et al. Strongyloidiasis–the most neglected of the neglected tropical diseases? Trans R Soc Trop Med Hyg 2009;103(10): 967–72.

13. Grove DI. Human strongyloidiasis. Adv Parasitol 1996;38:251–309.

14. Schad GA, Aikens LM, Smith G. *Strongyloides stercoralis*: is there a canonical migratory route through the host? J Parasitol 1989;75(5):740–9.

15. Mansfield LS, Alavi A, Wortman JA, et al. Gamma camera scintigraphy for direct visualization of larval migration in *Strongyloides stercoralis*-infected dogs. Am J Trop Med Hyg 1995;52(3):236–40.

16. Neva FA. Biology and immunology of human strongyloidiasis. J Infect Dis 1986; 153(3):397–406.

17. Freedman DO. Experimental infection of human subjects with *Strongyloides* species. Clin Infect Dis 1991;13(6):1221–6.

18. Czachor JS, Jonas AP. Transmission of *Strongyloides steracolis* person to person. J Travel Med 2000;7(4):211–2.

19. Said T, Nampoory MRN, Nair MP, et al. Hyperinfection strongyloidiasis: an anticipated outbreak in kidney transplant recipients in Kuwait. Transplant Proc 2007; 39(4):1014–5.

20. Ben-Youssef R, Baron P, Edson F, et al. *Stronglyoides stercoralis* infection from pancreas allograft: case report. Transplantation 2005;80(7):997–8.

21. Senephansiri P, Laummaunwai P, Laymanivong S, et al. Status and risk factors of *Strongyloides stercoralis* infection in rural communities of Xayaburi Province, Lao PDR. Korean J Parasitol 2017;55(5):569–73.

22. Widjana DP, Sutisna P. Prevalence of soil-transmitted helminth infections in the rural population of Bali, Indonesia. Southeast Asian J Trop Med Public Health 2000;31(3):454–9.

23. Hall A, Conway D, Anwar K, et al. *Strongyloides stercoralis* in an urban slum community in Bangladesh: factors independently associated with infection. Trans R Soc Trop Med Hyg 1994;88:527–30.

24. Bundy DA, Hall A, Medley GF, et al. Evaluating measures to control intestinal parasitic infections. World Health Stat Q 1992;45(2–3):168–79.

25. Lindo JF, Robinson RD, Terry SI, et al. Age-prevalence and household clustering of *Strongyloides stercoralis* infection in Jamaica. Parasitology 1995;110(Pt 1): 97–102.

26. Paula FM, Costa-Cruz JM. Epidemiological aspects of strongyloidiasis in Brazil. Parasitology 2011;138(11):1331–40.

27. Khieu V, Schär F, Forrer A, et al. High prevalence and spatial distribution of *Strongyloides stercoralis* in rural Cambodia. PLoS Negl Trop Dis 2014;8(6): e2854.

28. Schär F, Odermatt P, Khieu V, et al. Evaluation of real-time PCR for *Strongyloides stercoralis* and hookworm as diagnostic tool in asymptomatic schoolchildren in Cambodia. Acta Trop 2013;126(2):89–92.

29. Marques CC, da Penha Zago-Gomes M, Gonçalves CS, et al. Alcoholism and *Strongyloides stercoralis*: daily ethanol ingestion has a positive correlation with the frequency of Strongyloides larvae in the stools. PLoS Negl Trop Dis 2010;4(6):e717.

30. Krolewiecki AJ, Leon S, Scott PA, et al. Effect of chronic ethanol consumption on protective T-helper 1 and T-helper 2 immune responses against the parasites Leishmania major and *Strongyloides stercoralis* in mice. Alcohol Clin Exp Res 2001;25(4):571–8.

31. Jaleta TG, Zhou S, Bemm FM, et al. Different but overlapping populations of *Strongyloides stercoralis* in dogs and humans-dogs as a possible source for zoonotic strongyloidiasis. PLoS Negl Trop Dis 2017;11(8):e0005752.

32. Beknazarova M, Whiley H, Ross K. Mass drug administration for the prevention human strongyloidiasis should consider concomitant treatment of dogs. PLoS Negl Trop Dis 2017;11(8):e0005735.

33. Salvador F, Sulleiro E, Piron M, et al. Seroprevalence of *Strongyloides stercoralis* infection among HTLV-I infected blood donors in Barcelona, Spain: a cross-sectional study. Acta Trop 2017;176:412–4.

34. Gaus B, Toberer F, Kapaun A, et al. Chronic *Strongyloides stercoralis* infection. Larva currens as skin manifestation. Hautarzt 2011;62(5):380–3 [in German].

35. Grove DI. Strongyloidiasis in allied ex-prisoners of war in south-east Asia. Br Med J 1980;280(6214):598–601.

36. Hsieh YP, Wen YK, Chen ML. Minimal change nephrotic syndrome in association with strongyloidiasis. Clin Nephrol 2006;66(6):459–63.

37. Jaka H, Koy M, Egan JP, et al. *Strongyloides stercoralis* infection presenting as an unusual cause of massive upper gastrointestinal bleeding in an immunosuppressed patient: a case report. Trop Doct 2013;43(1):46–8.

38. Hong IS, Zaidi SY, McEvoy P, et al. Diagnosis of *Strongyloides stercoralis* in a peritoneal effusion from an HIV-seropositive man. A case report. Acta Cytol 2004;48(2):211–4.

39. Atul S, Ajay D, Ritambhara N, et al. An unusual cause of malabsorption in an immunocompetent host. J Ayub Med Coll Abbottabad 2005;17(1):85–6.

40. Gulbas Z, Kebapci M, Pasaoglu O, et al. Successful ivermectin treatment of hepatic strongyloidiasis presenting with severe eosinophilia. South Med J 2004; 97(9):907–10.

41. Richter J, Müller-Stöver I, Strothmeyer H, et al. Arthritis associated with *Strongyloides stercoralis* infection in HLA B-27-positive African. Parasitol Res 2006; 99(6):706–7.
42. Dunlap NE, Shin MS, Polt SS, et al. Strongyloidiasis manifested as asthma. South Med J 1984;77(1):77–8.
43. Tiwari S, Rautaraya B, Tripathy KP. Hyperinfection of *Strongyloides stercoralis* in an immunocompetent patient. Trop Parasitol 2012;2(2):135–7.
44. Nutman TB. Human infection with *Strongyloides stercoralis* and other related *Strongyloides* species. Parasitology 2017;144(3):263–73.
45. Buonfrate D, Requena-Mendez A, Angheben A, et al. Severe strongyloidiasis: a systematic review of case reports. BMC Infect Dis 2013;13:78.
46. Jamil SA, Hilton E. The *Strongyloides* hyperinfection syndrome. N Y State J Med 1992;92(2):67–8.
47. Cahill KM, Shevchuk M. Fulminant, systemic strongyloidiasis in AIDS. Ann Trop Med Parasitol 1996;90(3):313–8.
48. Bank DE, Grossman ME, Kohn SR, et al. The thumbprint sign: rapid diagnosis of disseminated strongyloidiasis. J Am Acad Dermatol 1990;23(2 Pt 1):324–6.
49. Link K, Orenstein R. Bacterial complications of strongyloidiasis: streptococcus bovis meningitis. South Med J 1999;92(7):728–31.
50. Machado ER, Carlos D, Sorgi CA, et al. Dexamethasone effects in the *Strongyloides venezuelensis* infection in a murine model. Am J Trop Med Hyg 2011; 84(6):957–66.
51. Ghosh K, Ghosh K. *Strongyloides stercoralis* septicaemia following steroid therapy for eosinophilia: report of three cases. Trans R Soc Trop Med Hyg 2007; 101(11):1163–5.
52. Carvalho EM, Da Fonseca Porto A. Epidemiological and clinical interaction between HTLV-1 and *Strongyloides stercoralis*. Parasite Immunol 2004;26(11–12): 487–97.
53. Gotuzzo E, Moody J, Verdonck K, et al. Frequent HTLV-1 infection in the offspring of Peruvian women with HTLV-1-associated myelopathy/tropical spastic paraparesis or strongyloidiasis. Rev Panam Salud Publica 2007;22(4): 223–30.
54. Hayashi J, Kishihara Y, Yoshimura E, et al. Correlation between human T cell lymphotropic virus type-1 and *Strongyloides stercoralis* infections and serum immunoglobulin E responses in residents of Okinawa, Japan. Am J Trop Med Hyg 1997;56(1):71–5.
55. Montes M, Sanchez C, Verdonck K, et al. Regulatory T cell expansion in HTLV-1 and strongyloidiasis co-infection is associated with reduced IL-5 responses to Strongyloides stercoralis antigen. PLoS Negl Trop Dis 2009;3(6):e456.
56. Gotuzzo E, Arango C, de Queiroz-Campos A, et al. Human T-cell lymphotropic virus-I in Latin America. Infect Dis Clin North Am 2000;14(1):211–39, x-xi.
57. Marcos LA, Terashima A, Canales M, et al. Update on strongyloidiasis in the immunocompromised host. Curr Infect Dis Rep 2011;13(1):35–46.
58. Mokaddas EM, Shati S, Abdulla A, et al. Fatal strongyloidiasis in three kidney recipients in Kuwait. Med Princ Pract 2009;18(5):414–7.
59. Weiser JA, Scully BE, Bulman WA, et al. Periumbilical parasitic thumbprint purpura: *Strongyloides* hyperinfection syndrome acquired from a cadaveric renal transplant. Transpl Infect Dis 2011;13(1):58–62.
60. Buonfrate D, Formenti F, Perandin F, et al. Novel approaches to the diagnosis of *Strongyloides stercoralis* infection. Clin Microbiol Infect 2015;21(6):543–52.

61. Requena-Méndez A, Chiodini P, Bisoffi Z, et al. The laboratory diagnosis and follow up of strongyloidiasis: a systematic review. PLoS Negl Trop Dis 2013; 7(1):e2002.
62. Joseph L, Gyorkos TW, Coupal L. Bayesian estimation of disease prevalence and the parameters of diagnostic tests in the absence of a gold standard. Am J Epidemiol 1995;141(3):263–72.
63. Krolewiecki AJ, Ramanathan R, Fink V, et al. Improved diagnosis of Strongyloides stercoralis using recombinant antigen-based serologies in a community-wide study in northern Argentina. Clin Vaccine Immunol 2010; 17(10):1624–30.
64. Siddiqui AA, Berk SL. Diagnosis of Strongyloides stercoralis infection. Clin Infect Dis 2001;33(7):1040–7.
65. Sato Y, Kobayashi J, Toma H, et al. Efficacy of stool examination for detection of Strongyloides infection. Am J Trop Med Hyg 1995;53(3):248–50.
66. Repetto SA, Durán PA, Lasala MB, et al. High rate of strongyloidosis infection, out of endemic area, in patients with eosinophilia and without risk of exogenous reinfections. Am J Trop Med Hyg 2010;82(6):1088–93.
67. Dreyer G, Fernandes-Silva E, Alves S, et al. Patterns of detection of Strongyloides stercoralis in stool specimens: implications for diagnosis and clinical trials. J Clin Microbiol 1996;34(10):2569–71.
68. Rivasi F, Pampiglione S, Boldorini R, et al. Histopathology of gastric and duodenal Strongyloides stercoralis locations in fifteen immunocompromised subjects. Arch Pathol Lab Med 2006;130(12):1792–8.
69. Verweij JJ, Canales M, Polman K, et al. Molecular diagnosis of Strongyloides stercoralis in faecal samples using real-time PCR. Trans R Soc Trop Med Hyg 2009;103(4):342–6.
70. Mejia R, Vicuña Y, Broncano N, et al. A novel, multi-parallel, real-time polymerase chain reaction approach for eight gastrointestinal parasites provides improved diagnostic capabilities to resource-limited at-risk populations. Am J Trop Med Hyg 2013;88(6):1041–7.
71. Cimino RO, Jeun R, Juarez M, et al. Identification of human intestinal parasites affecting an asymptomatic peri-urban Argentinian population using multi-parallel quantitative real-time polymerase chain reaction. Parasit Vectors 2015; 8:380.
72. Easton AV, Oliveira RG, O'Connell EM, et al. Multi-parallel qPCR provides increased sensitivity and diagnostic breadth for gastrointestinal parasites of humans: field-based inferences on the impact of mass deworming. Parasit Vectors 2016;9:38.
73. Llewellyn S, Inpankaew T, Nery SV, et al. Application of a multiplex quantitative PCR to assess prevalence and intensity of intestinal parasite infections in a controlled clinical trial. PLoS Negl Trop Dis 2016;10(1):e0004380.
74. Moore TA, Ramachandran S, Gam AA, et al. Identification of novel sequences and codon usage in Strongyloides stercoralis. Mol Biochem Parasitol 1996; 79(2):243–8.
75. Taniuchi M, Verweij JJ, Noor Z, et al. High throughput multiplex PCR and probe-based detection with Luminex beads for seven intestinal parasites. Am J Trop Med Hyg 2011;84(2):332–7.
76. Buonfrate D, Requena-Mendez A, Angheben A, et al. Accuracy of molecular biology techniques for the diagnosis of Strongyloides stercoralis infection-A systematic review and meta-analysis. PLoS Negl Trop Dis 2018;12(2):e0006229.

77. O'Connell EM, Nutman TB. Molecular diagnostics for soil-transmitted helminths. Am J Trop Med Hyg 2016;95:508–13.
78. Fernández-Soto P, Sánchez-Hernández A, Gandasegui J, et al. Strong-LAMP: a LAMP assay for *Strongyloides* spp. Detection in stool and urine samples. Towards the diagnosis of human strongyloidiasis starting from a rodent model. PLoS Negl Trop Dis 2016;10(7):e0004836.
79. Krolewiecki AJ, Koukounari A, Romano M, et al. Transrenal DNA-based diagnosis of *Strongyloides stercoralis* (Grassi, 1879) infection: Bayesian latent class modeling of test accuracy. PLoS Negl Trop Dis 2018;12(6):e0006550.
80. Buonfrate D, Sequi M, Mejia R, et al. Accuracy of five serologic tests for the follow up of *Strongyloides stercoralis* infection. PLoS Negl Trop Dis 2015;9(2): e0003491.
81. Ramanathan R, Burbelo PD, Groot S, et al. A luciferase immunoprecipitation systems assay enhances the sensitivity and specificity of diagnosis of *Strongyloides stercoralis* infection. J Infect Dis 2008;198(3):444–51.
82. Ravi V, Ramachandran S, Thompson RW, et al. Characterization of a recombinant immunodiagnostic antigen (NIE) from *Strongyloides stercoralis* L3-stage larvae. Mol Biochem Parasitol 2002;125(1–2):73–81.
83. Ramachandran S, Thompson RW, Gam AA, et al. Recombinant cDNA clones for immunodiagnosis of strongyloidiasis. J Infect Dis 1998;177(1):196–203.
84. Pak BJ, Vasquez-Camargo F, Kalinichenko E, et al. Development of a rapid serological assay for the diagnosis of strongyloidiasis using a novel diffraction-based biosensor technology. PLoS Negl Trop Dis 2014;8(8):e3002.
85. Bisoffi Z, Buonfrate D, Sequi M, et al. Diagnostic accuracy of five serologic tests for *Strongyloides stercoralis* infection. PLoS Negl Trop Dis 2014;8(1):e2640.
86. Anderson NW, Klein DM, Dornink SM, et al. Comparison of three immunoassays for detection of antibodies to *Strongyloides stercoralis*. Clin Vaccine Immunol 2014;21(5):732–6.
87. Toledo R, Muñoz-Antoli C, Esteban J-G. Strongyloidiasis with emphasis on human infections and its different clinical forms. Adv Parasitol 2015;88:165–241.
88. Checkley AM, Chiodini PL, Dockrell DH, et al. Eosinophilia in returning travelers and migrants from the tropics: UK recommendations for investigation and initial management. J Infect 2010;60(1):1–20.
89. Thwaites GE, Day NPJ. Approach to fever in the returning traveler. N Engl J Med 2017;376(6):548–60.
90. Mitchell T, Lee D, Weinberg M, et al. Impact of enhanced health interventions for United States-bound refugees: evaluating best practices in migration health. Am J Trop Med Hyg 2018;98(3):920–8.
91. Naidu P, Yanow SK, Kowalewska-Grochowska KT. Eosinophilia: a poor predictor of *Strongyloides* infection in refugees. Can J Infect Dis Med Microbiol 2013; 24(2):93–6.
92. O'Connell EM, Nutman TB. Eosinophilia in infectious diseases. Immunol Allergy Clin North Am 2015;35(3):493–522.
93. Ásbjörnsdóttir KH, Means AR, Werkman M, et al. Prospects for elimination of soil-transmitted helminths. Curr Opin Infect Dis 2017;30(5):482–8.
94. Henriquez-Camacho C, Gotuzzo E, Echevarria J, et al. Ivermectin versus albendazole or thiabendazole for *Strongyloides stercoralis* infection. Cochrane Database Syst Rev 2016;(1):CD007745.
95. Supattamongkol Y, Premasathian N, Bhumimuang K, et al. Efficacy and safety of single and double doses of ivermectin versus 7-day high dose albendazole for chronic strongyloidiasis. PLoS Negl Trop Dis 2011;5(5):e1044.

96. Repetto SA, Ruybal P, Batalla E, et al. Strongyloidiasis outside endemic areas: long-term parasitological and clinical follow-up after Ivermectin treatment. Clin Infect Dis 2018;66(10):1558–65.
97. Anselmi M, Buonfrate D, Guevara Espinoza A, et al. Mass administration of Ivermectin for the elimination of onchocerciasis significantly reduced and maintained low the prevalence of *Strongyloides stercoralis* in Esmeraldas, Ecuador. PLoS Negl Trop Dis 2015;9(11):e0004150.
98. Vargas P, Krolewiecki AJ, Echazú A, et al. Serologic monitoring of public health interventions against *Strongyloides stercoralis*. Am J Trop Med Hyg 2017;97(1): 166–72.
99. Kearns T, Currie B, Cheng A, et al. *Strongyloides* seroprevalence before and after an ivermectin mass drug administration in a remote Australian Aboriginal community. PLoS Negl Trop Dis 2017;11(5):19.
100. Barrett J, Broderick C, Soulsby H, et al. Subcutaneous ivermectin use in the treatment of severe *Strongyloides stercoralis* infection: two case reports and a discussion of the literature. J Antimicrob Chemother 2016;71(1):220–5.

Neurocysticerosis
An Individualized Approach

Christina M. Coyle, MD, MS*

KEYWORDS

- Neurocysticercosis • Cysticercosis • Tapeworm • *Taenia solium* • Seizures

KEY POINTS

- Infectious Diseases Society of America/American Society of Tropical Medicine and Hygiene (IDSA/ASTMH) recently published evidence-based guidelines for management.
- Dual therapy with albendazole and praziquantel for multiple parenchymal cysts (>2) should be used, and enhanced steroid dosing should be considered.
- Management of subarachnoid disease requires more intense antiparasitic therapy and anti-inflammatory therapy, but optimal management is still being defined.
- Endoscopic removal of the third and lateral intraventricular neurocysticercosis is the preferred approach when feasible.

INTRODUCTION

Neurocysticercosis (NCC) is an infection of the central nervous system by the larval stage of the pork tapeworm *Taenia solium*. The combination of modern diagnostic tests, use of antiparasitic drugs, improved anti-inflammatory treatments, and minimally invasive neurosurgery has improved outcomes in patients with NCC. Despite these advances, NCC is still the most common helminthic neurologic infection and a major public health problem in most of the world. Millions of individuals are estimated to be infected, many of whom become symptomatic at some point in their lives.[1] This tapeworm is endemic in most low-income countries where pigs are raised and continues to be one of the most important causes of seizures in the world.[2] Mortality in parenchymal NCC is limited to epilepsy-related deaths, unless there is a high burden of cysts, whereas extraparenchymal NCC still carries high mortalities, mainly due to intracranial hypertension, which requires aggressive management.[3,4]

Disclosure Statement: The author has no relationship with a commercial company that has a direct financial interest in subject matter or materials discussed in the article or with a company making a competing product.

Department of Medicine, Division of Infectious Disease, Albert Einstein College of Medicine, 1300 Morris Park Avenue, Bronx, NY 10461, USA

* 334 Weaver Street, Larchmont, NY 10538.

E-mail address: Christina.coyle@einstein.yu.edu

Infect Dis Clin N Am 33 (2019) 153–168
https://doi.org/10.1016/j.idc.2018.10.007
0891-5520/19/© 2018 Elsevier Inc. All rights reserved.

id.theclinics.com

NCC is endemic in most Latin American countries, sub-Saharan Africa, and large regions of Asia, including the Indian subcontinent, most of southeast Asia, and China.[1] With increases in immigration from endemic regions and travel, numbers of patients with NCC are increasing in countries where local transmission is low.[5–9]

NCC is complex in both the clinical presentation and the treatment approach, which depends on the number of cysts, location in the brain, stage of degeneration, and host inflammatory response.[3] Disease in the brain parenchyma behaves very differently than NCC involving the extraparenchymal space. Clinical presentation and therapeutic interventions for each location are different; therefore, principles for managing parenchymal disease cannot be applied to extraparenchymal disease. Clinical manifestations can vary from completely asymptomatic infection to severe disease and death. Extraparenchymal NCC has a worse prognosis than parenchymal disease and if not managed appropriately has a high mortality.[4,10,11]

LIFE CYCLE OF THE PARASITE

The human can act as both intermediate and definitive host. Humans acquire the adult tapeworm after ingesting infected pigs with cysticerci or larvae in tissue. Cysticerci or larvae attach to the small intestine of humans by a scolex, or head, which extends into segments referred to as proglottids. The distal segments are mature, each containing about 50,000 to 60,000 ova. In areas where pigs are not corralled and there is poor sanitation, they ingest feces containing ova, which develop into cysticerci in their tissue. After humans accidently ingest human feces contaminated with ova, they hatch into oncospheres, which invade the blood vessels of the intestine and disseminate into subcutaneous tissue, muscle, and brain. Studies from Peru suggest that cysticercosis is spread person to person, because there is a significant human cysticercosis seroprevalence gradient surrounding tapeworm carriers.[12]

IMMUNOLOGIC DIAGNOSIS

Diagnosis is usually based on neuroimaging methods, epidemiology, and reliable immune diagnostic tests. The enzyme-linked immunoelectrotransfer blot (EITB) assay, which uses lentil lectin purified glycoprotein antigens to detect antibodies to *T solium*, has a sensitivity approaching 98% for patients with 2 or more live parasites in the nervous system and does not cross-react with heterologous infections.[13,14] The sensitivity in the serum is slightly higher than cerebrospinal fluid (CSF) for parenchymal disease.[15,16] A negative serology in patients with greater than a single cyst should lead to a workup of alternative diagnoses. Conversely, in the setting of a single cyst, the EITB's sensitivity drops to 50% to 60%.[16,17] Therefore, when evaluating a single cyst, a negative EITB does not exclude NCC. Similarly, the sensitivity of the EITB is poor in patients with calcified cysticerci.[16,17] EITB should be used to establish the diagnosis of NCC because it is superior to commercially available antibody detection enzyme-linked immunosorbent assay (ELISA), which have poorer sensitivity.[18,19]

APPROACH TO PARENCHYMAL DISEASE
Imaging

When approaching neuroimaging of parenchymal disease, the clinician should stage the cysts. Computerized axial tomography (CAT) scan can detect calcifications better, whereas magnetic resolution imaging (MRI) is frequently superior at detecting disease in the extraparenchymal space.

Staging is based on the involution of the cysts. Live vesicular cysts are rounded lesions with fluid within the cyst that are isointense with CSF on computed tomography (CT) imaging and do not enhance after the administration of contrast. The tapeworm scolex can be frequently visualized as an internal asymmetric nodule within a cyst referred to as "hole with dot" sign (**Fig. 1**).[20–23] This sign is best visualized on the fluid-attenuated inversion recovery (FLAIR) technique on MRI (**Fig. 2**).[24] Diffusion-weighted images and fast imaging employing steady-state acquisition (FIESTA) may enhance the diagnostic accuracy of MRI because they allow the recognition of the scolices in cases that are not visualized with conventional sequences.[21,23,25] Eventually the immune response detects the parasite, leading to a host inflammatory response, and the cyst begins to degenerate, which can be reflected in changes on imaging. The cyst borders become poorly defined and enhance after the administration of contrast. On CT, the cyst will appear as isointense fluid with ring enhancement of the lesion, whereas MRI will reveal cyst fluid which is isointense, ring enhancement on post-contrast T-1 weighted images, and lack of a scolex (**Fig. 3**).[21] This stage is referred to as the colloidal stage, and it is common to see perilesional edema, which is best visualized on FLAIR technique on MRI.[22,24] Unusual radiographic presentations can occur, such as large cysts with fluid levels within thought to represent the inflammatory response (**Fig. 4**), which can mimic brain abscess. Cysts that are close together can appear as multi-septated cysts (**Fig. 5**). As the cyst involutes entirely, it transforms into a small nodular lesion referred to as the granular stage. CT and MRI demonstrate enhancement of the nodular lesion after contrast medium administration.[21,24] Calcified cysticerci are clearly visible on CT as nonenhancing hyperdense nodules.[21] Although conventional MRI sequences are not as sensitive as CT to detect calcified cysticerci, the sequences might improve with the use of susceptibility image protocols. Patients with calcification on CT scan can have persistent corresponding

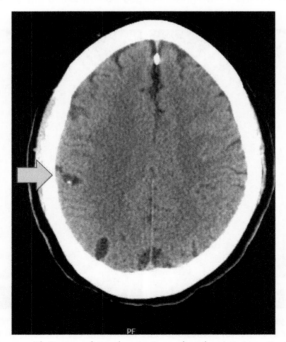

Fig. 1. Axial CAT scan with 2 parenchymal cysts. Arrowhead points to cyst with "dot in hole."

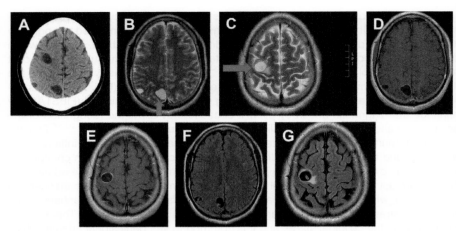

Fig. 2. (*A*) Three cystic lesions on CAT scan. (*B, C*) Corresponding cysts on T2-weighted images on MRI. Scoleces can be seen in cysts with arrows. (*D, E*) Corresponding cysts on T1 postgadolinium with thin rim of enhancement. Vesicular cyst that is beginning to develop inflammation. (*F, G*) Corresponding cysts on FLAIR images. Scoleces are clear in all 3 cysts.

enhancement on MR for prolonged periods.[26] Intermittent perilesional brain edema associated with calcified lesions are well described and often associated with corresponding clinical symptoms.[27] Perilesional edema appears as a bright signal using MRI FLAIR or T2 imaging. It is almost always accompanied by enhancement around the calcified focus on the T1-weighted images postgadolinium (**Fig. 6**).[28]

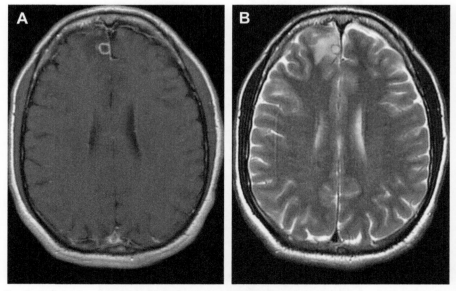

Fig. 3. Colloidal cyst. (*A*) A colloidal cyst seen on MRI T1 postgadolinium reveals enhancing cyst with irregular borders. (*B*) Perilesional edema around the cyst seen on the T2-weighted FLAIR images.

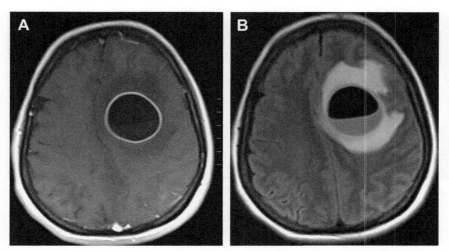

Fig. 4. A young woman from Honduras presented with hemiparesis. EITB was positive. (*A*) Large cyst with peripheral enhancement on MRI T1-weighted postgadolinium images and a fluid level layering within the cyst. (*B*) MRI FLAIR images reveal fluid layering within.

Clinical Manifestations

Recurrent seizures are most often the main or sole manifestation of parenchymal brain cysticercosis. Headaches can be commonly reported, and less commonly, focal findings can be seen due to mass effect usually secondary to edema. A rare form of parenchymal disease referred to as cysticercotic encephalitis presents with raised

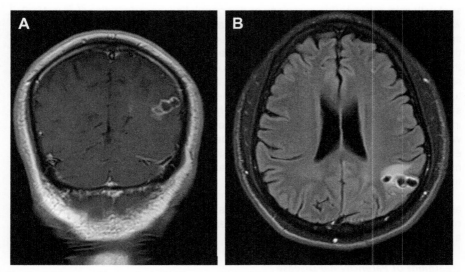

Fig. 5. A 34-year-old man from Haiti presented with new onset grand-mal seizures. (*A*) MRI T1-weighted postgadolinium images represent cyst that appears to be multiseptations with peripheral enhancement. (*B*). MRI FLAIR images reveal 3 separate cysts and peripheral edema.

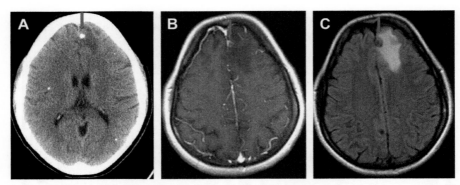

Fig. 6. A 42-year-old woman who immigrated from Guatemala 5 years ago presented with new onset seizures. (*A*) CAT scan reveals multiple calcified leions. Frontal calcified leions (*arrow*) revels perilesional edema. (*B*) Postgadolinium T1-weighted MRI sequence reveals ring enhancing lesion (*arrow*) corresponding to calcified lesion. Perilesional edema surrounds it. (*C*) MRI FLAIR images reveal calcified lesion in center of edema, which appears bright.

intracranial pressure due to diffuse cerebral edema secondary to numerous dying parenchymal cysts.

Up to one-third of all adult onset seizures in endemic regions are thought to be due to NCC.[2,29–31] Seizures are a very frequent manifestation in patients with degenerating cysts, but have also been reported in patients with nonenhancing vesicular cysts.[3,32,33] There is now increasing evidence that calcified NCC, once thought to be inactive disease, plays a large role in both cause and maintenance of seizure and epilepsy in endemic populations.[27] In hospitalized individuals with seizures in endemic regions, approximately 25%-50% have characteristic calcified lesions by CT examination. Calcified brain lesions are common in CT studies of persons who present with seizures in endemic regions and in population-based studies.[27,28] In 1998, it was first noted that patients with nodular calcification on CT had persistent corresponding enhancement on MR for up to a year after evidence of complete calcification. An early report of perilesional edema around calcified lesions was incorrectly thought to be reactivation.[26,34] It has become increasingly recognized that calcified lesions can provoke perilesional edema and is associated with recurrent seizures in up to 35% to 50% of cases.[27,28,35,36] Many experts have hypothesized antigen is either sporadically released or recognized by the host eliciting an inflammatory response in the brain seen as enhancement on MRI on T1-weighted postgadolinium images with or without intermittent perilesional edema.[27] Recurrence of the perilesional edema, usually around the same calcified lesion, has been reported. Calcified lesions may also be associated with hippocampal changes, which may predispose individuals to recurrent seizures.[37]

When undertaking treatment of parenchymal disease, it is important to stage and assess the burden of disease (number of cysts) and take into consideration location of cyst. MRI should be ordered to rule out extraparenchymal disease in addition to a CAT scan.[38]

Treatment of Parenchymal Disease

Viable and multiple enhancing lesions

Both praziquantel and albendazole have cystidal activity as single antiparasitic agents in NCC. Treatment with praziquantel has generally been less effective than albendazole.[39] In open-label studies, radiologic response rates with albendazole (generally dosed at 15 mg/kg/d in 2 daily doses for 1–2 weeks) have tended to be better than those with praziquantel (generally dosed at 50 mg/kg/d in 3 daily doses) for 14 days. The recommended daily dose of albendazole is 1,200 mg/day. Two high-quality placebo-controlled trials examining albendazole treatment in viable NCC demonstrated superior radiologic resolution in those who received albendazole over placebo.[40,41] Garcia and colleagues[40] noted there was a significant reduction in the numbers of generalized seizures; however, the overall number of seizures between the 2 groups was not significant. Similarly, Carpio and colleagues[39,41] demonstrated a decrease in the number of recurrent focal seizures with generalizations in a subgroup analysis, but despite more seizure-free patients in the albendazole group at 12 months, it was not significant.

Albendazole and praziquantel as dual therapy for parenchymal disease has been examined in both a phase I/II study and a randomized controlled study.[42,43] A randomized controlled trial examining albendazole (15 mg/kg) and higher-dose albendazole (22 mg/kg) and albendazole (15 mg/kg plus praziquantel 50 mg/kg) each for 10 days found resolution of viable cysts on MRI at 180 days was significantly higher in the combination group compared with the standard-dose and high-dose albendazole group among those individuals with 3 or more cysts.[43] Based on these observations, the Infectious Diseases Society of America/American Society of Tropical Medicine and Hygiene (IDSA/ASTMH) guidelines recommend administering albendazole (15 mg/kg/d divided in 2 doses) 10 to 14 days for 1 to 2 viable cysts and dual therapy with albendazole (15 mg/kg/d in 2 divided doses) and praziquantel (50 mg/kg/d) for 10 to 14 days in those with 3 or more parenchymal cysticerci.[38] Treatment of patients with cysticercotic encephalitis should be aimed at controlling the intracranial hypertension with corticosteroids, and antiparasitic drugs should be avoided.

Adequate control of the inflammatory response as cysts degenerate during treatment is critical. Viable parenchymal cysts induce little inflammation; however, the host initiates a robust inflammatory response to degenerating cysts as a response to treatment, which frequently results in worsening of neurologic symptoms, especially seizures the month after treatment.[44,45] Corticosteroids have been used to suppress this response. There is only one study examining dosing and length of administration of steroids during and after treatment with antiparasitics.[46] Garcia and colleagues[47] conducted an open-label randomized trial comparing 6 mg/d dexamethasone for 10 days with enhanced dosing at 8 mg/d for 28 days followed by a 2-week taper for patients with viable parenchymal NCC receiving albendazole treatment. Increased dexamethasone dosing resulted in fewer seizures in the first 21 days as well as over the first 180 days, but the study was underpowered due to slow enrollment.[47] Optimal dosing of steroids has not been established, but this study suggests that ongoing inflammation occurs beyond the 2-week albendazole treatment period, and improved steroid coverage continued after the cessation of antiparasitics may be preferable.

The IDSA/ASTMH guidelines recommend that patients with multiple enhancing lesions be treated using the same guidelines for viable cystic lesions.[38] The exception is the single enhancing lesion (SEL).

Single Enhancing Lesion

Patients with SEL, a common form of NCC reported in India, typically present with seizure or headache. The enhancing lesion represents the parasite transitioning from viable to dead parasite and host inflammatory response. The role of antiparasitic drugs in patients with SEL has been controversial. Several randomized trials have examined optimal management. A meta-analysis suggested that patients have a more rapid radiologic resolution and fewer seizures over 6 months if treated with corticosteroids and a short course of albendazole (15 mg/kg/d for 7 days).[48] IDSA/ASTMH guidelines recommend treatment with a 1-week course of albendazole along with steroids for SEL, but this was not a strong recommendation.[38]

Calcified Lesions

Calcified lesions do not require antiparasitic therapy.

Subarachnoid disease

Small, cystic, subarachnoid cysticerci located within the cortical sulci generally behave similar to parenchymal brain cysts as opposed to cysts that develop in the Sylvian fissure or basal cisterns, where they grow abnormally and can reach large sizes.[4,24] Neurocysticercosis in the subarachnoid space (SANCC) may require longer incubations before symptoms develop.[4] Cysts in these locations are proliferative, lack a scolex in many instances, and are referred to as racemose cysticercosis (**Fig. 7**). In these locations, the cysts continually grow and can elicit an exuberant inflammatory host response, and manifestations are usually severe.[4] This inflammatory reaction is characterized by CSF pleocystosis, elevated protein concentration, and low glucose.[19] Hydrocephalus, the most common complication of SANCC, is thought to be due to chronic arachnoiditis and resultant fibrosis involving the arachnoid villi, the occlusion of foramina of Luschka and Magendie by thickened leptomeninges, and the parasite's mass effect on the ventricular system.[4,49]

Clinical Manifestations

Intracranial hypertension, the main symptom of SANCC, is the major source of morbidity and mortality among NCC patients.[4] Cranial nerves can become trapped within the dense exudates formed by arachnoiditis, or they can be compressed by large cysts located in the cisterns leading to focal deficits. Patients can present with headaches that are confused with migraines over weeks to months, delaying diagnosis. Cognitive dysfunction has also been described.[4] Chronic papilledema secondary to increased intracranial pressure can lead to optic nerve damage and atrophy. Last, stroke is a recognized complication of NCC, occurring in 2% to 12% of cases

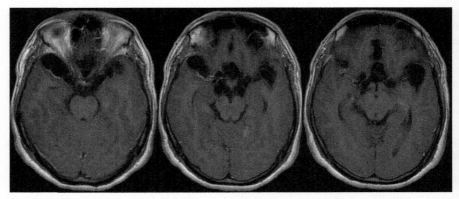

Fig. 7. A 42-year-old man from Cuenca, Ecuador arrived in the United States 18 years ago. He reported headaches for 2 months associated with nausea and blurry vision. T1-weighted images postgadolinium reveal multiple cystic lesions tracking along the subarachnoid space with enhancement.

and are mostly in the form of small lacunar infarcts, but larger vessels can be involved leading to major stroke syndromes.[50–53] Hemorrhagic cerebrovascular events in the setting of SANCC have been reported, but with less frequency than ischemic events.[54,55]

Imaging

MRI is the modality of choice to examine the basilar cisterns, mainly the suprasellar, perimesencephalic, magna, and Sylvian fissures. Findings may be subtle and are usually not well-defined on CT. The cystic masses are multiloculated on MRI and can result in cisternal expansion and deformity displacing neighboring structures and can behave as mass-occupying lesions.[24,56] They are related to local inflammatory reaction, which can cause leptomeningeal thickening and fibrosis.[55] Fibrous arachnoiditis, responsible for the development of hydrocephalus, is seen by CT or MRI as abnormal leptomeningeal enhancement at the base of the brain.

Neuroimaging appearance of cysticercosis-related cerebral infarcts is the same as that of cerebral infarcts from other causes. The cause-and-effect relationship between NCC and a cerebral infarct is usually supported by CT or MRI evidence of a meningeal cyst adjacent to the infarct or by CSF findings compatible with active arachnoiditis.[57,58] Angiographic findings in subarachnoid NCC include segmental narrowing or even occlusion of the major intracranial arteries in patients with cysticercotic-related cerebral infarcts.[58] Angiography may be normal in patients with small vessel angiitis.[58]

Basal subarachnoid NCC is associated with spinal involvement in about 60% of cases; therefore, patients with SANCC should have their spine evaluated by imaging.[59]

Treatment

Increasingly, physicians in nonendemic regions are faced with patients presenting with SANCC without much experience in treating this form of disease.[5] SANCC is particularly difficult to treat because it does not respond to the typical course of antiparasitic therapy. The inflammatory response, which ensues after initiating therapy, can result in worsening hydrocephalus or stroke if not adequately covered by steroids. Detection of circulating parasitic antigens in serum by ELISA with monoclonal antibodies has been used in clinical and field studies. Circulating antigens are present in the serum of patients with subarachnoid NCC, and serum concentrations rapidly decrease after successful treatment and may help to define treatment endpoints.[60] Patients with subarachnoid disease require a longer period of antiparasitic therapy with albendazole or preferably with dual therapy with albendazole and praziquantel. Endpoints for treatment have not been defined, but experts think that longer courses of therapy are required with adequate steroids and a slow taper to control the inflammatory response due to killing of the parasite (**Fig. 8**). Antibody to tumor necrosis factor has recently used successfully as a steroid-sparing agent (Theodore Nash, personal communication, 2017). An MRI should be repeated every 3 months to follow response to treatment. Many experts think that therapy should be continued until disappearance of cysts on MRI and serum antigen along with improvement of CSF pleocytosis.

VENTRICULAR NEUROCYSTICERCOSIS
Clinical Manifestations

Clinical manifestations of ventricular NCC are secondary to obstruction of CSF flow due to obstructing or migrating cysts, which can be complete or intermittent, and

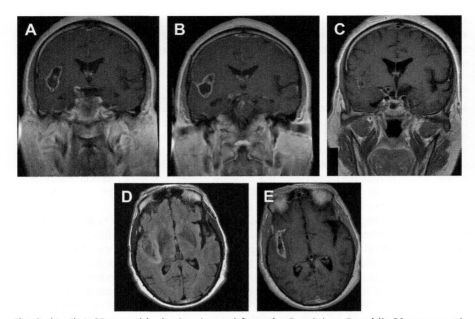

Fig. 8. (*A, B*) A 67-year-old who immigrated from the Dominican Republic 20 years previously now presented with headache. MRI coronal T1-weighted images postgadolinium reveal subarachnoid disease in the right Sylvian fissure with enhancement before treatment. (*C*) MRI coronal T1-weighted images postgadolinium on treatment with albendazole and praziquantel and steroids for 3 months reveal lesion is smaller and there is less enhancement. Antiparasitics are continued, and steroids continued to be tapered. The patient developed dysarthria 1 month later during steroid taper. (*E*) MRI axial T1-weighted images postgadolinium reveal worsening enhancement and edema is seen on (*D*) FLAIR images.

the associated ventriculitis that ensues.[3,61] Unattached cysts may cause acute or episodic symptoms due to transient obstruction of unattached, mobile cysts secondary to positional changes in the head referred to as Bruns syndrome.[62] Degenerating cysts elicit an inflammatory response, which results in acute or chronic ventriculitis. Ependymitis and subsequent adhesions, frequently in the aqueduct of Sylvius, result in CSF flow obstruction and hydrocephalus. Other complications include locked-in ventricles and lateral ventricle entrapment.[21,61,63] Inflamed cysts cause mass effect, enlargement, and obstruction of the foramina of Luschka and Magendie, and less commonly, the foramina of Monroe.[8,9,20]

Symptoms due to hydrocephalus are the most frequent manifestations.[61] In a recent review of one referral center's experience, symptoms due to acute or chronic obstruction resulting in hydrocephalus occurred in 73.9% of the patients.[61] Symptoms included headache, nausea, vomiting, dizziness, and confusion, as well as acute onset of syncope or coma. Greater than half of patients had symptoms with change of head position.[61]

Imaging

This form of NCC may be challenging to diagnose on CT, especially if coexisting parenchymal lesions are absent. Because many intraventricular neurocysticercosis cysts are isodense and isointense to CSF, it may be the presence of ventricular deformity, distention, and associated hydrocephalus that suggests IVNCC on CT.

Intraventricular and cisternal cysts are clearer on MRI by use of FLAIR, FIESTA, CISS (constructive interference in steady stage), or BFFE (balanced fast field echo) protocols (**Fig. 9**).[3,21,64,65] The wall of the cyst may occasionally be seen as a thin linear structure on T1-weighted imaging or may demonstrate contrast enhancement.

Treatment

Endoscopic management and open microsurgery in select cases have become mainstays of treatment in intraventricular disease. Medical therapy alone has been associated with poor outcomes in the literature.[66–70] Most patients treated with medical therapy alone receive a shunt procedure before medical therapy, but shunt therapy has also been associated with failure in this setting.[68,71,72] Administration of steroids, to decrease inflammation, leads to better outcomes.[72] Endoscopic therapy has replaced surgery for third and lateral ventricle cysts in centers with experience.[66,73] Many experts think enhancement on the MRI suggests the cyst is degenerating and inflamed associated with ventriculitis. These cysts may not be ideal candidates for removal because the cyst may become adherent to the wall of the ventricle with a risk of bleeding. Rupture of the cyst does not result in ventriculitis. Approach to fourth ventricular cysts should be individualized depending on the experience of the neuroendoscopist and the dilation of the fourth ventricle. Treatment with cyst removal, endoscopically or by open procedure, has led to better neurologic outcomes than shunt therapy alone.[38] Therefore, shunting should be regarded as an alternative strategy when the cyst is adherent or inflamed.[38] The recent ASTMH/IDSA guidelines suggest that patients undergoing shunting also be treated with antiparasitic drugs and steroids.[38] Despite being shunted, patients can still develop neurologic decompensation (**Fig. 10**). Dying cysts in the fourth ventricle can lead to ventriculitis, shunt failure, and/or edema around the fourth ventricle with ensuing nerve ischemia and impending herniation.

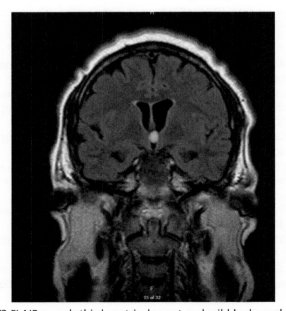

Fig. 9. Coronal T2 FLAIR reveals third ventricular cyst and mild hydrocephalus.

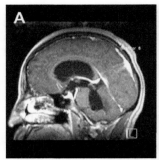
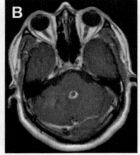
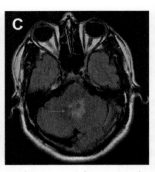

Fig. 10. (*A*) A 33-year-old from Ecuador presented with increased intracranial pressure due to a fourth ventricular cyst and hydrocephalus. The patient underwent a ventriculoperitoneal shunt and was treated with antiparasitic therapy and steroids. Fourth ventricular cyst (*arrow*) seen on sagittal MRI imaging. During tapering of steroids, the patient developed double vision and worsening inflammation seen as intense enhancement on the T1-weighted postgadolinium MRI around cyst in the fourth ventricle (*B*) and edema seen on the FLAIR MRI images (*C*). Patient developed permanent ocular nerve palsy.

SUMMARY

NCC is the most common neurologic parasitic infection of the central nervous system. It is a pleomorphic disease, and clinical manifestations are dependent on location of cysts, burden of disease, and host inflammatory response. Therapy needs to be individualized. Dual therapy with albendazole and praziquantel for multiple (>2 lesions) viable and enhancing cystic lesions should be used in parenchymal disease. Enhanced steroid dosing should be considered. Subarachnoid NCC requires longer courses of treatment with adequate steroid coverage at initiation and during tapering. Neuroendoscopy has replaced open microsurgery in the management of ventricular disease when appropriate. IDSA/ASTMH guidelines have been recently published.

REFERENCES

1. Coyle CM, Mahanty S, Zunt JR, et al. Neurocysticercosis: neglected but not forgotten. PLoS Negl Trop Dis 2012;6(5):e1500.
2. Ndimubanzi PC, Carabin H, Budke CM, et al. A systematic review of the frequency of neurocyticercosis with a focus on people with epilepsy. PLoS Negl Trop Dis 2010;4(11):e870.
3. Garcia HH, Nash TE, Del Brutto OH. Clinical symptoms, diagnosis, and treatment of neurocysticercosis. Lancet Neurol 2014;13(12):1202–15.
4. Fleury A, Carrillo-Mezo R, Flisser A, et al. Subarachnoid basal neurocysticercosis: a focus on the most severe form of the disease. Expert Rev Anti Infect Ther 2011; 9(1):123–33.
5. Serpa JA, Graviss EA, Kass JS, et al. Neurocysticercosis in Houston, Texas: an update. Medicine (Baltimore) 2011;90(1):81–6.
6. Serpa JA, White AC Jr. Neurocysticercosis in the United States. Pathog Glob Health 2012;106(5):256–60.
7. Cantey PT, Coyle CM, Sorvillo FJ, et al. Neglected parasitic infections in the United States: cysticercosis. Am J Trop Med Hyg 2014;90(5):805–9.
8. Fabiani S, Bruschi F. Neurocysticercosis in Europe: still a public health concern not only for imported cases. Acta Trop 2013;128(1):18–26.

9. Del Brutto OH. Neurocysticercosis among international travelers to disease-endemic areas. J Travel Med 2012;19(2):112–7.

10. Garcia HH, Gonzalez AE, Gilman RH. Cysticercosis of the central nervous system: how should it be managed? Curr Opin Infect Dis 2011;24(5):423–7.

11. Nash TE, Garcia HH. Diagnosis and treatment of neurocysticercosis. Nat Rev Neurol 2011;7(10):584–94.

12. Lescano AG, Garcia HH, Gilman RH, et al. Taenia solium cysticercosis hotspots surrounding tapeworm carriers: clustering on human seroprevalence but not on seizures. PLoS Negl Trop Dis 2009;3(1):e371.

13. Wilkins PP, Allan JC, Verastegui M, et al. Development of a serologic assay to detect Taenia solium taeniasis. Am J Trop Med Hyg 1999;60(2):199–204.

14. Tsang VC, Brand JA, Boyer AE. An enzyme-linked immunoelectrotransfer blot assay and glycoprotein antigens for diagnosing human cysticercosis (Taenia solium). J Infect Dis 1989;159(1):50–9.

15. Michelet L, Fleury A, Sciutto E, et al. Human neurocysticercosis: comparison of different diagnostic tests using cerebrospinal fluid. J Clin Microbiol 2011;49(1):195–200.

16. Rodriguez S, Dorny P, Tsang VC, et al. Detection of Taenia solium antigens and anti-T. solium antibodies in paired serum and cerebrospinal fluid samples from patients with intraparenchymal or extraparenchymal neurocysticercosis. J Infect Dis 2009;199(9):1345–52.

17. Rodriguez S, Wilkins P, Dorny P. Immunological and molecular diagnosis of cysticercosis. Pathog Glob Health 2012;106(5):286–98.

18. Garcia HH, Castillo Y, Gonzales I, et al. Low sensitivity and frequent cross-reactions in commercially available antibody detection ELISA assays for Taenia solium cysticercosis. Trop Med Int Health 2018;23(1):101–5.

19. Garcia HH, O'Neal SE, Noh J, et al. Laboratory diagnosis of neurocysticercosis/Taenia solium. J Clin Microbiol 2018;56(9) [pii:e00424-18].

20. Suss RA, Maravilla KR, Thompson J. MR imaging of intracranial cysticercosis: comparison with CT and anatomopathologic features. AJNR Am J Neuroradiol 1986;7(2):235–42.

21. Lerner A, Shiroishi MS, Zee CS, et al. Imaging of neurocysticercosis. Neuroimaging Clin N Am 2012;22(4):659–76.

22. Garcia HH, Del Brutto OH. Imaging findings in neurocysticercosis. Acta Trop 2003;87(1):71–8.

23. Del Brutto OH, Nash TE, White AC Jr, et al. Revised diagnostic criteria for neurocysticercosis. J Neurol Sci 2017;372:202–10.

24. Garcia HH, Del Brutto OH, Nash TE, et al. New concepts in the diagnosis and management of neurocysticercosis (Taenia solium). Am J Trop Med Hyg 2005;72(1):3–9.

25. Neyaz Z, Patwari SS, Paliwal VK. Role of FIESTA and SWAN sequences in diagnosis of intraventricular neurocysticercosis. Neurol India 2012;60(6):646–7.

26. Sheth TN, Pillon L, Keystone J, et al. Persistent MR contrast enhancement of calcified neurocysticercosis lesions. AJNR Am J Neuroradiol 1998;19(1):79–82.

27. Nash TE, Pretell EJ, Lescano AG, et al. Perilesional brain oedema and seizure activity in patients with calcified neurocysticercosis: a prospective cohort and nested case-control study. Lancet Neurol 2008;7(12):1099–105.

28. Nash TE, Del Brutto OH, Butman JA, et al. Calcific neurocysticercosis and epileptogenesis. Neurology 2004;62(11):1934–8.

29. Medina MT, Aguilar-Estrada RL, Alvarez A, et al. Reduction in rate of epilepsy from neurocysticercosis by community interventions: the Salama, Honduras study. Epilepsia 2011;52(6):1177–85.

30. Montano SM, Villaran MV, Ylquimiche L, et al. Neurocysticercosis: association between seizures, serology, and brain CT in rural Peru. Neurology 2005;65(2): 229–33.

31. Del Brutto OH, Santibáñez R, Idrovo L, et al. Epilepsy and neurocysticercosis in Atahualpa: a door-to-door survey in rural coastal Ecuador. Epilepsia 2005;46(4): 583–7.

32. Garcia-Noval J, Moreno E, de Mata F, et al. An epidemiological study of epilepsy and epileptic seizures in two rural Guatemalan communities. Ann Trop Med Parasitol 2001;95(2):167–75.

33. Garcia-Noval J, Allan JC, Fletes C, et al. Epidemiology of Taenia solium taeniasis and cysticercosis in two rural Guatemalan communities. Am J Trop Med Hyg 1996;55(3):282–9.

34. Sheth TN, Lee C, Kucharczyk W, et al. Reactivation of neurocysticercosis: case report. Am J Trop Med Hyg 1999;60(4):664–7.

35. Nash T. Edema surrounding calcified intracranial cysticerci: clinical manifestations, natural history, and treatment. Pathog Glob Health 2012;106(5):275–9.

36. Nash TE, Pretell J, Garcia HH. Calcified cysticerci provoke perilesional edema and seizures. Clin Infect Dis 2001;33(10):1649–53.

37. Del Brutto OH, Issa NP, Salgado P, et al. The Association Between Neurocysticercosis and Hippocampal Atrophy is Related to Age. Am J Trop Med Hyg 2017; 96(1):243–8.

38. White AC Jr, Coyle CM, Rajshekhar V, et al. Diagnosis and Treatment of Neurocysticercosis: 2017 Clinical Practice Guidelines by the Infectious Diseases Society of America (IDSA) and the American Society of Tropical Medicine and Hygiene (ASTMH). Clin Infect Dis 2018;66(8):1159–63.

39. Carpio A, Kelvin EA, Bagiella E, et al. Effects of albendazole treatment on neurocysticercosis: a randomised controlled trial. J Neurol Neurosurg Psychiatry 2008; 79(9):1050–5.

40. Garcia HH, Pretell EJ, Gilman RH, et al. A trial of antiparasitic treatment to reduce the rate of seizures due to cerebral cysticercosis. N Engl J Med 2004;350(3): 249–58.

41. Romo ML, Wyka K, Carpio A, et al. The effect of albendazole treatment on seizure outcomes in patients with symptomatic neurocysticercosis. Trans R Soc Trop Med Hyg 2015;109(11):738–46.

42. Garcia HH, Lescano AG, Gonzales I, et al. Cysticidal efficacy of combined treatment with praziquantel and albendazole for parenchymal brain cysticercosis. Clin Infect Dis 2016;62(11):1375–9.

43. Garcia HH, Gonzales I, Lescano AG, et al. Efficacy of combined antiparasitic therapy with praziquantel and albendazole for neurocysticercosis: a double-blind, randomised controlled trial. Lancet Infect Dis 2014;14(8):687–95.

44. Sotelo J, Escobedo F, Rodriguez-Carbajal J, et al. Therapy of parenchymal brain cysticercosis with praziquantel. N Engl J Med 1984;310(16):1001–7.

45. Ramos-Zuniga R, Pérez-Gómez HR, Jáuregui-Huerta F, et al. Incidental consequences of antihelmintic treatment in the central nervous system. World Neurosurg 2013;79(1):149–53.

46. Cuello-Garcia CA, Roldán-Benítez YM, Pérez-Gaxiola G, et al. Corticosteroids for neurocysticercosis: a systematic review and meta-analysis of randomized controlled trials. Int J Infect Dis 2013;17(8):e583–92.

47. Garcia HH, Gonzales I, Lescano AG, et al. Enhanced steroid dosing reduces seizures during antiparasitic treatment for cysticercosis and early after. Epilepsia 2014;55(9):1452–9.
48. Otte WM, Singla M, Sander JW, et al. Drug therapy for solitary cysticercus granuloma: a systematic review and meta-analysis. Neurology 2013;80(2):152–62.
49. Estanol B, Kleriga E, Loyo M, et al. Mechanisms of hydrocephalus in cerebral cysticercosis: implications for therapy. Neurosurgery 1983;13(2):119–23.
50. Del Brutto OH. Cysticercosis and cerebrovascular disease: a review. J Neurol Neurosurg Psychiatry 1992;55(4):252–4.
51. Levy AS, Lillehei KO, Rubinstein D, et al. Subarachnoid neurocysticercosis with occlusion of the major intracranial arteries: case report. Neurosurgery 1995; 36(1):183–8 [discussion: 188].
52. Alarcon F, Hidalgo F, Moncayo J, et al. Cerebral cysticercosis and stroke. Stroke 1992;23(2):224–8.
53. Alarcon F, Vanormelingen K, Moncayo J, et al. Cerebral cysticercosis as a risk factor for stroke in young and middle-aged people. Stroke 1992;23(11):1563–5.
54. Viola GM, White AC Jr, Serpa JA. Hemorrhagic cerebrovascular events and neurocysticercosis: a case report and review of the literature. Am J Trop Med Hyg 2011;84(3):402–5.
55. Amaral L, Maschietto M, Maschietto R, et al. Ununsual manifestations of neurocysticercosis in MR imaging: analysis of 172 cases. Arq Neuropsiquiatr 2003; 61(3A):533–41.
56. Del Brutto OH, Sotelo J, Aguirre R, et al. Albendazole therapy for giant subarachnoid cysticerci. Arch Neurol 1992;49(5):535–8.
57. Barinagarrementeria F, Cantu C. Neurocysticercosis as a cause of stroke. Stroke 1992;23(8):1180–1.
58. Barinagarrementeria F, Cantu C. Frequency of cerebral arteritis in subarachnoid cysticercosis: an angiographic study. Stroke 1998;29(1):123–5.
59. Callacondo D, Garcia HH, Gonzales I, et al. High frequency of spinal involvement in patients with basal subarachnoid neurocysticercosis. Neurology 2012;78(18): 1394–400.
60. Garcia HH, Gonzalez AE, Gilman RH, et al. Circulating parasite antigen in patients with hydrocephalus secondary to neurocysticercosis. Am J Trop Med Hyg 2002;66(4):427–30.
61. Nash TE, Ware JM, Mahanty S. intraventricular neurocysticercosis: experience and long-term outcome from a tertiary referral center in the United States. Am J Trop Med Hyg 2018;98(6):1755–62.
62. Sinha S, Sharma BS. Intraventricular neurocysticercosis: a review of current status and management issues. Br J Neurosurg 2012;26(3):305–9.
63. Zee CS, Segall HD, Destian S, et al. MRI of intraventricular cysticercosis: surgical implications. J Comput Assist Tomogr 1993;17(6):932–9.
64. Govindappa SS, Narayanan JP, Krishnamoorthy VM, et al. Improved detection of intraventricular cysticercal cysts with the use of three-dimensional constructive interference in steady state MR sequences. AJNR Am J Neuroradiol 2000; 21(4):679–84.
65. Mont'Alverne Filho FE, Machado Ldos R, Lucato LT, et al. The role of 3D volumetric MR sequences in diagnosing intraventricular neurocysticercosis: preliminar results. Arq Neuropsiquiatr 2011;69(1):74–8.
66. Bergsneider M, Holly LT, Lee JH, et al. Endoscopic management of cysticercal cysts within the lateral and third ventricles. J Neurosurg 2000;92(1):14–23.

67. Zee CS, Segall HD, Apuzzo ML, et al. Intraventricular cysticercal cysts: further neuroradiologic observations and neurosurgical implications. AJNR Am J Neuroradiol 1984;5(6):727–30.

68. Rangel-Castilla L, Serpa JA, Gopinath SP, et al. Contemporary neurosurgical approaches to neurocysticercosis. Am J Trop Med Hyg 2009;80(3):373–8.

69. Proano JV, Madrazo I, García L, et al. Albendazole and praziquantel treatment in neurocysticercosis of the fourth ventricle. J Neurosurg 1997;87(1):29–33.

70. Cuetter AC, Garcia-Bobadilla J, Guerra LG, et al. Neurocysticercosis: focus on intraventricular disease. Clin Infect Dis 1997;24(2):157–64.

71. Bandres JC, White AC Jr, Samo T, et al. Extraparenchymal neurocysticercosis: report of five cases and review of management. Clin Infect Dis 1992;15(5): 799–811.

72. Kelley R, Duong DH, Locke GE. Characteristics of ventricular shunt malfunctions among patients with neurocysticercosis. Neurosurgery 2002;50(4):757–61 [discussion: 761–2].

73. Bergsneider M, Holly LT, Lee JH, et al. Endoscopic management of cysticercal cysts within the lateral and third ventricles. Neurosurg Focus 1999;6(4):e7.

Sound Around the World
Ultrasound for Tropical Diseases

Daniel Kaminstein, MD, DTM&H[a],*, Tom Heller, MD[b],
Francesca Tamarozzi, DVM, MD, MSc, PhD[c]

KEYWORDS

- Ultrasound • POCUS • Tropical disease • FASH • Schistosomiasis
- Echinococcosis • Practical application

KEY POINTS

- The use of point-of-care-ultrasound (POCUS) in the hands of clinicians has significant implications for the diagnosis and treatment of many tropical diseases.
- POCUS involves the integration of findings on ultrasound imaging with the physician's knowledge about the patients and the tropical disease that they are suffering from.
- Recent ultrasound protocols have been designed and implemented by physicians caring for patients in resource-limited settings where advanced diagnostic capabilities are not available.

 Video content accompanies this article at http://www.id.theclinics.com/.

WHY ULTRASOUND AND WHY NOW?

Any article that purports to argue for the benefits of ultrasound (US) for tropical disease must first make the argument for why US should be used by clinicians at all.

As far back as the 1980s, clinicians were beginning to realize the benefit that US could provide in patients suffering from blunt trauma.[1] The initial clinical application of point-of-care US (POCUS), was the focused assessment with sonography for trauma (FAST) examination. This was a systematic assessment of critically ill patients with an acute injury, who were hypotensive from potential hemorrhage. The location of blood loss was less clear by history and physical examination alone, so the US assessment allowed clinicians to quickly and reliably identify and differentiate peritoneal bleeding from thoracic cavity bleeding and pericardial bleeding. This meant that

Disclosure Statement: The authors have no commercial or financial conflicts of interest.
[a] Department of Emergency Medicine, Medical College of Georgia, Augusta University, Augusta, GA 30912, USA; [b] Lighthouse Clinic, Kamuzu Central Hospital, Area 33, P.O. Box 106, Lilongwe, Malawi; [c] Center for Tropical Diseases, IRCSS, Sacro Cuore Don Calabria Hospital, Via Don A Sempreboni 5, Negrar, Verona 37024, Italy
* Corresponding author. 1120 15th Street, Augusta, GA 30912.
E-mail address: dakaminstein@augusta.edu

Infect Dis Clin N Am 33 (2019) 169–195
https://doi.org/10.1016/j.idc.2018.10.008
0891-5520/19/© 2018 Elsevier Inc. All rights reserved.

id.theclinics.com

decisions about emergent surgery or further imaging could be made more accurately at the bedside.

Today's world of trauma surgery looks different than it did almost 40 years ago but the value of the US to provide rapid, reproducible information that is not readily apparent by history and physical examination alone has not changed.

Granted, the environment encountered in a major urban trauma center is different from that of a clinic based in a small town in, for example, East Africa. Still, many of the same limitations are present for clinicians in both areas: need for rapid assessment and decision making with limited information, overwhelmed systems, and patient needs that often outstrip the resources available. US can be a valuable tool in both these situations to help clinicians take better care of their patients.

If US has been around for decades, why is it only in the past few years that it has been discussed for tropical medicine applications and used in resource-limited settings? In reality, as this article explores, US has been used to target specific tropical diseases since the early 1990s. For several reasons it was never widely adopted in clinical practice in much of the world.

Among the big limitations were cost and size of US machines. Even 10 years ago most US machines were too large and too expensive to be easily transported and maintained in tropical environments. Much like consumer electronics, however, US systems have been shrinking both in size and price. Portable systems paved the way for clinicians everywhere to ask how US could be specifically applied in situations where other advanced imaging tests were not available. Today, high-quality tablet-based systems can run off of solar power and provide excellent images. Prices may still be prohibitive for the average clinician but, as more clinicians adopt US in their practice and more companies start to produce portable systems, the price will rapidly decline.

This leads back to the original question—Why US and why now? Today there is a strong evidence base regarding the benefits of US in tropical environments with a technology that is increasingly accessible to most clinicians.

WHAT IS CLINICAL ULTRASOUND OR POINT-OF-CARE ULTRASOUND?

The term POCUS is used to differentiate traditional diagnostic US that is performed by radiologists from US examinations performed by a clinician at the bedside. The latter has different questions from and a different approach to the information obtained from an US compared with the radiologist interpreting US study of patients they may never meet. Both types of study are valuable but need to be applied in specific situations with specific goals in mind.

POCUS is by definition performed by a clinician at the bedside. It is by design structured to answer patient-specific management questions. Rather than asking, "What do I see when I evaluate the abdomen with an US?" a clinician might ask, "Is there free fluid in the abdomen?" The answer to this second question is more straightforward compared to the first and often can be answered with a dichotomous answer of yes or no. The physician then needs to integrate this yes/no answer with what is already known about the patient and make a decision about a management plan.

Thus, POCUS has 4 essential components when integrating US into patient care:

1. Image indication—clinicians must correctly identify patients who would benefit from an US examination and determine which examination type should be performed.

2. Image acquisition—the clinician must be able to acquire the appropriate US images at the bedside.
3. Image interpretation—once the correct image is acquired, the clinician must be able to appropriately identify the image as either normal or abnormal.
4. Clinical integration—the clinician must then be able to apply the specific US findings and use these to make appropriate management decisions in the context of the patient (**Fig. 1**).

None of these steps is different from what clinicians do every day when performing a history and physical examination. There is a tendency, however, when applying US imaging technology, to expect that it will provide an answer. Clinical US should not be thought of as a technology that can in isolation provide a definitive diagnosis. Rather, US imaging, just like the physical examination, is used by a clinician to refine a differential diagnosis and inform the management plan based on each individual patient. Faced with a patient who is suspected of having HIV-associated extrapulmonary tuberculosis (EPTB), US does not provide a definitive answer if the patient has

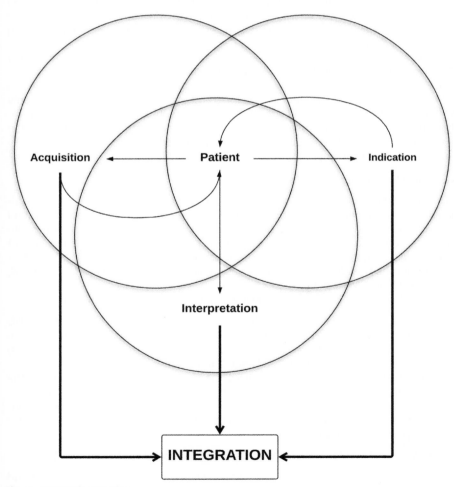

Fig. 1. POCUS in practice.

tuberculosis (TB) or not. Rather, the imaging protocol, as discussed later, sets up a series of easy-to-answer questions. The answers to these questions in conjunction with the patient's history, physical examination, risk factors, available laboratory tests, and clinical presentation are combined to allow the clinician to decide if the patient is likely to have EPTB. It is in this context that US applications are discussed for 4 tropical infectious diseases applications and implications reflected on for the care of these patients in resource-limited settings.

ULTRASOUND USE FOR TROPICAL INFECTIOUS DISEASES
Schistosomiasis

In 1978, ultrasonography was already being explored as a way to help characterize the morphologic features of liver fibrosis from schistosomiasis.[2] Although the practical implications of this were initially unclear, it was not long until the clinical utility of these image findings was elucidated. In 1984, Cerri and colleagues[3] published a case series of 103 patients demonstrating that the degree of liver fibrosis in patients with schistosomiasis could be reliably graded by US. Other studies suggested that US might be better than liver biopsy at characterizing the focality of lesions in schistosomiasis.[4] US provided a way to evaluate patients infected with schistosomiasis without having to perform a direct pathologic evaluation of the liver.

Since that time, more than 60 studies have been published regarding the efficacy of US in detecting pathology from schistosomiasis that otherwise would be clinically silent.[5-7] US has also proved useful in evaluating patients' response to treatment.[8] In 1998, it was shown that US grading of fibrosis had predictive value for which patients would mostly likely experience variceal bleeding.[9] US findings could thus directly influence the clinical management of patients. It demonstrated that not only could the extent of disease be graded but also this grading could be used to predict clinically important disease severity.

Niamey-Belo-Horizonte Protocol

Based on these early studies, an initial protocol for the optimal use of US in the evaluation of schistosomiasis was proposed. In 1991, a group of experts met in Cairo and an initial protocol was proposed but was not reproducible enough to be put into routine practice. In 1996 a second meeting in Niamey, Niger, finalized the current World Health Organization (WHO) protocol that is still in use today (**Fig. 2**).[10] Most of the published studies on schistosomiasis using US have followed the protocol, as outlined in the WHO publication[5,6]

The WHO protocol for intestinal schistosomiasis consists of 3 main parts:

- Pictorial assessment—involves the grading of liver fibrosis by comparing US findings to a standardized image pattern (IP) (**Fig. 3**). The IPs are presented in increasing degrees of severity of fibrosis (**Fig. 4**A, for example of liver fibrosis) and also account for the mix between 2 main pattern types.
- Quantitative measurements—involves the assessment of fibrosis through the quantitative measurement of the wall thickness of segmental portal branches
- Assessing portal hypertension—done by evaluating the main portal vein, measurement of the spleen size, evaluating for collateral vessels, and assessing for the presence of ascites

The WHO protocol for *Schistosoma haematobium* consists of 4 main parts:

- Evaluation of the urinary bladder—assessing shape of the urinary bladder and evaluating for bladder wall thickening/irregularities/polyps

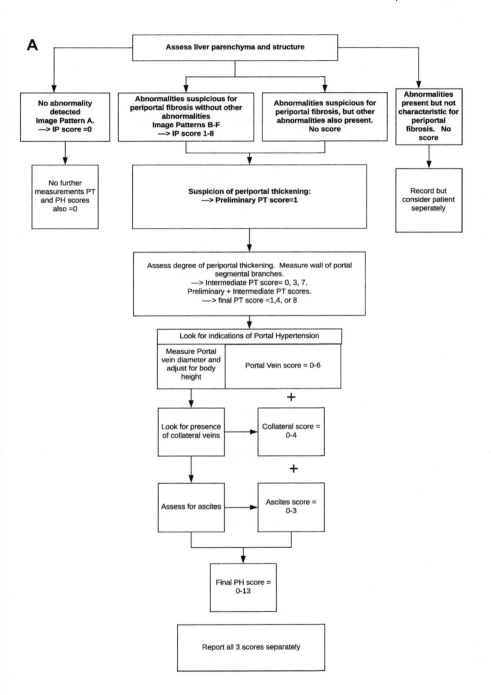

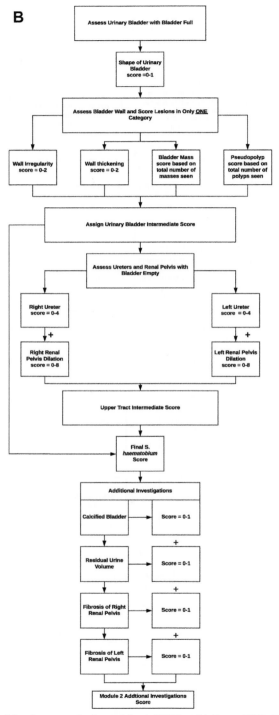

Fig. 2. (*A*) Protocol for S mansoni adapted from WHO guidelines. (*B*) Protocol for S heamatobium adapted from WHO guidelines. IP, image pattern; PH, portal hypertension; PT, periportal thickening.

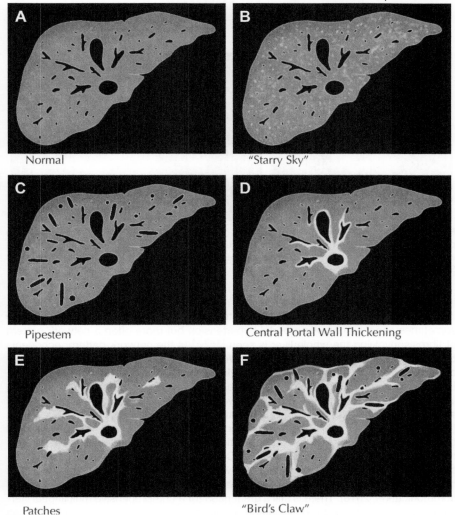

Fig. 3. IP for *S mansoni* liver involvement. (*A*) Normal (*B*) Starry sky. (*C*) Pipe stem. (*D*) Central portal wall thickening. (*E*) Patches. (*F*) Bird claw.

- Evaluation of the ureters—assessing for ureteral dilation
- Evaluation of the renal pelvis—grading degree of hydronephrosis (see **Fig. 4**B, for example of hydronephrosis) based on parenchymal thickness
- Additional investigations—assessing bladder volume, residual urine after voiding, and fibrosis of the renal pelvis

For both urogenital schistosomiasis and intestinal schistosomiasis, multiple measurements are required. The total score is based on all these measurements. The WHO protocols focus on the 2 dominant species of the parasite. There is far less information about the US appearance of the other species.

Schistosoma japonicum

The species, *S japonicum*, often causes a markedly different US appearance in adults compared with *S mansoni*.[11,12] Clinically, infection induced by *S japonicum* tends to be

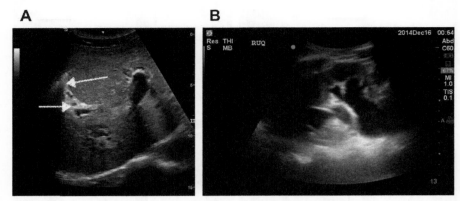

Fig. 4. (*A*) Transverse view of the liver with curvilinear probe shows extensive pipe-stem periportal fibrosis surrounding the portal vein and its branches (*arrows*). (*B*) Long-axis view of the right kidney showing extensive renal pelvis dilation in a patient infected with *S haematobium*.

more severe and to manifest itself with high rates of morbidity much earlier in childhood compared with the other species of schistosomiasis. Periportal fibrosis patterns are sometimes seen with resulting portal hypertension but more often a network pattern of fibrosis involving the whole liver is seen.[11,13,14] In the network pattern, echogenic bands separate lobules of normal looking liver tissue (Video 1). These bands seem specific for *S japonicum* infection and are not related anatomically to the portal venous system.[11,12] The network of bands can appear in a variety of patterns from thin and indistinct to thick echogenic bands.[15] Network patterns are seen more often in adults and do not appear to be reversible after treatment.[11,12,15] US seems better at detecting this early network fibrosis pattern compared with CT.[16] There is still much research to be done regarding why the US characteristics of this parasite and the clinical implications. There were recommendations at the Cairo meeting to standardize a grading classification system for *S japonicum* but these were never adopted because they were not believed sufficient to monitor dynamic changes in morbidity[15] (J. Richter, personal communication, 2018). There is still a great need for a comprehensive multilingual literature review and consensus on an image classification system for *S japonicum* that can be accessible to the clinician but also practical for ongoing field research.

Schistosoma mekongi

Little has been published about the US characteristics of *S mekongi*. This is most likely due to the geographic distribution of the parasite and the lower total number of infected individuals with ready access to US evaluation. In contrast to *S japonicum*, *S mekongi* does not seem to have a unique fibrosis pattern on US.[12,17] The pattern of *S mekongi* liver fibrosis seems similar to the pattern displayed in *S mansoni* infections (**Fig. 5**). The reason for this is unclear, especially given that *S japonicum* and *S mekongi* have similar size eggs. As with *S japonicum*, more research is needed to determine if there are characteristic findings that differentiate this species.

Moving Forward

There has been little modification to the Naimey protocols since first introduced more than 20 years ago. Although not yet incorporated into the WHO protocols, there have been several recent changes proposed to both the urogenital and

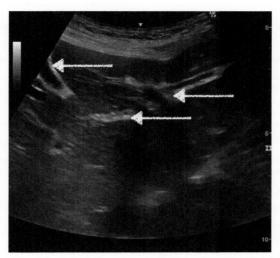

Fig. 5. Transverse view of the liver in a patient infected with *S mekongi*. This image demonstrates periportal fibrosis and fibrosis around the gallbladder (*arrows*), mirroring the pattern described for *S mansoni*.

intestinal schistosomiasis scoring systems.[5,6] These changes are aimed at simplifying the protocols and eliminating measurements that were not found helpful in risk-stratifying disease severity. One example of this is the elimination of measuring wall thickness in branch portal vessels in the intestinal scoring system. Those measurements were never well adopted and have not been found to help in predicting severe pathology[5] (**Box 1**).

Summary for the Treating Clinician

The WHO protocols, even with the proposed changes, are not specifically targeted at the clinician practicing at the bedside. There is still extensive measurement and expertise involved in obtaining all images. Additionally, little is published about how the findings can influence treatment decisions. Almost all studies focus on screening of outpatient populations, so guidance for the clinician on how these might be incorporated in the clinic setting is limited. From the treating clinician standpoint at the bedside, the WHO protocols (see **Fig. 2**) can be overwhelming and time consuming.

For the clinician at the bedside, there are some key points that can help in clinical decision making: identifying early reversible fibrotic changes in *S mansoni* (WHO patterns B–D) can be important, especially in children. Patients with these patterns are most likely to benefit from treatment with praziquantel and show reversal of fibrosis.[8] Patients with advanced fibrotic disease (WHO patterns E and F) are at the highest risk of variceal bleeding and are the most likely to benefit from endoscopic evaluation.[9] In *S haematobium*, patients with significant hydronephrosis should be considered high risk for needing more advanced urologic intervention as well as those with bladder masses or polyps (and thus a higher risk for carcinoma) that can be easily distinguished by US.

Small studies have hinted at promising results in the evaluation of bedside US findings of both urogenital and intestinal schistosomiasis when examinations are performed by novice sonographers after short training sessions.[18] This is an encouraging sign that modified versions of the WHO protocols can be easily learned and applied by clinicians. Several other articles on POCUS suggest the utility of US for

---

Box 1

Proposed changes to World Health Organization protocols for intestinal and urogenital schistosomiasis

Recommended improvements to the urogenital (S haematobium) protocol (Akpata 2015)[6]

1. Bladder score simplification
   Grade 0: bladder wall, which is less then to 5-mm thick
   Grade 1: any area of bladder wall 5-mm to 7-mm thick
   Grade 2: any area of the bladder wall of 8-m m to 9-mm thick
   Grade 3: an area of the bladder wall (including tumor or polyp) >10-mm thick

2. Define minimal bladder filling required for US examination based on height.

3. Renal pelvis dilation refined to improve sensitivity. Smaller dilations between 0 mm and 10 mm are broken up to allow more subtle signs of hydronephrosis to be identified.

4. Remove kidney and bladder fibrosis evaluation.

5. Add findings of bladder calcifications, calculi, and sludge (bladder snow).

6. Add measurement of distal ureteral wall irregularities and thickening.

7. Add evaluation for scrotal abnormalities (hydrocele and testicular mass).

8. Add evaluation for prostatic abnormalities.

Potential changes to intestinal schistosomiasis protocol (el Scheich 2014)[5]

1. Omit all quantitative measurements except for central portal vein diameter.

2. Additional assessment of liver parenchyma and measurements of the liver size are relegated to additional investigations and not part of primary score.

3. Grade IP with a first-choice/second-choice system to allow for patterns that do not strictly fall into a single category.

4. Replace portal vein score by portal vein quotient based on patient height (portal vein/height).

5. Add gallbladder findings to the score (external protuberances, tenderness sludge, or calculi).

6. Measure spleen length and/or depth.

7. Add portal flow velocity and direction using Doppler US if available.

8. Add intestinal wall thickening using high-frequency probe.

Other factors to include:
   Publications should include how many patients have been screened for coinfection with hepatitis B virus, hepatitis C virus, and hepatitis D virus.
   Evaluate for changes in US findings after therapy.
   Assessing postprandial gallbladder contractility in patients who have gallbladder involvement noted by US

---

schistosomiasis.[19,20] There remains a need for protocols targeted toward the application of POCUS in the care of infected patients in both the clinic and hospital settings. Although clinicians often perform modified versions of the WHO protocol, there is little to no evidence to guide them on how their findings should be applied.

ECHINOCOCCOSIS

The use of US for the diagnosis of human cystic echinococcosis (CE) started in the late 1960s in the clinical setting and represented a significant advancement in the diagnosis and follow-up of patients with this infection. Prior to this, radiographs could only visualize calcified cysts in the abdomen; US allowed for the visualization of the cysts and their defining characteristics.[21] The introduction of portable US machines allowed, in the mid-1980s, the screening of populations in rural areas.[21] Today, US is the imaging modality of choice for the diagnosis and staging of CE cysts in the abdomen, where a vast majority of the lesions are found.[22] MRI and CT are used in particular instances when cysts are not accessible by US and before surgery to assess the relative topography of cysts and nearby structures. The performance of CT imaging, however, in identifying features diagnostic for CE and for cyst staging is poor, whereas MRI has similar performance characteristics.[23] Serology tests are not standardized; their performances depend on many factors, the most important of which is the cyst stage; therefore, interpretation of their results should be done with caution and always in the light of US results.[24] Thus, for CE diagnosis and clinical management in both high-resource and low-resource settings, the most appropriate imaging technique, that is, US, is also the most accessible.

CE cysts may evolve spontaneously from unilocular fluid-filled to semisolid with calcified wall, passing through other morphologically different stages.[25,26] This morphologic heterogeneity corresponds with different cysts' activity states, and, of great practical importance, correlates with different response rates to nonsurgical treatments.[26–31] Clinical management decision making for uncomplicated liver CE is based on diagnosis and staging of CE cysts using imaging (stage-specific approach); it is, therefore, important for treating clinicians to understand the basics of an US-based classification of CE cysts.

Several US classifications have been used in the past; the most recent one in use was introduced by the WHO Informal Working Group on Echinococcosis (IWGE) in 2003 and refined in 2010.[22,32] The WHO-IWGE classification encompasses 6 CE stages: CE1 (unilocular fluid-filled cysts) and CE2 (multiloculated fluid-filled cysts with daughter vesicles) cysts are classified as active cysts; CE3a and CE3b cysts (cysts with detached inner parasitic layers and multiloculated cysts with daughter vesicles in a solid matrix, respectively) are classified in the transitional group; and CE4 and CE5 cysts (cysts with solid content without or with egg-shell wall calcifications, respectively) are classified as inactive. CE3 cysts are further differentiated into CE3a (with detached endocyst) and CE3b (predominantly solid with daughter vesicles). This distinction is of great practical importance because CE3a cysts activity is variable whereas CE3b are active cysts: this difference is also reflected in their different response to nonsurgical treatments.[27,33] CE3a cysts respond well to medical therapy with albendazole and to classic percutaneous treatments, such as puncture, aspiration of cyst fluid, injection of scolicidal agent, and reaspiration (PAIR); whereas, a majority of CE3b cysts that initially respond to albendazole relapse within 2 years from the end of treatment, and relapse is almost invariably observed after PAIR. The WHO-IWGE classification also encompasses an imaging type named cystic lesion (CL): this is not a CE stage, but rather a temporary definition for a CL without clear-cut features of CE or non-CE etiology, requiring further work-up.

The stage-specific approach is recommended by the WHO-IWGE for uncomplicated hepatic CE cysts. In all other instances (extrahepatic locations and/or complications), surgery is generally the advised procedure, but consultation with a physician experienced in the clinical management of CE is strongly advised before definitive management decisions are made.

Uniloculated fluid-filled cysts (CE1 and CE3a) tend to respond well to full medical treatment course with albendazole and classic percutaneous treatment, such as PAIR.[33] Albendazole should be administered every day, avoiding the interrupted administration scheme.[22,33] Although the length of standard albendazole therapy is not well defined, 3 months to 6 months is generally suggested.

The use of PAIR in the treatment of specific stages of CE is a relatively new approach to management of CE. Surgery for cyst removal was and is the traditional approach with all the associated risks of the surgery itself plus the very real risk of spillage of cyst fluid during the procedure with significant associated complications.[29] The use of a percutaneous approach with a needle is also done under US guidance (Video 2). Thus, US plays a part not only in the diagnosis and prognosis of patients with CE but also in treatment.

No matter what invasive procedure is used in the treatment of CE cysts, prophylaxis against secondary CE that may result from spillage of cyst fluid requires treatment with albendazole from 1 day to 1 week before the procedure to 1 month after.[34] The use of a scolicidal agent in percutaneous procedures requires that the treating physicians verify that there is no communication between the cyst and the biliary tree to avoid the risk of inducing chemical sclerosing cholangitis when the scolicidal agent is infused. A recent study has suggested the potential safety and efficacy of US-guided percutaneous evacuation of the cyst fluid in CE1 and CE3a cysts complemented by a full course of albendazole therapy, without the use of the scolicidal agent.[35] More studies are needed to confirm the effectiveness of this modified procedure and to allow this being recommended in all cases as a replacement of classic PAIR. What is exciting about this is that the advanced imaging that was required prior to injecting scolicidal agent may not be needed, thus expanding the potential for US to be used by more practitioners in the treatment of appropriately staged CE cysts.

Inactive cysts (CE4 and CE5) do not require treatment and only need to be monitored over time (watch-and-wait approach). Reactivation (ie, passing from CE4/5 to CE3b stage) is infrequent in cysts that are first diagnosed in these stages (ie, cysts that became inactive spontaneously), and albendazole treatment does not prevent reactivation; therefore, it is imperative to avoid overtreatment of these patients, with attendant side effects and costs.[26,31,36]

The reliability of the WHO-IWGE classification in the hands of clinicians familiar with CE was preliminary evaluated by Solomon and colleagues[37] with good results. It is still seldom reported, however, in published articles addressing the diagnosis and clinical management of CE.[38] This is reflected in that the WHO-IWGE recommendations for the clinical management of CE are still not well adopted worldwide.[39–41] Also, the inclusion of CL as a type of CE diagnosis rather than as a suspect case is a common problem in both literature and clinical practice. This situation is partly due to the lack of prospective randomized clinical trials on the treatment of CE. Treatment recommendations still rely largely on data from retrospective case series and expert experience. The new WHO-IWGE steering group is currently working on a practical technical manual with front-line treating clinicians the target audience. This document will be addressed to all physician specialists potentially involved in the diagnosis and management of patients with CE and include a more detailed and stringent description of US features pathognomonic for CE and case definitions.

Summary for the Treating Clinician

Because clinical management decision making for uncomplicated liver CE is based on diagnosis first and then staging of CE cysts using imaging (stage-specific approach), it is important for treating clinicians to know the US-based classification of CE cysts (**Table 1**). In all other instances (extrahepatic locations and/or complications), consultation with a physician experienced in the clinical management of CE is strongly advised. At the bedside, US allows clinicians to identify CE cysts or cysts that are highly suspicious for CE and decide which require treatment by

Table 1
Characterization and treatment recommendations based on cystic echinococcosis stage-specific approach

Cystic Echinococcosis Stage	Ultrasound Image	Description per World Health Organization Informal Working Group on Echinococcosis	Imaging Tips	Recommended Treatment (in Asymptomatic, Uncomplicated Hepatic Cystic Echinococcosis)
CE1	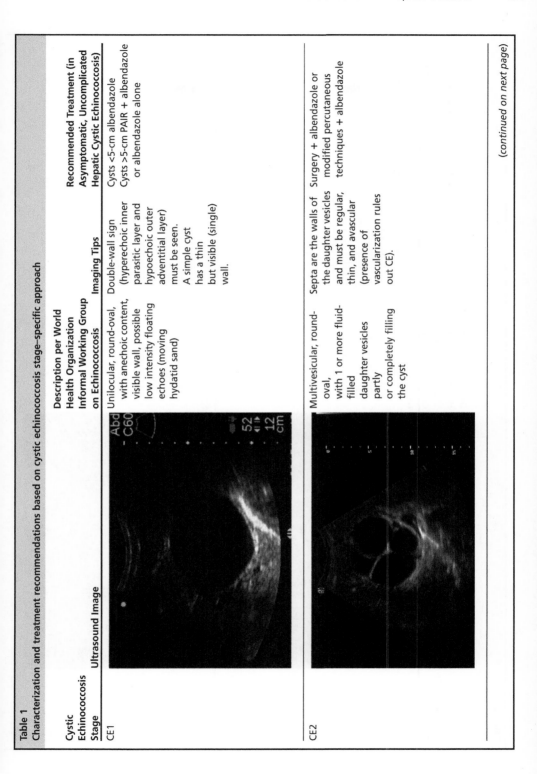	Unilocular, round-oval, with anechoic content, visible wall, possible low intensity floating echoes (moving hydatid sand)	Double-wall sign (hyperechoic inner parasitic layer and hypoechoic outer adventitial layer) must be seen. A simple cyst has a thin but visible (single) wall.	Cysts <5-cm albendazole Cysts >5-cm PAIR + albendazole or albendazole alone
CE2		Multivesicular, round-oval, with 1 or more fluid-filled daughter vesicles partly or completely filling the cyst	Septa are the walls of the daughter vesicles and must be regular, thin, and avascular (presence of vascularization rules out CE).	Surgery + albendazole or modified percutaneous techniques + albendazole

(continued on next page)

Table 1
(continued)

Cystic Echinococcosis Stage	Ultrasound Image	Description per World Health Organization Informal Working Group on Echinococcosis	Imaging Tips	Recommended Treatment (in Asymptomatic, Uncomplicated Hepatic Cystic Echinococcosis)
CE3a		Unilocular, roundoval, with anechoic content and detached inner parasitic layers (water-lily sign)	The detached inner parasitic membrane is visible as a continuous hyperechoic thin, regular, avascular layer floating in the anechoic cyst content.	Cysts <5-cm albendazole Cysts >5-cm PAIR + albendazole
CE3b		Round-oval with 1 or more round anechoic daughter vesicles in an echoic content (disrupted membranes)	Cyst with heterogeneous structure. Folded inner parasitic layer is seen in a matrix containing one or more round daughter vesicles.	Surgery + albendazole or modified percutaneous techniques + albendazole

CE4

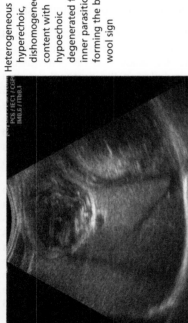

Heterogeneous hyperechoic, dishomogeneous content with hypoechoic degenerated folded inner parasitic layers forming the ball of wool sign

Cyst with heterogeneous structure. In the solid component, the hypoechoic folded inner parasitic layer is seen in a hyperechoic avascular matrix.

Watch and wait

CE5

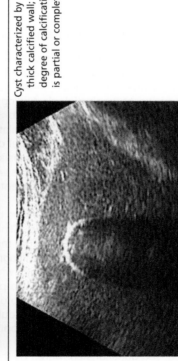

Cyst characterized by thick calcified wall; degree of calcification is partial or complete.

Eggshell calcification of the cyst walls can create dramatic shadows. In CE, the calcification is always in the wall and never originates from the central matrix component.

Watch and wait

chemotherapy alone, PAIR, surgery or a combination of the two, or further diagnostic work-up. Particularly important is the need to avoid treatment in cysts with completely solid content (CE4–CE5). These cysts require no intervention but are often removed exposing patients to unnecessary risk with no clear benefit. **Table 1** summarizes the recommended stage-specific approach based on US findings. Although the nuances of more advanced disease and noncharacteristic liver cysts can complicate the presentation of CE, a clinician trained in basic bedside US can identify the majority of potential CE cysts and make treatment and referral decisions based on these findings.

US for both CE and schistosomiasis have a proved track record for population-based studies.[42,43] US for both of these diseases was initially developed as a screening tool for community surveys, where these parasitic diseases were often asymptomatic. The WHO protocols were designed with the goal of screening in mind. The clinician can adapt the protocols for their use on the evaluation and treatment of individual patients but where US is at its best for both these diseases is when screening large populations. In more recent years, US protocols for dealing with the resurgence of HIV-associated TB have been derived not from challenges of population screening but from individual patient care challenges. As such, newer US studies that have emerged rely less on a precise identification of disease and focus more on helping the clinician risk-stratify the individual patient they are caring for.

FOCUSED ASSESSMENT WITH SONOGRAPHY FOR HIV-ASSOCIATED TUBERCULOSIS

The FASH protocol is an excellent example of a POCUS protocol derived out of clinical need in resource-limited settings, where imaging is not widely available, and in high-prevalence settings, where a condition, in this case HIV-associated TB, is frequently seen.[44,45] Most of the pathophysiologic findings included in the protocol are well described as characteristic of EPTB in the sub-Saharan setting. In areas of high TB burden, pleural effusion, especially when unilateral, and pericardial effusion have been described as highly suggestive of pleural or pericardial EPTB and as such are included in WHO guidelines for clinical diagnosis of EPTB.[46] Detection of abdominal lymphadenopathy and splenic microabscesses were characterized as typical findings for disseminated TB in South African HIV patients, although these findings had been previously described in imaging literature.[47,48]

Because all these findings are easily identified by US, a logical consequence was to look for a confluence of these findings by US. Clinicians in rural hospital in South Africa developed a POCUS protocol for EPTB.[49] The main goal in the initial description was not whether the FASH findings would be diagnostic for EPTB, because this was assumed from the published evidence, but whether clinicians can be taught the FASH technology in short courses.[50] After this publication, the diagnostic relevance of the findings summarized in the FASH protocol has been repeatedly shown in various settings.[51–55] Initially mainly used in adult patients, recent publications have confirmed its utility also in pediatric patient populations in settings with high HIV/TB prevalence.[56,57]

In brief, the focused questions answered by the FASH protocol aim to identify features that are suggestive of TB. They are

1. Is a pericardial effusion present?
2. Is a pleural effusion present?
3. Is ascites present? In the absence of other causal diseases, such as cardiac failure and cirrhosis, it can suggest TB peritonitis.

4. Are enlarged abdominal lymph nodes present?
5. Are hypoechoic focal lesions in the spleen present (eg, splenic microabscesses are frequently seen in disseminated miliary TB) (**Table 2**)?

FASH US should be considered for all patients with a high clinical probability of disseminated and EPTB. Patients with HIV infection belong to this group, in particular, patients with low CD4 counts. Recent studies of the FASH examination in India highlight that FASH in patients who are HIV negative is not nearly as diagnostic, emphasizing the point that the physician must be able to integrate their US findings with the patient's presentation.[55] The FASH examination is not meant to replace traditional TB diagnostics but to augment a clinician's medical decision making, especially in instances where patients are likely to be smear negative (HIV) and where GeneXpert (Cepheid Inc, Sunnyvale, CA) is not readily available. The patient should be screened for clinical symptoms of TB, and persistent fever, weight loss, and night sweats are suggestive systemic symptoms. In any suspected TB case and irrespective of the FASH results, a sputum examination (microscopy and if possible GeneXpert or culture) should be done. When FASH findings are recognized, the following diagnostic and therapeutic considerations ensue.

Table 2
Focused assessment with sonography for HIV-associated tuberculosis questions and probe location

FASH Question	Probe Location	Pearls	Pitfalls
Is there a pericardial effusion?	Subxiphoid—position 2 on **Fig. 6**	Follow the inferior vena cava from the liver back toward the heart if having trouble with the view.	Not pushing hard enough and angling the probe toward the back rather than up into the chest
Is a pleural effusion present?	Right upper quadrant and left upper quadrant—positions 1 and 3 in **Fig. 6**	Visualize the diaphragm located directly above the spleen/liver and look for effusion above the diaphragm.	Mistaking ascites for pleural effusion or vice versa
Is ascites present?	Right upper quadrant—positions 1 and 4 in **Fig. 6**	Use the liver as primary target—Morison pouch in the right upper quadrant is where dependent fluid collects in a supine patient.	A dilated gallbladder or full inferior vena cava can occasionally be mistaken for free fluid in the right upper quadrant.
Are abdominal lymph nodes visible?	Position 2	Visualize the aorta in both short and long axis to look for lymph nodes scattered around the aorta.	There are usually multiple enlarged lymph nodes rather than just 1 and they may be matted together.
Are splenic lesions present?	Position 3	Splenic lesions are best sign using a high-frequency linear probe because they may be subtle when viewed with a convex probe.	Mistaking large splenic masses for a TB microabscess Splenic lesions in the FASH examination are small and hypoechoic.

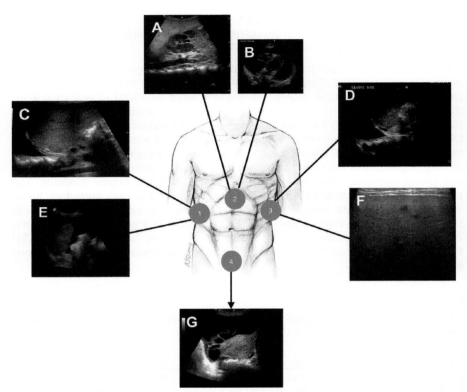

Fig. 6. Abnormal images in the FASH examination by probe location. (*A*) Periaortic lymph nodes. (*B*) TB pericardial effusion. (*C*) Right pleural effusion. (*D*) Left pleural effusion. (*E*) Ascites around the liver. (*F*) Splenic lesions. (*G*) Pelvic ascites. (1) Right Upper Quadrant; (2) Subxiphoid; (3) Left Upper Quadrant; (4) Pelvis.

Pericardial Effusion

In a setting where TB has a high prevalence (such as sub-Saharan Africa), pericardial TB is the most frequent cause of pericardial effusion.[58] Nevertheless, other differential diagnoses, such as malignancies, for example, Kaposi sarcoma (KS) or lymphoma, should be considered, especially in patients with suggestive lesions in other parts of the body. In an HIV-infected patient with a pericardial effusion, empirical anti-TB treatment is warranted, particularly in the presence of severe immunosuppression.[46]

Pleural Effusion

A pleural effusion in HIV-positive patients is suggestive of TB, especially when unilateral. Possible differential diagnoses of pleural effusions, particularly in bilateral effusions, are generalized KS, other malignancies, and congestive heart failure possibly due to HIV cardiomyopathy. US can be used to guide thoracentesis and fluid is usually exudative.

Ascites

Ascites needs to be interpreted in light of other clinical and laboratory findings. Providers should attempt to assess for other causes, such as liver cirrhosis (US of the liver and spleen shows nodular surface, decreased vascular markings, and splenomegaly due to portal hypertension), for example, due to chronic hepatitis B infection, renal failure, and cardiac failure. US can be used to guide ascites aspiration for laboratory investigation and culture. Ascites in isolation without other supporting findings, such as lymph nodes or spleen abscesses, is not strongly suggestive of EPTB.

Enlarged Lymph Nodes

In high TB prevalence settings, TB treatment without laboratory confirmation is indicated for HIV-positive patients with enlarged abdominal lymph nodes, especially when further diagnostic work-up delays or prevents treatment and may lead to morbidity or mortality.

Spleen Abscesses

Multiple hypoechoic lesions in the spleen representing small TB abscesses are characteristic, and disseminated TB should be assumed and treated. Differential diagnoses, such as other infections, for example, brucellosis, melioidosis, leishmaniasis, or disseminated malignancy (eg, lymphoma), should be included in the differential diagnosis but are much less likely.[59] In an HIV-positive patient with low CD4 counts, there should be a low threshold to start anti-TB treatment on clinical grounds (**Fig. 6**).

In recent years, the FASH protocol has become one of the most widely used POCUS protocols in South Africa and other HIV/TB settings.[60,61] One study assessed the diagnostic value of FASH in comparison to the most widely available imaging modality, the chest radiograph (CXR). It showed that in a significant proportion of patients with FASH findings, abnormalities suggestive of TB are also visible on the CXR, but approximately 25% of HIV patients with positive FASH findings have a normal CXR.[62] These cases are difficult to diagnose without the FASH US. Additionally, although CXR can be assumed the most widely available image modality, even this modality is out of reach for many clients in resource-poor settings.[63] FASH US with a portable US machine often can be considered more easily available in many settings because it requires less infrastructure, equipment, and radiation protection.

A point recognized early, which must be considered in the interpretation of FASH findings, is that treated lesions might initially persist or even increase in size as a result of immune reconstitution inflammatory syndrome. This might be pronounced when a patient starts antiretroviral therapy at the same time. A case series of HIV/TB coinfected patients who had serial US examinations showed that in a large majority of patients treated for EPTB, characteristic US findings disappeared by month 3 of treatment. Persistence beyond this time suggests treatment complications, like TB resistance, severe immune reconstitution inflammatory syndrome, and nonadherence or an alternative diagnosis.[64]

Thus, US can also help treating physicians with medical decision making beyond the initial EPTB diagnosis. Patients with continued positive US findings while on treatment require careful evaluation for adherence and possible drug resistance. These US measurements are more accessible than a CD4 count, and viral load and can help the clinician at the bedside take the best possible care of a patient. This is where clinical US in low-resource settings is at its best. It helps with the initial diagnosis of the patient but can also help refine treatment strategies in patients during their ongoing care without the need for advanced testing or expensive laboratory facilities.

CARDIAC EVALUATION IN RESOURCE-LIMITED SETTINGS

Bedside cardiac US is not considered a specific US examination type for tropical disease. It is included in this review, however, for several reasons. Many studies looking at the most common US abnormalities and most useful US examination types in resource-limited settings have identified basic cardiac US images as having high clinical utility.[61,65] The distinction should be emphasized between bedside cardiac US performed by a clinician and traditional echocardiography performed in an echocardiography laboratory by a cardiologist or echocardiography technician. As noted at the beginning of this article, the bedside US examinations are focused on asking and answering clinical questions with relatively straightforward US images. Much like the FASH examination, the basic cardiac US can help clinicians with making appropriate management decisions in high-risk patients.

The sequalae of many tropical infectious disease has specific cardiac manifestations that can be easily detected by relatively novice sonographers with some basic training.[65,66] The FASH examination, as described previously, looks for TB pericardial effusions, which is 1 component of a basic cardiac evaluation. HIV, even if well controlled, predisposes patients to acute and chronic cardiac conditions.[67,68] Schistosomiasis has been shown to cause pulmonary hypertension and the resulting dilation of the right ventricle is readily apparent by US.[69] Other conditions, such as rheumatic heart disease and resulting valvular pathology, can be identified by POCUS.[70]

The increasing recognition that noncommunicable diseases, such as coronary artery disease, hypertension, and diabetes, are becoming an increasing public health threat in low-resource settings also makes cardiac evaluation an important skill.

Traditional echocardiography is a complex skill and falls well outside the domain of the clinician providing care at the bedside. Advanced echocardiography is invaluable in many situations but unfortunately rarely available in low-resource settings that see a high burden of tropical diseases. One approach to the use of bedside cardiac US evaluation is to ask 3 basic questions that can help with the risk stratification of patients with suspected diseases.

These questions are

- Is a pericardial effusion present – yes or no?
- What is the estimated function of the left ventricle – normal or depressed?
- Is the right ventricle smaller than the left ventricle and are the left and right atria approximately the same size?

The answers to these 3 questions can be easily obtained by most clinicians using POCUS. Although the findings by cardiac US are not definitive for a specific disease state as they can be in schistosomiasis or echinococcosis, when integrated with the clinical presentation they can be extremely helpful in decisions about patient care. Using the 4 basic cardiac windows outlined in many POCUS publications, these 3 questions can be addressed without the need for extensive training required for a complete echocardiogram.[71]

Table 3 illustrates how the answer to 3 basic questions can provide a significant amount of information about both acute and chronic sequelae of tropical infectious diseases as well as some important noncommunicable diseases. Again, the goal of cardiac US in the hands of the clinician is to integrate the findings on US with the clinical characteristics of the patient. The clinical appearance of many patients with severe cardiac pathology in resource-limited settings can overlap significantly whereas their treatments may be very divergent. For example, a patient presenting with the inability to lay flat, severe dyspnea, and advanced HIV might be suffering from end-stage cardiomyopathy or a massive pericardial effusion. The clinical findings of these patients and even cardiomegaly on CXR might look similar. A rapid US can quickly distinguish a massive pericardial effusion from a severely depressed ejection fraction. The treatment of these diseases is dramatically different, and US can help with both the diagnostic decisions

Table 3	
Pathology seen by bedside cardiac ultrasound and implications for differential diagnosis	
Pathology	**Associated Disease**
Pericardial effusion	• TB • Dengue • Acute Chagas cardiomyopathy • Endomyocardial fibrosis
Depressed left ventricular function	• HIV-associated cardiomyopathy • Postpartum cardiomyopathy • Hypertensive heart disease • Chagas cardiomyopathy • Ischemic heart disease • Rheumatic aortic valvular disease
Dilated right ventricle	• Acute pulmonary embolism • Chronic pulmonary hypertension (often from schistosomiasis)
Dilated left or right atrium	• Acute or chronic rheumatic valvular (mitral commonly) • Tricuspid regurgitation from elevated pulmonary artery pressures (seen in conjunction with dilated right ventricle) • Endomyocardial fibrosis

and, in the case of a pericardial effusion, with real-time needle guidance for pericardiocentesis. The US can also, as in FASH, gauge a patient's response to treatment. If a patient is placed on an inotrope to help with depressed EF, the US can quickly assess if there has been an improvement in left ventricular function. This again is the power of US in the hands of the clinician; it is not a static imaging tool, it is something that can be brought to the bedside of the patient and used dynamically to make initial treatment decisions and measure the response to a treatment and adjust treatments in real time.

TEACHING TROPICAL ULTRASOUND

One of the pressing questions, as US techniques and technology become more clinically relevant and clinician focused, is how to make it accessible in the settings where it is most needed. This is more than just supplying the equipment; it is primarily a question about training clinicians to use US.

Two of the central components of appropriately using US at the bedside depend on clinicians being able to obtain the appropriate images and to interpret them correctly. As a result, US is frequently described as a user-dependent imaging modality. The utility of the technology is based on the assumption that the end users can recreate the images that are described in the research studies. This is not always the case, and US expertise requires years of training and thousands of US studies. If this is true, then how can clinicians be equipped to use US safely and effectively?

There are several recent studies that help to provide insight about how this might be accomplished and where it is best to target US training to make the most impact. Heller and colleagues[50] described FASH training for clinicians soon after the examination was developed. They were able to show that the FASH examination could be taught easily and most of the findings could be reproduced reliably after a short period of time. This is a model that has proved effective in other targeted US training for novice sonographers in similar settings.[18,65] The key is targeted training of limited examination types and US views.

So, 1 component of teaching US is to train clinicians in a narrow spectrum of US applications that are targeted at the most relevant findings/diseases that they are likely to encounter. Several studies have looked at the highest-yield imaging modalities in low-resource settings. Based on several of these articles using different methodologies, there is a clear pattern of examination types that emerge. In settings of high HIV prevalence, the FASH examination is extremely important for clinicians to use. Other high-yield imaging modalities include cardiac and deep vein thrombosis assessment.

Because this article is focused primarily on US for tropical infectious diseases, it does not address the obstetric uses of US. Although many tropical diseases have significant implications for the fetus if acquired while the mother is pregnant, the US findings of placental abnormalities or microcephaly are advanced enough in terms of image acquisition and image interpretation to fall well outside the range of traditional POCUS.

The utility of US for third-trimester evaluation of fetal head position, placental position, fetal heart rate, and assessing for multiparity clearly has benefits. Decades of experience and many studies have shown that this is useful information, especially when making decisions in low-resource settings about who needs to be referred to the health care setting for delivery. Although this topic is not discussed in depth, it is mentioned because it is clearly one of the most useful application of US in the hands of clinicians when caring for patients in low-resource settings.

One question that comes up frequently in the discussion of US trainings is where clinicians can go for training and whether or not there is a standardized curriculum or accreditation that exists for clinical US as a whole or specifically for US in tropical diseases? Clinical US, especially its use in resource-limited settings, is an evolving field. The answer in regard to accreditation/certification is complex and beyond the scope of this article because it is specialty-specific and country-specific (and often health system–specific). The short answer is that currently there is no universally recognized standard for clinicians to receive accreditation.

Over the past 10 years, many application-specific courses have been described that target either a specific disease or group of clinicians.[50,65,70,72–74] These are extremely helpful in demonstrating the utility of focused US training but such courses are not currently widely available to the average clinician. Courses such as these are ongoing but often based on prior relationships between an US expert and a hospital or health system and not available to those outside the health system. Several paid continuing medical educaiton courses exist through the University of Pavia (Pavia, Italy) and the Center for Ultrasound Education at Augusta University (Augusta, GA) that are open to all but are given only once a year. Thus, there exists a clear need for making training more available and accessible to clinicians throughout the world.

SUMMARY

A significant body of literature is summarized in this article that supports the utility of US in detecting pathology caused by several tropical infectious diseases. That an imaging modality can detect pathology should not be all the surprising; there are several articles and textbooks discuss a more extensive list of tropical diseases where US has been used.[19,20]

What is more valuable is how US can be the primary imaging modality for the clinician at the bedside caring for the patient with a suspected for tropical diseases. This article summarizes the most up-to-date literature in the diseases where both evidence and clinical experience have proved the value of this modality. With moving into an increasing digital age and portable age, this technology will be increasingly accessible to a wide variety of clinicians. Rather than view this as a potential threat, tropical medicine advocates leverage this imaging technology and combine it with knowledge of these diseases to help those on the front lines take the best possible care of their patients.

Diagnostic and Therapeutic Implications for the Clinician

POCUS is not something new. It was part of the WHO protocols for schistosomiasis and echinococcus developed over the past 20 years. Neither protocol was initially designed for the clinician at the bedside taking care of patients because there were not many physicians who were doing this. The protocols were targeted at researchers performing community screening. As US has become the imaging modality of choice for those seeking to care for patients in resource-limited settings, these protocols have been applied more broadly. This article attempts to distill current protocols into key points that are most useful for the physician and patient at the bedside. The FASH examination points forward to a new era of US application, designed primarily to be used in the clinical context and taught to clinicians who are on the front lines.

The Bottom Line

For schistosomiasis—being able to identify patients with high-risk features of advanced hepatic involvement and advanced renal and bladder involvement can be valuable in both treatment and prognosis. The exact grading has quite a bit of value on its own, but for the average clinician even knowing that a patient with grade D fibrosis is at much higher risk for esophageal varices then a patient with grade B fibrosis can be lifesaving.

In CE, again, the clinician should be aware of several key take-home points—the staging of cysts has important treatment implications. US can be the primary modality to make decisions on the treatment (or, in cases of CE4 and CE5 cysts, no treatment) that is most appropriate. It is also part of the treatment modality when PAIR is used. Clinicians less experienced with CE can use cyst appearance by ultrasound to decide on the optimal treatment approach.

For cardiac US—the utility of cardiac US in patients with tropical diseases is extensive. For the average clinician, simply being able to assess for pericardial effusion, contraction of the left ventricle, and relative chamber size helps significantly with risk-stratifying patients based on the most likely etiology of their disease.

There is still a long way to go to US being the stethoscope of clinicians in low-resource settings, but increasing portability and decreasing cost mean that the reality is closer than it has ever been. Understanding of how best to use it will also continue to evolve and, just as the FASH examination has shown, it will likely be clinicians in the field seeking to better care for patients with complex diseases who are making innovations in this modality.

SUPPLEMENTARY DATA

Supplementary data related to this article can be found online at https://doi.org/10.1016/j.idc.2018.10.008.

REFERENCES

1. Halbfass HJ, Wimmer B, Hauenstein K, et al. Ultrasonic diagnosis of blunt abdominal injuries. Fortschr Med 1981;99(41):1681–5 [in German].
2. Abdel-Wahab MF A-LZ, El-Kady NM, Arafa NM. The use of ultrasonography in diagnosis of different schistosomal-syndromes. Proceedings of the Third International Workshop on Diagnostic Ultrasound Imaging. Cairo, Egypt, 1978. p. 458–63.
3. Cerri GG, Alves VA, Magalhaes A. Hepatosplenic schistosomiasis mansoni: ultrasound manifestations. Radiology 1984;153(3):777–80.

4. Voieta I, de Queiroz LC, Andrade LM, et al. Imaging techniques and histology in the evaluation of liver fibrosis in hepatosplenic schistosomiasis mansoni in Brazil: a comparative study. Mem Inst Oswaldo Cruz 2010;105(4):414–21.

5. el Scheich T, Holtfreter MC, Ekamp H, et al. The WHO ultrasonography protocol for assessing hepatic morbidity due to Schistosoma mansoni. Acceptance and evolution over 12 years. Parasitol Res 2014;113(11):3915–25.

6. Akpata R, Neumayr A, Holtfreter MC, et al. The WHO ultrasonography protocol for assessing morbidity due to Schistosoma haematobium. Acceptance and evolution over 14 years. Systematic review. Parasitol Res 2015;114(4):1279–89.

7. Doehring-Schwerdtfeger E, Kardorff R. Ultrasonography in schistosomiasis in Africa. Mem Inst Oswaldo Cruz 1995;90(2):141–5.

8. Berhe N, Myrvang B, Gundersen SG. Reversibility of schistosomal periportal thickening/fibrosis after praziquantel therapy: a twenty-six month follow-up study in Ethiopia. Am J Trop Med Hyg 2008;78(2):228–34.

9. Richter J, Correia Dacal AR, Vergetti Siqueira JG, et al. Sonographic prediction of variceal bleeding in patients with liver fibrosis due to Schistosoma mansoni. Trop Med Int Health 1998;3(9):728–35.

10. Richter J HC, Campagne G, Berquist N. Ultrasound in Schistosomiasis. A practical guide to the standardized use of ultrasonography for the assessment of schistosomiasis-related morbidity. WHO-document. 2000:1-51.

11. Kardorff R, Olveda RM, Acosta LP, et al. Hepatosplenic morbidity in schistosomiasis japonica: evaluation with Doppler sonography. Am J Trop Med Hyg 1999; 60(6):954–9.

12. Hatz CF. The use of ultrasound in schistosomiasis. Adv Parasitol 2001;48:225–84.

13. Cai WM, Qiu DC, Hatz C. Studies on ultrasonographic diagnosis of schistosomiasis japonica in China–a review of selected Chinese studies. Acta Trop 1992; 51(1):37–43.

14. Cheung H, Lai YM, Loke TK, et al. The imaging diagnosis of hepatic schistosomiasis japonicum sequelae. Clin Radiol 1996;51(1):51–5.

15. Ohmae H, Sy OS, Chigusa Y, et al. Imaging diagnosis of schistosomiasis japonica–the use in Japan and application for field study in the present endemic area. Parasitol Int 2003;52(4):385–93.

16. Hamada M, Ohta M, Yasuda Y, et al. Hepatic calcification in schistosomiasis japonica. J Comput Assist Tomogr 1982;6(1):76–8.

17. Ohmae H, Sinuon M, Kirinoki M, et al. Schistosomiasis mekongi: from discovery to control. Parasitol Int 2004;53(2):135–42.

18. Barsky M, Kushner L, Ansbro M, et al. A feasibility study to determine if minimally trained medical students can identify markers of chronic parasitic infection using bedside ultrasound in rural Tanzania. World J Emerg Med 2015;6(4):293–8.

19. Brunetti E, Heller T, Richter J, et al. Application of ultrasonography in the diagnosis of infectious diseases in resource-limited settings. Curr Infect Dis Rep 2016;18(2):6.

20. Belard S, Tamarozzi F, Bustinduy AL, et al. Point-of-care ultrasound assessment of tropical infectious diseases–a review of applications and perspectives. Am J Trop Med Hyg 2016;94(1):8–21.

21. Macpherson CN, Bartholomot B, Frider B. Application of ultrasound in diagnosis, treatment, epidemiology, public health and control of Echinococcus granulosus and E. multilocularis. Parasitology 2003;127(Suppl):S21–35.

22. Brunetti E, Kern P, Vuitton DA. Expert consensus for the diagnosis and treatment of cystic and alveolar echinococcosis in humans. Acta Trop 2010;114(1):1–16.

23. Stojkovic M, Rosenberger K, Kauczor HU, et al. Diagnosing and staging of cystic echinococcosis: how do CT and MRI perform in comparison to ultrasound? PLoS Negl Trop Dis 2012;6(10):e1880.
24. Lissandrin R, Tamarozzi F, Piccoli L, et al. Factors influencing the serological response in hepatic echinococcus granulosus infection. Am J Trop Med Hyg 2016;94(1):166–71.
25. Rogan MT, Hai WY, Richardson R, et al. Hydatid cysts: does every picture tell a story? Trends Parasitol 2006;22(9):431–8.
26. Solomon N, Kachani M, Zeyhle E, et al. The natural history of cystic echinococcosis in untreated and albendazole-treated patients. Acta Trop 2017;171:52–7.
27. Hosch W, Junghanss T, Stojkovic M, et al. Metabolic viability assessment of cystic echinococcosis using high-field 1H MRS of cyst contents. NMR Biomed 2008; 21(7):734–54.
28. Stojkovic M, Zwahlen M, Teggi A, et al. Treatment response of cystic echinococcosis to benzimidazoles: a systematic review. PLoS Negl Trop Dis 2009;3(9):e524.
29. Golemanov B, Grigorov N, Mitova R, et al. Efficacy and safety of PAIR for cystic echinococcosis: experience on a large series of patients from Bulgaria. Am J Trop Med Hyg 2011;84(1):48–51.
30. Rinaldi F, De Silvestri A, Tamarozzi F, et al. Medical treatment versus "Watch and Wait" in the clinical management of CE3b echinococcal cysts of the liver. BMC Infect Dis 2014;14:492.
31. Piccoli L, Tamarozzi F, Cattaneo F, et al. Long-term sonographic and serological follow-up of inactive echinococcal cysts of the liver: hints for a "watch-and-wait" approach. PLoS Negl Trop Dis 2014;8(8):e3057.
32. Group WIW. International classification of ultrasound images in cystic echinococcosis for application in clinical and field epidemiological settings. Acta Trop 2003; 85(2):253–61.
33. Junghanss T, da Silva AM, Horton J, et al. Clinical management of cystic echinococcosis: state of the art, problems, and perspectives. Am J Trop Med Hyg 2008; 79(3):301–11.
34. Akhan O, Yildiz AE, Akinci D, et al. Is the adjuvant albendazole treatment really needed with PAIR in the management of liver hydatid cysts? A prospective, randomized trial with short-term follow-up results. Cardiovasc Intervent Radiol 2014; 37(6):1568–74.
35. Firpo G, Vola A, Lissandrin R, et al. Preliminary Evaluation of percutaneous treatment of echinococcal cysts without injection of scolicidal agent. Am J Trop Med Hyg 2017;97(6):1818–26.
36. Stojkovic M, Rosenberger KD, Steudle F, et al. Watch and wait management of inactive cystic echinococcosis - does the path to inactivity matter - analysis of a prospective patient cohort. PLoS Negl Trop Dis 2016;10(12):e0005243.
37. Solomon N, Fields PJ, Tamarozzi F, et al. Expert reliability for the World Health Organization standardized ultrasound classification of cystic echinococcosis. Am J Trop Med Hyg 2017;96(3):686–91.
38. Tamarozzi F, Nicoletti GJ, Neumayr A, et al. Acceptance of standardized ultrasound classification, use of albendazole, and long-term follow-up in clinical management of cystic echinococcosis: a systematic review. Curr Opin Infect Dis 2014;27(5):425–31.
39. Nabarro LE, Amin Z, Chiodini PL. Current management of cystic echinococcosis: a survey of specialist practice. Clin Infect Dis 2015;60(5):721–8.
40. Muhtarov M, Rainova I, Tamarozzi F. Treatment of hepatic cystic echinococcosis in patients from the Southeastern Rhodope Region of Bulgaria in 2004-2013:

comparison of current practices with expert recommendations. Am J Trop Med Hyg 2016;94(4):900–5.

41. Chebli H, Laamrani El Idrissi A, Benazzouz M, et al. Human cystic echinococcosis in Morocco: ultrasound screening in the Mid Atlas through an Italian-Moroccan partnership. PLoS Negl Trop Dis 2017;11(3):e0005384.

42. Tamarozzi F, Hou A, Morales ML, et al. Prevalence and risk factors for human cystic echinococcosis in the Cusco Region of the Peruvian Highlands diagnosed using focused abdominal ultrasound. Am J Trop Med Hyg 2017;96(6):1472–7.

43. Tamarozzi F, Akhan O, Cretu CM, et al. Prevalence of abdominal cystic echinococcosis in rural Bulgaria, Romania, and Turkey: a cross-sectional, ultrasound-based, population study from the HERACLES project. Lancet Infect Dis 2018;18(7):769–78.

44. Maru DS, Schwarz R, Jason A, et al. Turning a blind eye: the mobilization of radiology services in resource-poor regions. Global Health 2010;6:18.

45. Abdool Karim SS, Churchyard GJ, Karim QA, et al. HIV infection and tuberculosis in South Africa: an urgent need to escalate the public health response. Lancet 2009;374(9693):921–33.

46. WHO. WHO: improving the diagnosis and treatment of smear- negative pulmonary and extrapulmonary tuberculosis among adults and adolescents: recommendations for HIV-prevalent and resource-constrained settings 2006. 2006.

47. Heller T, Goblirsch S, Wallrauch C, et al. Abdominal tuberculosis: sonographic diagnosis and treatment response in HIV-positive adults in rural South Africa. Int J Infect Dis 2010;14(Suppl 3):e108–12.

48. Monill-Serra JM, Martinez-Noguera A, Montserrat E, et al. Abdominal ultrasound findings of disseminated tuberculosis in AIDS. J Clin Ultrasound 1997;25(1):1–6.

49. Heller T, Wallrauch C, Goblirsch S, et al. Focused assessment with sonography for HIV-associated tuberculosis (FASH): a short protocol and a pictorial review. Crit Ultrasound J 2012;4(1):21.

50. Heller T, Wallrauch C, Lessells RJ, et al. Short course for focused assessment with sonography for human immunodeficiency virus/tuberculosis: preliminary results in a rural setting in South Africa with high prevalence of human immunodeficiency virus and tuberculosis. Am J Trop Med Hyg 2010;82(3):512–5.

51. Giordani MT, Tamarozzi F, Kaminstein D, et al. Point-of-care lung ultrasound for diagnosis of Pneumocystis jirovecii pneumonia: notes from the field. Crit Ultrasound J 2018;10(1):8.

52. Giordani MT, Brunetti E, Binazzi R, et al. Extrapulmonary mycobacterial infections in a cohort of HIV-positive patients: ultrasound experience from Vicenza, Italy. Infection 2013;41(2):409–14.

53. Goblirsch S, Bahlas S, Ahmed M, et al. Ultrasound findings in cases of extrapulmonary TB in patients with HIV infection in Jeddah, Saudi Arabia. Asian Pac J Trop Dis 2014;4(1):14–7.

54. von Hahn T, Bange FC, Westhaus S, et al. Ultrasound presentation of abdominal tuberculosis in a German tertiary care center. Scand J Gastroenterol 2014;49(2):184–90.

55. Weber SF, Saravu K, Heller T, et al. Point-of-care ultrasound for extrapulmonary tuberculosis in india: a prospective Cohort Study in HIV-positive and HIV-negative presumptive tuberculosis patients. Am J Trop Med Hyg 2018;98(1):266–73.

56. Belard S, Heller T, Orie V, et al. Sonographic findings of abdominal tuberculosis in children with pulmonary tuberculosis. Pediatr Infect Dis J 2017;36(12):1224–6.

57. Belard S, Heuvelings CC, Banderker E, et al. Utility of point-of-care ultrasound in children with pulmonary tuberculosis. Pediatr Infect Dis J 2018;37(7):637–42.

58. Heller T, Lessells RJ, Wallrauch C, et al. Tuberculosis pericarditis with cardiac tamponade: management in the resource-limited setting. Am J Trop Med Hyg 2010;83(6):1311–4.
59. Heller T, Belard S, Wallrauch C, et al. Patterns of hepatosplenic brucella abscesses on cross-sectional imaging: a review of clinical and imaging features. Am J Trop Med Hyg 2015;93(4):761–6.
60. van Hoving DJ, Lamprecht HH, Stander M, et al. Adequacy of the emergency point-of-care ultrasound core curriculum for the local burden of disease in South Africa. Emerg Med J 2013;30(4):312–5.
61. Heller T, Mtemang'ombe EA, Huson MA, et al. Ultrasound for patients in a high HIV/tuberculosis prevalence setting: a needs assessment and review of focused applications for Sub-Saharan Africa. Int J Infect Dis 2017;56:229–36.
62. Heller T, Goblirsch S, Bahlas S, et al. Diagnostic value of FASH ultrasound and chest X-ray in HIV-co-infected patients with abdominal tuberculosis. Int J Tuberc Lung Dis 2013;17(3):342–4.
63. Pedrazzoli D, Lalli M, Boccia D, et al. Can tuberculosis patients in resource-constrained settings afford chest radiography? Eur Respir J 2017;49(3) [pii: 1601877].
64. Heller T, Wallrauch C, Brunetti E, et al. Changes of FASH ultrasound findings in TB-HIV patients during anti-tuberculosis treatment. Int J Tuberc Lung Dis 2014; 18(7):837–9.
65. Stanley A, Wajanga BM, Jaka H, et al. The impact of systematic point-of-care ultrasound on management of patients in a resource-limited setting. Am J Trop Med Hyg 2017;96(2):488–92.
66. Stolz LA, Muruganandan KM, Bisanzo MC, et al. Point-of-care ultrasound education for non-physician clinicians in a resource-limited emergency department. Trop Med Int Health 2015;20(8):1067–72.
67. Vos A, Tempelman H, Deville W, et al. HIV and risk of cardiovascular disease in sub-Saharan Africa: rationale and design of the Ndlovu Cohort Study. Eur J Prev Cardiol 2017;24(10):1043–50.
68. Barnes RP, Lacson JC, Bahrami H. HIV infection and risk of cardiovascular diseases beyond coronary artery disease. Curr Atheroscler Rep 2017;19(5):20.
69. Colley DG, Bustinduy AL, Secor WE, et al. Human schistosomiasis. Lancet 2014; 383(9936):2253–64.
70. Sippel S, Muruganandan K, Levine A, et al. Review article: use of ultrasound in the developing world. Int J Emerg Med 2011;4:72.
71. Shah S, Price D. Partners in health manual of ultrasound for resource- limited settings. In: Shah S, editorvol. 1, 1st edition. Boston: Partners in Health; 2011. Available at: https://act.pih.org/page/-/img/haiti/PIH_Manual_of_Ultrasound_for_Resource-Limited_Settings_1st_Edition.pdf. Accessed August 7, 2018.
72. Shah S, Noble VE, Umulisa I, et al. Development of an ultrasound training curriculum in a limited resource international setting: successes and challenges of ultrasound training in rural Rwanda. Int J Emerg Med 2008;1(3):193–6.
73. Kimberly HH, Murray A, Mennicke M, et al. Focused maternal ultrasound by midwives in rural Zambia. Ultrasound Med Biol 2010;36(8):1267–72.
74. Training in diagnostic ultrasound: essentials, principles and standards. Report of a WHO Study Group. World Health Organ Tech Rep Ser 1998;875:i-46, back cover.

New Tools to Test Stool

Managing Travelers' Diarrhea in the Era of Molecular Diagnostics

Eric J. Eckbo, MD[a], Cédric P. Yansouni, MD, DTM&H[b],
Jeffrey M. Pernica, MD, DTM&H[c], David M. Goldfarb, MD[d,e,*]

KEYWORDS

- Travelers' diarrhea • Enteric infections • Molecular testing • Multiplex PCR
- Diagnostics • *Shigella* • Enterotoxigenic *Escherichia coli*

KEY POINTS

- Travelers' diarrhea affects up to 60% of visitors to tropical and subtropical regions.
- A vast majority of cases are caused by bacteria, and disease is generally self-limited.
- Treatment of mild disease should be avoided; self-administration of a macrolide or fluoro-quinolone antibiotic for moderate to severe disease can reduce the duration of symptoms by approximately 1 day.
- Any exposure to antimicrobials during travel is strongly associated with new colonization by multidrug-resistant gram-negative bacteria among returning travelers.
- Multiplex testing panels provide results for a broader range of potential pathogens compared with traditional diagnostics. Clinicians are now challenged with the decision as to whether to treat or monitor, especially in cases of multiple organisms detected in a single specimen.

Disclosures: E.J. Eckbo has no commercial or financial conflicts of interest and no funding disclosures. C.P. Yansouni, J.M. Pernica, and D.M. Goldfarb have received investigator-initiated funding from bioMérieux, Inc for research on diarrheal diagnostics.
^a Department of Pathology and Laboratory Medicine, Division of Medical Microbiology, University of British Columbia, Vancouver General Hospital, 899 West 12th Avenue, Vancouver, British Columbia V5Z 1M9, Canada; ^b J.D. MacLean Centre for Tropical Diseases, McGill University Health Centre, 1001 Boulevard Decarie, Montreal, Quebec H4A 3J1, Canada; ^c Department of Pediatrics, Division of Infectious Diseases, McMaster University, Hamilton Health Sciences Centre, 1280 Main Street West, Hamilton, Ontario L8S 4K1, Canada; ^d Department of Pathology and Laboratory Medicine, Division of Medical Microbiology, University of British Columbia, Vancouver, British Columbia, Canada; ^e Department of Pediatrics, Division of Infectious Diseases, University of British Columbia, Vancouver, British Columbia, Canada
* Corresponding author. British Columbia Children's Hospital, 4500 Oak Street, Vancouver, British Columbia V6H 3N1, Canada.
E-mail address: david.goldfarb@cw.bc.ca

Infect Dis Clin N Am 33 (2019) 197–212
https://doi.org/10.1016/j.idc.2018.10.012
0891-5520/19/© 2018 Elsevier Inc. All rights reserved.

id.theclinics.com

INTRODUCTION

Enteric infections are the most common illnesses experienced by travelers, with diarrhea affecting up to 33% to 60% of visitors to tropical and subtropical regions either during their trip or on return.[1,2] Newly arrived immigrants and refugees are also frequently afflicted by acute or chronic gastrointestinal infections.[3,4] Although often self-limiting, these infections can be associated with significant morbidity and even mortality, particularly in immunosuppressed or otherwise vulnerable patients. Recently conducted cohort and case-control studies using sensitive molecular techniques have shed new light on the importance of certain pathogens in terms of causality and sequelae. These newer diagnostic techniques are increasingly available for routine clinical practice, allowing clinicians to provide pathogen-specific therapy and management. Rather than summarizing current evidence-based guidelines for the management of travelers' diarrhea (TD),[5,6] this review aims to provide insight into how advances in clinical diagnostics are changing understanding of the etioepidemiology and interpretation of test results for clinical decision making.

DEFINITIONS AND EPIDEMIOLOGY

TD can generally be defined as a change in baseline stool frequency and quality to 3 unformed stools within a 24-hour period in a traveler, accompanied by symptoms, such as abdominal cramping, nausea, vomiting, fever, and hematochezia.[7] Most episodes of diarrhea are self-limited and resolve within 1 day to 7 days of symptom onset.[8] Symptomatic episodes lasting greater than 14 days can be considered persistent and are caused by a different spectrum of pathogens and/or pathologies.

The predominating risk for TD derives from the location of travel (**Fig. 1**). High-risk destinations include South/Southeast Asia, Middle East, Africa, Mexico, and South/Central America.[8,10]

Male and female travelers are equally affected by TD. Infants, children, and young adults are at increased risk for TD, as are low-budget travelers.[10–13] The routinely provided advice of "boil it, cook it, peel it, or forget it" has not been found particularly effective in actually preventing diarrhea in practice.[14,15] Episodes of TD do not protect against future bouts of illness, and travelers can experience multiple episodes in a single trip.[10]

Most episodes of TD manifest and resolve within the first week of travel; however, approximately 20% of travelers experience continuation or new onset of symptoms

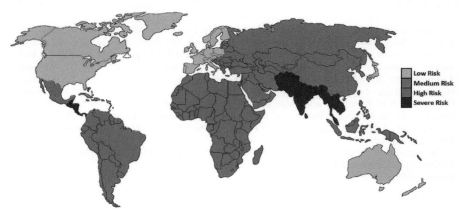

Fig. 1. Global risk map of TD. (*Data from* Refs.[1,8,9])

after returning home.[16] Recent advances in clinical diagnostics may allow for timely and analytically sensitive detection of potential enteric pathogens. The introduction of broad syndromic testing panels has, however, created challenges in the interpretation of results. Traditional microbiologic work-up of stool specimens had low sensitivity and could detect only a limited number of pathogens; in contrast, current molecular diagnostics target a much broader range of pathogens and are able to detect microorganisms present at extremely low levels, which raises the issue of what truly constitutes a pathologic enteric infection. The travel medicine clinician has become tasked with evaluating the relevance of organisms identified in large testing panels performed on returning travelers and, furthermore, is challenged with the decision of whether to treat with targeted antimicrobials.

MOLECULAR DIAGNOSTICS: NEW TOOLS FOR UNDERSTANDING OLD INFECTIONS

Traditional diagnostics for bacterial stool pathogens have typically involved culture of isolates on selective agar plates and enrichment broth media. Clinicians may not be aware of the organisms that are identified in a laboratory's standard stool culture, because these can vary between institutions. Certain organisms are more fastidious and may be difficult to culture in the laboratory, particularly if there are delays in transport, such as *Campylobacter* spp. Even for bacteria that grow readily, such as *Shigella* spp, large case-control studies have found that routine culture misses approximately half of clinically relevant cases when compared with molecular detection.[17] What is more, conventional culture-based microbiology approaches still widely used in most clinical microbiology laboratories (including reference centers) are unable to detect several travel-associated bacterial infections (eg, diarrheagenic *Escherichia coli*). Evaluation for parasitic pathogens has generally relied on stool concentration followed by visual identification of ova and parasites on a stained slide or alternatively, antigen-based testing. Prior to the implementation of molecular assays, viral diagnostics necessitated electron microscopy, cell culture, or immunoassays. These techniques have all proved complex and resource intensive, with results often taking several days to reach clinicians. Often, the yield of this extensive testing is very low.[18]

Several recent large prospective studies of diarrheal disease conducted in high burden countries and using sensitive and specific molecular diagnostic techniques have significantly advanced understanding of enteric infections. The Global Enteric Multicenter Study (GEMS), with initial results published in 2013, was a large-scale effort to evaluate the etiology and burden of diarrheal disease in the pediatric population across multiple sites in sub-Saharan Africa and South Asia. The 3-year prospective matched cohort study included 9439 children with diarrhea and 13,129 age-matched, gender-matched, location-matched, and time-matched controls. The study used conventional culture techniques for bacterial pathogens (with subsequent polymerase chain reaction [PCR] to detect diarrheagenic *E coli* from culture plates), immunoassays for most viral and parasitic targets, and PCR for norovirus.[19] The case-control study design allowed for the determination of the attributable fraction (AF) of moderate-to-severe diarrhea caused by each pathogen (adjusted for the others); comparisons of the various AFs made possible the establishment of a hierarchy of enteric pathogen importance. After the completion of this study, Liu and colleagues[20] performed a reanalysis of a large subset of 5304 paired case and control specimens from the GEMS study where broad quantitative PCR panel testing was applied. This testing and interpretation methodology resulted in a significant shift in estimated pathogen-specific burdens compared with the initial, more conventional testing methodology. For example, the total estimated burden of *Shigella* spp/enteroinvasive *E coli*

(EIEC) essentially doubled when using this approach, and the estimated relative burden of adenovirus 40/41 increased 5-fold. In the many children with moderate-to-severe diarrhea who had multiple enteropathogens detected, however, it was not possible to ascribe causality to a particular pathogen. A recent study sought to deal with this issue by prospectively following more than 400 young children in Bangladesh and performing serial enteric sample testing.[21] These children had stool samples collected and tested using a multiplex semiquantitative PCR panel each month as well as whenever they developed diarrhea; this way, the investigators were able to better ascribe causality of clinical illness by determining which pathogen(s) were found newly present or present in higher numbers at the onset of diarrhea. Using this analysis, it was found that there were certain pathogens—notably *Shigella* spp/EIEC, rotavirus, *Entamoeba histolytica*, and *Cryptosporidium* spp—that, when detected, were associated with the onset of diarrheal disease greater than 90% of the time. Although these findings may not be directly applicable to adult or even pediatric travelers to regions with the greatest burden of enteric illness, it is reasonable to assume that the enteropathogens most often associated with disease in endemic regions are probably common in travelers to those regions.

More recently, clinical microbiology laboratories in North America and Europe have also begun using multiplex panels based on nucleic acid amplification technologies. These panels have been designed to be highly sensitive, highly specific, and often simple to use with fast turnaround times. The multiplex nature of the panels allows for many potential pathogens to be tested for simultaneously. Syndromic based panels may provide alternate diagnoses in instances where clinicians did not specify them for testing; for example, a study conducted by Stockmann and colleagues[22] in 2015 demonstrated that an alternate enteric pathogen (ie, the potential cause of illness) was detected in 29% of samples submitted only for *Clostridium difficile* testing. Recent studies that have included multiplex testing of both asymptomatic travelers and travelers with diarrhea have revealed high rates of enteropathogen detection in both groups. In a Finnish study published in 2016, enteropathogens were detected in 61% of asymptomatic travelers and 83% of those with ongoing TD.[23] In a larger follow-up study of 459 travelers by the same research group, between 46% and 80% of asymptomatic travelers had at least 1 bacterial enteropathogen detected in their stool and between 17% and 44% had multiple bacterial pathogens detected depending on region of travel.[24] For patients with ongoing TD, 30% to 64% had multiple bacterial pathogens detected depending on region of travel. All travelers had stool samples tested prior to travel and only 4% had any targets detected. Clearly, a large proportion of travelers acquire bacterial enteropathogens during their trips, even if they do not develop overt diarrhea. Most travelers with diarrhea have mixed detections particularly when multianalyte molecular panels are used that include the various diarrheagenic *E coli*. **Table 1** summarizes the pathogen results of multiplex molecular testing studies conducted on patients with TD.

Bacteria account for up to 90% of infectious etiologies of TD (**Fig. 2**). The importance of bacterial pathogens as etiologic causes of TD is also supported by evidence demonstrating that prophylaxis with antibiotics, such as fluoroquinolones, is associated with a dramatic reduction in the risk of developing TD: relative risk = 0.12 (95% CI, 0.07–0.21).[6] Although there is always variability based on region of travel, the most common pathogen identified in past cohort studies is enterotoxigenic *Escherichia coli* (ETEC), followed by *Campylobacter jejuni*, *Shigella* spp, and *Salmonella*.[10,29,30] Viral pathogens causing TD include norovirus, rotavirus, and astrovirus.[10,13,30] Viral infections have generally been found at lower rates in studies of TD in returned travelers but higher rates have been found when testing is done at the

Table 1
Multiplex polymerase chain reaction detection rates in patients with travelers' diarrhea

Potential Pathogens	Polymerase Chain Reaction Detection Rate (%)
Viruses	
Adenovirus 40/41	0–1
Astrovirus	0–0.2
Norovirus Genogroup I/Genogroup II	3–34.4
Rotavirus	0–2.6
Sapovirus	3–3.9
Bacteria	
Campylobacter spp	2–31.2
C difficile	1–5
Plesiomonas shigelloides	1.5
Vibrio spp (non-cholerae)	0.8
Salmonella	1–8.4
EAEC	17–46
EPEC	26–47
ETEC	7–22
STEC (including O157:H7)	1–9
Shigella spp/EEIC	1–12.2
Yersinia enterocolitica	0–1
Vibrio cholerae	1.3
Bacteroides fragilis	7.1
Aeromonas spp	8.4
Helicobacter pylori	2.6
Parasites	
Cyclospora cayetanensis	0.5–1.3
Cryptosporidium spp	0.8–1.3
G lamblia	0.7–8
Entamoeba histolytica	0–1.6

Data from Refs.[23,25–28]

site of travel.[28] *Giardia lamblia* is the most common parasitic cause of TD.[10] *Entamoeba* presents a unique case of PCR-based methods increasing specificity of identification. Molecular-based assays are more specific for *Entamoeba histolytica*, which is indistinguishable from nonpathogenic species by microscopy (eg, *Entamoeba dispar*). Molecular methods seem to significantly increase the sensitivity of testing for enteric parasites, such as *Cryptosporidium* spp and *G lamblia*[31,32] compared with conventional microscopy, although (albeit less sensitive) immunochromatographic assays are also useful.[33]

An understanding of how causality can be demonstrated is required for the interpretation of primary data on enteric infections and extrapolation to other groups. Although the AF methodology used in seminal studies like GEMS has been key to better defining the burden of etiologic agents of diarrhea in endemic settings, it is important to make a distinction between a putative pathogen's AF and its causal relationship to diarrhea. Causality can be demonstrated by meeting specific criteria, such as those of Koch

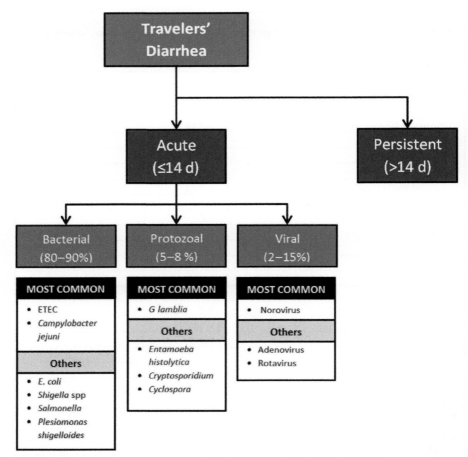

Fig. 2. Flowchart of acute diarrheal etiologies in travelers. (*Data from* Refs.[10,13,29,30])

or Hill, that depend on the chronicity and specificity of the syndrome in question.[34,35] In contrast, the AF of a given pathogen for diarrhea varies across settings. For example, *Giardia* has been demonstrated to meet criteria for causality of both acute[36] and chronic[37] gastrointestinal disease in adults from high-income settings. Yet, very large studies have repeatedly failed to show any epidemiologic association of *Giardia* with diarrhea in children from low-income countries.[19,38–40] Similarly, inconsistent AFs have been described for other pathogens, such as *Campylobacter* spp, across settings. Several factors are postulated to explain such differences, such as interactions with nutritional status, and the relative pathogenicity and ecological niches of entero-pathogens constituting the local landscape. For returning travelers with diarrhea, in whom exposure to enteropathogens is presumably less intense compared with those people living in diarrhea-endemic areas, the positive predictive value of molecular detection of an enteropathogen is likely to be relatively high, at least for pathogens for which a causal relationship to diarrhea has been well demonstrated.

As previously outlined, commercial molecular diagnostic panels for diarrhea are now used for diagnosis of TD. A travel clinic in Spain used a 15-target commercial multiplex PCR assay for evaluation of TD; in their cohort, 86 pathogens were detected in 67 of 185 stool specimens (36.2%) using the multiplex assay, whereas only 16 of 86 pathogens were detected using traditional methods. Furthermore, coinfections were found relatively common, occurring in 20 cases.[27] Another study published by Connor and colleagues[26] in 2018 assessing the utility of a commercial multiplex panel for detection of pathogens in TD found 207 pathogens in 327 specimens (63.4%) after excluding individuals believed to have postinfectious irritable bowel syndrome, a positivity rate that they note is higher than that seen in historical controls. Additionally, the use of the multiplex panel was associated with increased detection of viral pathogens and the identification of individuals with coinfections. Again, this points to the importance of test interpretation; results such as these could indicate asymptomatic carriage, resolved infection with detection of nonviable organisms, or a biphasic illness with pathogens representing differential incubation periods.[26] The benefits to patient care were demonstrated in an 2018 study conducted by Cybulski and colleagues,[41] investigating the use of a multiplex panel for the prospective evaluation of a large cohort of adults and children presenting with TD. The use of rapid molecular testing led to identification of a pathogen in 35.3% of patients compared with 6% in historical controls using conventional techniques (although in the historical cohort testing was somewhat limited). Furthermore, use of the rapid tests decreased collection-to-result time from 47 hours to 18 hours, the proportion of patients who received empiric antimicrobial treatment was significantly lower, and time-to-treatment was significantly shorter. The investigators noted that the proportion of patients receiving targeted treatment increased over the study period, likely indicative of clinicians' progressively increasing familiarity with the testing protocol.[41]

Traditionally, microbiological diagnostics have required collection of bulk stool samples for completion of testing. One of the many barriers to diagnosing diarrheal illness is the difficulty in obtaining and transporting bulk specimens.[42] Recent studies have shown that rectal flocked swabs show comparable performance to bulk stool samples in molecular testing assays that test for viral, bacterial, and protozoan targets.[42–45] Introduction of rectal swabs may provide a more convenient and acceptable method for patients to obtain samples for diagnostics. Clinicians should consult with their clinical microbiology laboratory to confirm which sample types are accepted and validated for testing.

IMPORTANT AND POTENTIALLY EMERGING PATHOGENS IN TRAVELERS' DIARRHEA
Diarrheagenic Escherichia coli

The diarrheagenic E coli strains generally include ETEC, enteropathogenic E coli (EPEC), enteroaggregative E coli (EAEC), EIEC (very similar to Shigella in terms of clinical presentation), and shiga toxin–producing E coli (STEC). Historically, ETEC has been considered the leading pathogen causing TD around the world. As outlined previously, several more recent large molecular diagnostic-based studies enrolling travelers from all major regions demonstrated a significantly higher proportion of patients with EPEC and EAEC detected.[23,26] Little is known, however, regarding their clinical significance, particularly in otherwise healthy adult travelers; there seem to be similar detection rates of EPEC and EAEC in those with diarrhea and in asymptomatic controls, although EAEC demonstrated a stronger association with diarrheal illness in 1 case-control study of TD.[28] The potential benefit of antibiotic therapy for the treatment of EPEC or EAEC has not been systematically investigated, in contrast to the management of Shigella spp and Campylobacter spp infections. Antibiotics should generally not be given to those with known STEC infections, because this may predispose to the development of hemolytic-uremic syndrome, which carries significant morbidity and mortality risk. Ideally, more data would be acquired in clinical trials before making recommendations regarding routine treatment of these pathogens when detected in travelers with diarrhea.

Clostridium difficile

Given the relatively frequent use of broad-spectrum antibiotics by travelers, it might be expected that they would be at increased risk for *C difficile* infection (CDI). The Geo-Sentinel Surveillance Network recently conducted a review of 187 cases of CDI between 1997 and 2015. Results showed CDI was diagnosed in travelers returning from all world regions; destinations in Asia accounted for 31% of cases, Central/South America or the Caribbean 30%, and Africa 24%.[46] Several recent studies of TD have included testing for *C difficile* toxin genes; there has been wide variability in the frequency of detection, which may be related to antimicrobial exposure during or after travel.[26–28]

Tropheryma whipplei

Tropheryma whipplei has historically been believed an extremely rare, primarily gastrointestinal bacterial infection that can occasionally spread to extraintestinal sites to cause disease, including the central nervous system. Recent studies of children in France and Ghana, however, revealed significantly higher rates of detection in acute diarrhea cases compared with asymptomatic controls.[47,48] Subsequent studies of travelers to Senegal and Hajj travelers/pilgrims were performed where stool samples were collected before and after travel and found what seem to be low rates of *T whipplei* acquisition. For the Senegal travelers, only 3.4% (n = 2) were negative before and positive after travel, whereas 6.8% were positive prior to travel.[49] For the Hajj travelers, among 129 pilgrims studied, none had *T whipplei* DNA detected in their stool prior to travel; only 1 had detection after travel, and that pilgrim did not report having diarrhea.[50] At present, it does not seem that *T whipplei* is a routine cause of TD, but larger studies in adults are required to further understand its potential contribution.

ACQUISITION OF ANTIMICROBIAL-RESISTANT BACTERIA DURING TRAVEL

In 1985, a consensus statement was released by the National Institutes of Health to address the question of antimicrobial prophylaxis for travelers to high-risk areas. The group concluded that the risks associated with mass administration outweigh the potential benefits in a disease that generally self-resolves and has no documented mortality. Rather than provide prophylaxis, the group recommended prompt initiation of antimicrobial therapy in travelers experiencing moderate to severe disease.[51] This recommendation remains supported by the Centers for Disease Control and Prevention *Yellow Book*.[10] Studies have shown reduction in duration of diarrhea and associated symptoms from 3 days to approximately 1 day with prompt antibiotic treatment.[52] The frequent treatment of diarrheal illness with antibiotics in many settings has likely contributed to the emergence of resistant organisms. Surveillance conducted in areas of Southeast Asia have shown widespread resistance of enteric pathogens to ampicillin, trimethoprim-sulfamethoxazole, chloramphenicol, and tetracycline.[53–55] Isolates of *Campylobacter* spp from Thailand have developed widespread resistance to fluoroquinolones, with rates approaching 96%.[55–57] Surveillance efforts in the United States have demonstrated introduction of fluoroquinolone-resistant *Shigella sonnei* from travelers into the domestic population, with subsequent outbreaks in high-risk groups.[58] Macrolides, specifically azithromycin, may represent 1 of the few remaining options for empiric treatment.[59] Studies

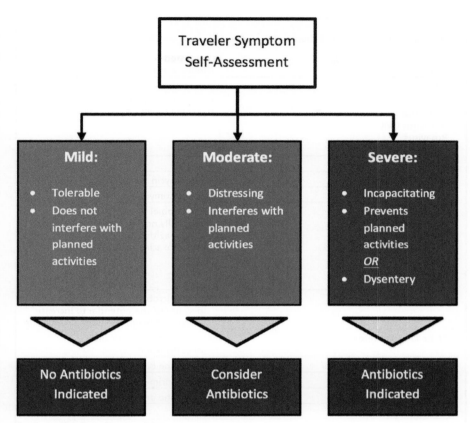

Fig. 3. Indications for empiric treatment.

in South Asia, however, have shown rapid emergence of macrolide resistance in human isolates in this region.[60] In addition to the risk of resistance in enteric pathogens, studies have shown that up to 80% of travelers who experience diarrhea and are treated with antibiotics return to their home country with colonization by extended-spectrum β-lactamase–producing *Enterobacteriaceae* that were not present prior to travel.[61–63] Consequently, there is now recognition that the modest benefit of antibiotic treatment of nonsevere TD must be balanced against the very real risk of new acquisition of antimicrobial-resistant organisms. It must be emphasized that in some regions of the world (eg, South Asia) it is not uncommon to encounter pathogens that are essentially resistant to all commonly used antibiotics. Although no study to date has yet demonstrated an increased rate of clinical infection with antimicrobial-resistant pathogens in newly colonized travelers returning from abroad, the acquisition of highly resistant organisms, and later risk of transmission in the community would be of great concern.

TREATMENT

Evidence accumulated over several decades has consistently shown the benefit of antimicrobial therapy in shortening the duration of TD and its associated morbidity. The risks and public health implications, however, have also been clearly

Table 2
Indicated agents for targeted therapy for moderate–severe diarrhea

Potential Pathogens	Suggested Treatment (Noninvasive Disease)
Viruses	
Adenovirus 40/41	No antimicrobial therapy indicated
Astrovirus	Possible benefit of probiotics
Norovirus GI/II	
Rotavirus	
Sapovirus	
Bacteria	
Campylobacter spp	Azithromycin
C difficile	Oral vancomycin
Plesiomonas shigelloides	Antimicrobial therapy
Aeromonas spp	generally not indicated
Vibrio spp (non-cholerae)	Consider azithromycin or
Salmonella—nontyphoidal	ciprofloxacin for nonresolving
EAEC	disease
EPEC	
ETEC	
STEC (including O157:H7)	No antimicrobial therapy indicated because of the potential to increase the risk of hemolytic-uremic syndrome
Shigella spp/enteroinvasive *E coli*	Azithromycin, ciprofloxacin, or ceftriaxone
Salmonella typhi/paratyphi	Ceftriaxone or ciprofloxacin
Yersinia enterocolitica	Trimethoprim-sulfamethoxazole
Vibrio cholerae	Doxycycline or azithromycin
Parasites	
Cyclospora cayetanensis	Trimethoprim-sulfamethoxazole
Cryptosporidium spp	Nitazoxanide
G lamblia	Metronidazole or tinidazole
Entamoeba histolytica	Metronidazole or tinidazole followed by a luminal agent (such as paromomycin)

demonstrated. In the spring of 2016, a group of experts convened to formulate guidelines for the prevention and treatment of TD; these guidelines were published in 2017 and are summarized in **Fig. 3**. As previously discussed, extensive antibiotic resistance has already been discovered in many enteric pathogens and geographic areas; consequently, the choice of antibiotic depends on the presenting symptoms and area of travel. Rifaximin is a nonabsorbable (ie, remains in the lumen of the gastrointestinal tract) antibiotic that has demonstrated efficacy against noninvasive diarrheagenic *E coli*. This drug should not be the empiric choice for travelers returning from areas with high rates of invasive pathogens, such as *Campylobacter* spp, *Salmonella*, and *Shigella* spp, or for patients with dysentery.[5] Empiric therapies for bloody and/or severe TD include fluoroquinolones or azithromycin for outpatient adults, and azithromycin for children. High rates of fluoroquinolone resistance in *Campylobacter* spp and other enteric pathogens in South and Southeast Asia make these agents unsuitable for patients who have traveled to these regions. Children can generally be treated empirically with azithromycin, although those under

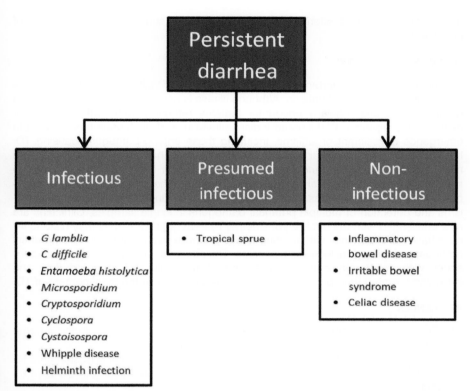

Fig. 4. Etiologies of persistent TD. (*Data from* Barrett J, Brown M. Travellers' diarrhoea. BMJ 2016;353:i1937; and Duplessis CA, Gutierrez RL, Porter CK. Review: chronic and persistent diarrhea with a focus in the returning traveler. Trop Dis Travel Med Vaccines 2017;3:9.)

3 months of age or with severe disease requiring hospitalization should be treated with an intravenous third-generation cephalosporin. Given the increased risk of carriage of antimicrobial-resistant organisms for those who take antibiotics for TD, some investigators have advocated against the routine use of standby antibiotics for TD.[64] **Table 2** provides a summary of recommended first-line antimicrobial agents for treatment of severe illness.[65,66] Treatment duration of 1 days to 3 days is generally sufficient.[66]

The emergence of syndromic testing panels, which provide clinicians with sensitive and rapid diagnostics for enteric pathogens, may provide a means by which to triage patients and reserve antimicrobial therapy for those with a treatable etiology of disease. Improved diagnostics combined with appropriate antimicrobial stewardship may help prolong the effectiveness of first-line agents and slow down the emergence of resistant organisms. In light of the emergence of drug resistance, several studies have demonstrated the efficacy of probiotics for the prevention of TD.[67,68] Additionally, some probiotics have shown efficacy in the treatment of diarrhea, but more research is needed, specifically in the context of TD.[69–71]

PERSISTENT TRAVELERS' DIARRHEA

Although a majority of travelers with diarrhea experience short-lived illness with no major sequelae, a minority present with nonresolving symptoms. Persistent TD is defined as disease that extends beyond 14 days. **Fig. 4** summarizes the etiologies of persistent TD.

SUMMARY

TD continues to inflict morbidity on a large proportion of visitors to tropical and sub-tropical international destinations. Although illness is usually self-limited and of short duration, clinicians regularly encounter patients returning home with ongoing or new-onset symptoms. Widespread indiscriminate use of antibiotics has resulted in emergence of resistant organisms, including those enteric pathogens causing TD. Implementation of molecular syndromic testing panels has provided clinicians with highly sensitive, specific, and rapid diagnostics, which can aid in the decision to initiate targeted antimicrobial or antiparasitic therapy. The secondary effect of multi-plex testing has been increased detection of previously uncommonly reported organisms and detection of multiple potential pathogens in single samples. Clinicians are now challenged with the decision of whether to treat organisms they may historically have had little experience with treating and to prioritize treatment of multiple potential pathogens detected in individual patients. Despite these challenges, early experiences with syndromic testing panels have shown quicker turnaround time and improved targeted therapy, which should prove beneficial in the management of TD.

REFERENCES

1. Greenwood Z, Black J, Weld L, et al. Gastrointestinal infection among international travelers globally. J Travel Med 2008;15(4):221–8.
2. Chen LH, Han PV, Wilson ME, et al. Self-reported illness among Boston-area international travelers: a prospective study. Travel Med Infect Dis 2016;14(6):604–13.
3. Maaßen W, Wiemer D, Frey C, et al. Microbiological screenings for infection control in unaccompanied minor refugees: the German Armed Forces Medical Service's experience. Mil Med Res 2017;4:13.
4. Wolf ER, Beste S, Barr E, et al. Health outcomes of international HIV-infected adoptees in the US. Pediatr Infect Dis J 2016;35(4):422–7.
5. Riddle MS, Connor BA, Beeching NJ, et al. Guidelines for the prevention and treatment of travelers' diarrhea: a graded expert panel report. J Travel Med 2017;24(suppl_1):S63–80.
6. Libman M, on behalf of CATMAT. Summary of the Committee to Advise on Tropical Medicine and Travel (CATMAT) Statement on Travellers' Diarrhea. Can Commun Dis Rep 2015;41(11):272–84.
7. Zwar NA, Torda A. Investigation of diarrhoea in a traveller just returned from India. BMJ 2011;342:d2978.
8. Barrett J, Brown M. Travellers' diarrhoea. BMJ 2016;353:i1937.
9. Steffen R, Hill DR, DuPont HL. Traveler's diarrhea: a clinical review. JAMA 2015;313(1):71–80.
10. Connor BA. Travelers' diarrhea. 2018 yellow book [Chapter 2] Travelers' Health. Atlanta (GA): CDC; 2018. Available at: https://wwwnc.cdc.gov/travel/yellowbook/2018/the-pre-travel-consultation/travelers-diarrhea.
11. Schindler VM, Jaeger VK, Held L, et al. Travel style is a major risk factor for diarrhoea in India: a prospective cohort study. Clin Microbiol Infect 2015;21(7):676.e1-4.
12. Steffen R. Epidemiology of traveler's diarrhea. Clin Infect Dis 2018;41(Suppl 8):S536–40.

13. Diemert DJ. Prevention and self-treatment of traveler's diarrhea. Clin Microbiol Rev 2006;19(3):583–94.
14. Shlim DR. Looking for evidence that personal hygiene precautions prevent traveler's diarrhea. Clin Infect Dis 2018;41(Suppl 8):S531–5.
15. Steffen R, Hill DR, DuPont HL, et al. Traveler's diarrhea: a clinical review. JAMA 2018;313(1):71–80.
16. Vilkman K, Pakkanen SH, Lääveri T, et al. Travelers' health problems and behavior: prospective study with post-travel follow-up. BMC Infect Dis 2016;16: 328.
17. Lindsay B, Ochieng JB, Ikumapayi UN, et al. Quantitative PCR for detection of Shigella improves ascertainment of Shigella burden in children with moderate-to-severe diarrhea in low-income countries. J Clin Microbiol 2013;51(6):1740–6.
18. Smieja M, Goldfarb DM. Molecular detection of diarrheal pathogens. Clin Microbiol Newsl 2016;38(17):137–45.
19. Kotloff KL, Nataro JP, Blackwelder WC, et al. Burden and aetiology of diarrhoeal disease in infants and young children in developing countries (the Global Enteric Multicenter Study, GEMS): a prospective, case-control study. Lancet 2013; 382(9888):209–22.
20. Liu J, Platts-Mills JA, Juma J, et al. Use of quantitative molecular diagnostic methods to identify causes of diarrhoea in children: a reanalysis of the GEMS case-control study. Lancet 2016;388(10051):1291–301.
21. Taniuchi M, Sobuz SU, Begum S, et al. Etiology of diarrhea in Bangladeshi infants in the first year of life analyzed using molecular methods. J Infect Dis 2013; 208(11):1794–802.
22. Stockmann C, Rogatcheva M, Harrel B, et al. How well does physician selection of microbiologic tests identify Clostridium difficile and other pathogens in paediatric diarrhoea? Insights using multiplex PCR-based detection. Clin Microbiol Infect 2015;21(2):179.e9-15.
23. Lääveri T, Antikainen J, Pakkanen SH, et al. Prospective study of pathogens in asymptomatic travellers and those with diarrhoea: aetiological agents revisited. Clin Microbiol Infect 2016;22(6):535–41.
24. Lääveri T, Vilkman K, Pakkanen SH, et al. A prospective study of travellers' diarrhoea: analysis of pathogen findings by destination in various (sub)tropical regions. Clin Microbiol Infect 2018;24(8):908.e9-16.
25. Antikainen J, Kantele A, Pakkanen SH, et al. A quantitative polymerase chain reaction assay for rapid detection of 9 pathogens directly from stools of travelers with diarrhea. Clin Gastroenterol Hepatol 2013;11(10):1300–7.e3.
26. Connor BA, Rogova M, Whyte O. Use of a multiplex DNA extraction PCR in the identification of pathogens in travelers' diarrhea. J Travel Med 2018;25(1). https://doi.org/10.1093/jtm/tax087.
27. Zboromyrska Y, Hurtado JC, Salvador P, et al. Aetiology of traveller's diarrhoea: evaluation of a multiplex PCR tool to detect different enteropathogens. Clin Microbiol Infect 2014;20(10):O753–9.
28. Lertsethtakarn-Ketwalha P, Silapong S, Sakpaisal P, et al. Travelers' diarrhea in Thailand: a quantitative analysis using TaqMan® Array Card. Clin Infect Dis 2018;67(1):120–7.
29. Shah N, DuPont HL, Ramsey DJ. Global etiology of travelers' diarrhea: systematic review from 1973 to the present. Am J Trop Med Hyg 2009;80(4):609–14.
30. Gascón J. Epidemiology, etiology and pathophysiology of traveler's diarrhea. Digestion 2018;73(Suppl. 1):102–8.

31. Nazeer JT, El Sayed Khalifa K, von Thien H, et al. Use of multiplex real-time PCR for detection of common diarrhea causing protozoan parasites in Egypt. Parasitol Res 2013;112(2):595–601.

32. Mero S, Kirveskari J, Antikainen J, et al. Multiplex PCR detection of Cryptosporidium sp, Giardia lamblia and Entamoeba histolytica directly from dried stool samples from Guinea-Bissauan children with diarrhoea. Infect Dis (Lond) 2017; 49(9):655–63.

33. Kabir M, Ahmed E, Hossain B, et al. Giardia/Cryptosporidium QUIK CHEK® Assay is more Specific than qPCR for Rapid Point-of-care Diagnosis of Cryptosporidiosis in Infants in Bangladesh. Clin Infect Dis 2018;67(12):1897–903.

34. Lowe AM, Yansouni CP, Behr MA. Causality and gastrointestinal infections: Koch, Hill, and Crohn's. Lancet Infect Dis 2008;8(11):720–6.

35. Rasmussen SA, Jamieson DJ, Honein MA, et al. Zika virus and birth defects — Reviewing the evidence for causality. N Engl J Med 2016;374(20):1981–7.

36. Nash TE, Herrington DA, Losonsky GA, et al. Experimental human infections with Giardia lamblia. J Infect Dis 1987;156(6):974–84.

37. Hanevik K, Wensaas K-A, Rortveit G, et al. Irritable bowel syndrome and chronic fatigue 6 years after giardia infection: a controlled prospective cohort study. Clin Infect Dis 2014;59(10):1394–400.

38. Hanevik K. Editorial commentary: giardia lamblia–pathogen or commensal? Clin Infect Dis 2016;63(6):798–9.

39. Donowitz JR, Alam M, Kabir M, et al. A prospective longitudinal cohort to investigate the effects of early life giardiasis on growth and all cause diarrhea. Clin Infect Dis 2016;63(6):792–7.

40. Platts-Mills JA, Babji S, Bodhidatta L, et al. Pathogen-specific burdens of community diarrhoea in developing countries: a multisite birth cohort study (MAL-ED). Lancet Glob Health 2015;3(9):e564–75.

41. Cybulski JRJ, Bateman AC, Bourassa L, et al. Clinical impact of a multiplex gastrointestinal PCR panel in patients with acute gastroenteritis. Clin Infect Dis 2018. https://doi.org/10.1093/cid/ciy357.

42. Goldfarb DM, Steenhoff AP, Pernica JM, et al. Evaluation of anatomically designed flocked rectal swabs for molecular detection of enteric pathogens in children admitted to hospital with severe gastroenteritis in Botswana. J Clin Microbiol 2014;52(11):3922–7.

43. Kabayiza J-C, Andersson ME, Welinder-Olsson C, et al. Comparison of rectal swabs and faeces for real-time PCR detection of enteric agents in Rwandan children with gastroenteritis. BMC Infect Dis 2013;13:447.

44. Bassis CM, Moore NM, Lolans K, et al. Comparison of stool versus rectal swab samples and storage conditions on bacterial community profiles. BMC Microbiol 2017;17(1):78.

45. Gustavsson L, Westin J, Andersson LM, et al. Rectal swabs can be used for diagnosis of viral gastroenteritis with a multiple real-time PCR assay. J Clin Virol 2011; 51(4):279–82.

46. Michal Stevens A, Esposito DH, Stoney RJ, et al. Clostridium difficile infection in returning travellers. Journal of Travel Medicine 2017;24(3):taw066.

47. Vinnemeier CD, Klupp EM, Krumkamp R, et al. Tropheryma whipplei in children with diarrhoea in rural Ghana. Clin Microbiol Infect 2016;22(1):65.e61–3.

48. Raoult D, Fenollar F, Rolain JM, et al. Tropheryma whipplei in children with gastroenteritis. Emerg Infect Dis 2010;16(5):776–82.

49. Gautret P, Lagier JC, Benkouiten S, et al. Does Tropheryma whipplei contribute to travelers' diarrhea?: a PCR analysis of paired stool samples in French travelers to Senegal. Travel Med Infect Dis 2014;12(3):264–7.
50. Gautret P, Benkouiten S, Parola P, et al. Occurrence of Tropheryma whipplei during diarrhea in Hajj pilgrims: a PCR analysis of paired rectal swabs. Travel Med Infect Dis 2014;12(5):481–4.
51. Travelers' diarrhea. NIH consensus development conference. JAMA 1985; 253(18):2700–4.
52. Ericsson CD. Travelers' diarrhea. Epidemiology, prevention, and self-treatment. Infect Dis Clin North Am 1998;12(2):285–303.
53. Nguyen TV, Le PV, Le CH, et al. Antibiotic resistance in diarrheagenic Escherichia coli and Shigella strains isolated from children in Hanoi, Vietnam. Antimicrob Agents Chemother 2005;49(2):816–9.
54. Isenbarger DW, Hoge CW, Srijan A, et al. Comparative antibiotic resistance of diarrheal pathogens from Vietnam and Thailand, 1996-1999. Emerg Infect Dis 2002;8(2):175–80.
55. Hoge CW, Gambel JM, Srijan A, et al. Trends in antibiotic resistance among diarrheal pathogens isolated in Thailand over 15 years. Clin Infect Dis 1998;26(2): 341–5.
56. Mason CJ, Sornsakrin S, Seidman JC, et al. Antibiotic resistance in Campylobacter and other diarrheal pathogens isolated from US military personnel deployed to Thailand in 2002-2004: a case-control study. Trop Dis Travel Med Vaccines 2017;3:13.
57. Sanders JW, Isenbarger DW, Walz SE, et al. An observational clinic-based study of diarrheal illness in deployed United States military personnel in Thailand: presentation and outcome of Campylobacter infection. Am J Trop Med Hyg 2002; 67(5):533–8.
58. Bowen A, Hurd J, Hoover C, et al. Importation and domestic transmission of Shigella sonnei resistant to ciprofloxacin - United States, May 2014-February 2015. MMWR Morb Mortal Wkly Rep 2015;64(12):318–20.
59. Tribble DR, Sanders JW, Pang LW, et al. Traveler's diarrhea in Thailand: randomized, double-blind trial comparing single-dose and 3-day azithromycin-based regimens with a 3-day levofloxacin regimen. Clin Infect Dis 2007;44(3):338–46.
60. Mukherjee P, Dutta S, Mukhopadhyay AK. Development and evaluation of a PCR assay for rapid detection of azithromycin resistant. Gut Pathog 2017;9:37.
61. Reuland EA, Sonder GJ, Stolte I, et al. Travel to Asia and traveller's diarrhoea with antibiotic treatment are independent risk factors for acquiring ciprofloxacin-resistant and extended spectrum β-lactamase-producing Enterobacteriaceae-a prospective cohort study. Clin Microbiol Infect 2016;22(8):731.e1-7.
62. Kantele A, Lääveri T, Mero S, et al. Antimicrobials increase travelers' risk of colonization by extended-spectrum betalactamase-producing Enterobacteriaceae. Clin Infect Dis 2015;60(6):837–46.
63. Kantele A, Mero S, Kirveskari J, et al. Fluoroquinolone antibiotic users select fluoroquinolone-resistant ESBL-producing Enterobacteriaceae (ESBL-PE) - Data of a prospective traveller study. Travel Med Infect Dis 2017;16:23–30.
64. Vilkman K, Lääveri T, Pakkanen SH, et al. Stand-by antibiotics encourage unwarranted use of antibiotics for travelers' diarrhea: a prospective study. Travel Med Infect Dis 2018. [Epub ahead of print].
65. Shane AL, Mody RK, Crump JA, et al. 2017 Infectious Diseases Society of America Clinical Practice Guidelines for the Diagnosis and Management of Infectious Diarrhea. Clin Infect Dis 2017;65(12):1963–73.

66. Gilbert DN. The Sanford guide to antimicrobial therapy 2017. 47th edition. Sperryville (VA): Antimicrobial Therapy; 2017.
67. McFarland LV. Meta-analysis of probiotics for the prevention of traveler's diarrhea. Travel Med Infect Dis 2007;5(2):97–105.
68. Sazawal S, Hiremath G, Dhingra U, et al. Efficacy of probiotics in prevention of acute diarrhoea: a meta-analysis of masked, randomised, placebo-controlled trials. Lancet Infect Dis 2006;6(6):374–82.
69. Hempel S, Newberry SJ, Maher AR, et al. Probiotics for the prevention and treatment of antibiotic-associated diarrhea: a systematic review and meta-analysis. JAMA 2012;307(18):1959–69.
70. Szajewska H, Mrukowicz JZ. Probiotics in the treatment and prevention of acute infectious diarrhea in infants and children: a systematic review of published randomized, double-blind, placebo-controlled trials. J Pediatr Gastroenterol Nutr 2001;33(Suppl 2):S17–25.
71. Guandalini S. Probiotics for prevention and treatment of diarrhea. J Clin Gastroenterol 2011;45:S149–53.

The Rickettsioses
A Practical Update

Lucas S. Blanton, MD

KEYWORDS

- Spotted fever group rickettsioses • Rocky mountain spotted fever
- *Rickettsia rickettsii* • Epidemic typhus • *Rickettsia prowazekii* • Murine typhus
- *Rickettsia typhi* • Vector-borne disease

KEY POINTS

- Organisms in the genus *Rickettsia* are small, obligately intracellular, gram-negative bacilli that are transmitted to humans via hematophagous arthropod vectors (ie, ticks, lice, mites, and fleas).
- Pathogenic *Rickettsia* are found throughout the world and continue to emerge and reemerge as important causes of febrile illness.
- Rickettsioses present clinically as an undifferentiated febrile illness, and they are often accompanied by rash and an eschar.
- Serology is the mainstay of laboratory diagnosis, but serum should be tested during both the acute and convalescent phase, because antibodies are rarely present during early illness.
- Doxycycline is the treatment of choice for all rickettsioses; it should be initiated empirically when a rickettsial illness is suspected.

INTRODUCTION

Organisms of the genus *Rickettsia* occur throughout the world and are distributed among a variety of hematophagous arthropod vectors, which include ticks, lice, mites, and fleas.[1,2] Despite the prevalence of these organisms in nature, they are often overlooked as an important cause of illness throughout the world. This is in part because of their undifferentiated clinical manifestations, which are often indistinguishable from other acute febrile infectious diseases endemic to tropical and subtropical regions. Rickettsioses are also difficult to diagnose, because there are no rapid point-of-care tests available to establish the diagnosis during acute infection, and confirmation of diagnosis, when sought, is usually retrospective by use of serologic methods. Recognition of these diseases as a cause of acute febrile illness is important because, when

Disclosure: The author has no conflicts of interest to disclose.
Department of Internal Medicine, Division of Infectious Diseases, University of Texas Medical Branch, 301 University Boulevard, Galveston, TX 77555-0435, USA
E-mail address: lsblanto@utmb.edu

Infect Dis Clin N Am 33 (2019) 213–229
https://doi.org/10.1016/j.idc.2018.10.010
0891-5520/19/© 2018 Elsevier Inc. All rights reserved.

id.theclinics.com

proper treatment is administered, symptoms can be quickly alleviated. When highly pathogenic species are involved (eg, *Rickettsia rickettsii*), delay in treatment is associated with poor outcomes and death.[3,4] Because clinicians often fail to recognize rickettsioses as a potential cause of illness, it is difficult to know their full societal impact, but it has been shown that these illnesses can affect the productivity of those afflicted and cost a great deal to the health care system when not promptly recognized.[5,6] These pathogens also continue to emerge and reemerge as causes of illness throughout the world.[2] Even in the United States, reported tick-borne infections, such as spotted fever group (SFG) rickettsioses, have increased.[7] In addition, as the world becomes increasingly mobile, there is a risk of acquiring these diseases while traveling. Indeed, SFG rickettsioses have been increasingly recognized in travelers, especially those visiting sub-Saharan Africa, and murine typhus has been recognized in European travelers visiting southeast Asia and the United States.[8–11] This article updates readers on the epidemiology, manifestations, diagnosis, treatment, and prevention of diseases caused by organisms in the genus *Rickettsia*.

MICROBIOLOGY, TAXONOMY, AND PATHOGENESIS

Rickettsia are small (0.3–0.5 by 0.8–2.0 μm), obligately intracellular, gram-negative bacilli. They reside in the host cell cytosol and have active transport systems to use the host cell's adenosine triphosphate, amino acids, and phosphorylated sugars. These organisms have small (1.1–1.5 Mb) genomes that have evolved through extensive genome reduction as they have found their intracellular niche.[12] The species of the genus *Rickettsia* are divided into 4 groups or clades: a basal ancestral group, the SFG, the typhus group, and the transitional group.[13] All but the ancestral group contain pathogens capable of causing human disease. The SFG and typhus groups are the classic rickettsial clades, whereas the transitional group consists of members with features between the SFG and typhus group. With the advent of molecular methods in the last 2 decades, there has been a boom in the number of species and species candidates, especially within the SFG. At present, the SFG comprises a large number of species of which at least 15 cause disease; the typhus group is composed of *Rickettsia prowazekii* and *Rickettsia typhi*, and the transitional group is composed of *Rickettsia akari*, *Rickettsia australis*, and *Rickettsia felis*.

Rickettsiae are transmitted through a person's skin. Transmission of SFG species occur during the feeding of an infected tick. Organisms of the typhus group are transmitted via inoculation of infected louse or flea feces (*R prowazekii* and *R typhi*, respectively) onto a bite wound or mucous membranes. *R akari* is transmitted by *Liponyssoides sanguineus* mites. Once inoculated into the skin, organisms are phagocytized by dendritic cells and transported via lymphatics to local lymph nodes where they replicate. Organisms then enter the bloodstream and disseminate to infect the endothelium of the microcirculation. As disseminated endothelial infection occurs, damage ensues and leads to increased vascular permeability, which in turn results in manifestations such as rash and, when severe, interstitial pneumonia, meningoencephalitis, acute kidney injury, multiorgan failure, and death.[14]

EPIDEMIOLOGY
Spotted Fever Group Rickettsioses

The SFG rickettsiae are tick-transmitted rickettsioses (**Table 1**). These organisms infect various tick species throughout the world and therefore have a wide geographic distribution.[1] Ticks not only serve as vectors but also serve as reservoir hosts by passing the *Rickettsia* transstadially (from one life stage to the next) and transovarially (from

Table 1
Epidemiologic features of rickettsial diseases

Disease	Organism	Group	Distribution	Vector	Severity
Rocky Mountain spotted fever	*R rickettsii*	Spotted fever	Americas	Tick	++++
Mediterranean spotted fever	*Rickettsia conorii*	Spotted fever	Europe, Africa, Asia	Tick	+++
Siberian tick typhus	*Rickettsia sibirica*	Spotted fever	Eurasia, Africa	Tick	++
Japanese spotted fever	*Rickettsia japonica*	Spotted fever	Japan, eastern Asia	Tick	++
Flinders Island spotted fever	*Rickettsia honei*	Spotted fever	Australia, Asia	Tick	++
Far Eastern spotted fever	*Rickettsia heilongjiangensis*	Spotted fever	Eastern Asia	Tick	++
African tick bite fever	*Rickettsia africae*	Spotted fever	Sub-Saharan Africa, Caribbean islands	Tick	++
Maculatum disease	*Rickettsia parkeri*	Spotted fever	Americas	Tick	++
Tick-borne lymphadenopathy	*Rickettsia slovaca*	Spotted fever	Europe, Asia	Tick	+
Tick-borne lymphadenopathy	*Rickettsia raoultii*	Spotted fever	Europe, Asia	Tick	+
Unnamed	*Rickettsia massiliae*	Spotted fever	South America, Europe	Tick	+[a]
Pacific Coast tick fever	*Candidatus R. philippii*	Spotted fever	United States	Tick	+[a]
Unnamed	*Rickettsia aeschlimannii*	Spotted fever	Europe, Africa	Tick	+[a]
Unnamed	*Rickettsia monacensis*	Spotted fever	Europe	Tick	+[a]
Unnamed	*Rickettsia helvetica*	Spotted fever	Europe	Tick	+[a,b]
Asymptomatic or mild illness with seroconversion	*Rickettsia amblyommatis*	Spotted fever	Americas	Tick	±[b]
Typhus	*R prowazekii*	Typhus	South America, Africa, Eurasia	Body louse, ectoparasites of flying squirrels	++++
Murine typhus	*R typhi*	Typhus	Worldwide	Flea	+++
Rickettsialpox	*R akari*	Transitional	North America, Eurasia	Mouse mite	++
Queensland tick typhus	*R australis*	Transitional	Eastern Australia	Tick	++
Flea-borne spotted fever	*R felis*	Transitional	Worldwide	Flea	+

[a] Clinical data based on a limited number of patients reported in the literature.
[b] Implicated as a cause of subclinical infection with subsequent seroconversion.

infected female to egg progeny). The prevalence of rickettsiae infecting ticks is variable and depends on a variety of factors that affect their ability to be passaged and/or acquired through feeding on a rickettsemic host.[15] R rickettsii, considered the most pathogenic rickettsial species, is pathogenic to its tick vector, and, as a result, as few as 1 in 1000 Dermacentor ticks are infected with the agent. Therefore, in the case of R rickettsii, an amplifying mammalian host is required to maintain infection in nature.[16] In contrast, some agents (eg, Rickettsia africae) are less pathogenic, undergo efficient transovarial transmission, and are therefore more prevalent within their tick host. The presence of one rickettsial species within a tick can inhibit the transovarial transmission of another species.[17] Thus, the presence of one SFG species within a tick can interfere with the ability of another SFG agent to establish itself within a population (a phenomenon known as interference).

The names of diseases associated with an agent often reflect their region of discovery but often fail to encompass their full geographic range (see **Table 1**). For example, Rocky Mountain spotted fever (RMSF), although originally described in Idaho and attributed to ticks in Montana, is a disease of the entire Americas.[18] In the United States, RMSF occurs in the southeast and south central states, where it is transmitted by Dermacentor variabilis, and in the western mountainous states, where it is transmitted by Dermacentor andersoni.[1] An ongoing outbreak of RMSF on tribal lands of Arizona and in Sonora, Mexico, is attributed to the spillover of R rickettsii into Rhipicephalus sanguineus, which are ubiquitous among dogs and have the ability to cause peridomestic infestations.[3,19] In Central and South America, RMSF is transmitted by a variety of Amblyomma species (ie, Amblyomma cajennense, Amblyomma sculptum, Amblyomma mixtum, Amblyomma patinoi, Amblyomma tonelliae, and Amblyomma aureolatum).[20] Rickettsia parkeri and Candidatus R. philippii are other causes of SFG rickettsioses transmitted throughout the Americas and along the Pacific coast of the United States, respectively.[21–23] In the last decade, there has been a marked increase in the reporting of SFG rickettsioses in the United States,[24] but much of this increase is likely related to seroprevalence as a result of exposure to SFG species other than R rickettsii. Supporting evidence includes the very low case fatality rate nationally (0.3%) compared with that in Arizona, where R rickettsii is the predominant pathogen (10%); the paucity of confirmed SFG cases and the predominance of cases being diagnosed with single antibody titers; and the high prevalence of other SFG rickettsiae within ticks (especially R amblyommatis, which often infects the aggressive biting and highly prevalent tick, Amblyomma americanum).[25,26]

Mediterranean spotted fever (MSF) is caused by Rickettsia conorii and is transmitted by R sanguineus in Europe, Africa, and Asia. The disease's many other names (Marseilles fever, Kenya tick typhus, Astrakhan spotted fever, Israeli tick typhus, and Indian tick typhus) attest to its broad geographic distribution.[1] Experimentally, dogs have been shown to be a competent mammalian reservoir capable of transmitting R conorii to uninfected ticks.[27] Cases occur in the summer months when ticks are most active.[28] MSF has been reported to occur in people traveling to endemic areas.[29] R sanguineus also harbors Rickettsia massiliae. Long thought to be nonpathogenic, the organism has since been reported to cause disease with manifestations that are similar to MSF. Several cases have been reported in Europe and 1 in Argentina.[30] African tick bite fever (ATBF), caused by R africae, is transmitted by Amblyomma hebraeum and Amblyomma variegatum in sub-Saharan Africa. These ticks are highly aggressive, nondiscriminant biters, and exhibit a high prevalence of infection with R africae.[31] Consequently, it is a frequent cause of illness in travelers to sub-Saharan Africa.[11,29] Tick-borne lymphadenopathy (TIBOLA) is caused by Rickettsia slovaca and Rickettsia raoultii in Europe and Asia. It is transmitted by Dermacentor marginatus.

Unlike other SFG rickettsioses that peak during warmer months, it most frequently occurs during cooler months, when these ticks are most active.[32,33]

Typhus Group Rickettsioses

Louse-borne epidemic typhus, caused by *R prowazekii*, occurs when unhygienic conditions promote infestations of the body louse (*Pediculus humanus humanus*) (see **Table 1**). Such conditions occur when war, natural disasters, or famine promote the mass migration of people, crowding, and the inability to change and launder clothing.[34,35] The body louse lives in the clothes and becomes infected when taking a blood meal from a rickettsemic patient. *R prowazekii* infects the midgut epithelium of the louse, is shed in the louse feces, and is inoculated into louse-bitten skin by scratching or when rubbed into mucous membranes. The lice are not adapted to increased body temperatures. When a person is infected and febrile, lice leave for a new host and spread infection. Body lice infected with *R prowazekii* do not serve as a reservoir, because they succumb to infection. People who recover from typhus remain latently infected and may recrudesce in the setting of unknown factors that may be associated with waning immunity (eg, malnutrition, alcoholism, and advancing age). When conditions leave louse infestations unchecked, a single case of recrudescent typhus can start an epidemic. Typhus epidemics in the last few decades have occurred in Burundi and Rwanda.[36] The last reported outbreak occurred in a youth rehabilitation center in Rwanda, where the attack rate was 10%.[37] The disease also occurs at endemic levels in the highlands of Peru. A sylvatic cycle of typhus occurs in association with flying squirrels (*Glaucomys volans*), which serve as an extrahuman reservoir of *R prowazekii* in the eastern half of North America. The squirrels become rickettsemic without ill effect and humans become infected when in close contact with these squirrels and their ectoparasites. Infection is often sporadic but has occurred in clusters when squirrels infest the crawl spaces and walls of homes and cabins.[38]

Murine typhus, caused by *R typhi*, is also known as endemic typhus, because it occurs at endemic levels throughout much of the world, especially in tropical and subtropical seaboard regions where *Rattus* spp. serve as the primary reservoir. The rat flea (*Xenopsylla cheopis*) acquires *R typhi* from rickettsemic rats. Neither rats nor fleas are detrimentally affected by infection with *R typhi*. The fleas shed the organism in their feces. Humans become infected when the *Rickettsia*-laden flea feces are scratched into a flea bite wound or into mucous membranes. Urban areas and port cities with heavy shipping traffic are often rife with rats and murine typhus.[39] For this reason, the rat-flea cycle of transmission is often referred to as the urban cycle of transmission. In countries of southeast Asia, murine typhus has been implicated as the cause of febrile illness in as few as 0.4% to as many as 7%.[40,41] Specifically in Vietnam, murine typhus has been implicated as the cause of 33% of fevers when investigators excluded other febrile illnesses (ie, malaria, dengue, typhoid fever, and leptospirosis).[42] In the United States the peak incidence of murine typhus was in 1944, when 5401 cases were reported nationally. The use of dichlorodiphenyltrichloroethane (DDT) on rat harborages during the mid-1940s resulted in a dramatic decline in reported cases. By the mid-1950s, fewer than 100 cases were being reported annually.[43] Although it is unknown what the effects of DDT were on murine typhus elsewhere, the pesticide saw wide use throughout the world in the decades following World War II and may have altered the incidence elsewhere.[44] Since the 1940s, murine typhus has remained endemic in southern California and in south Texas, where it is likely transmitted by the cat flea (*Ctenocephalides felis*), with opossums being the amplifying host.[45,46] In Texas, the disease is being increasingly recognized in municipalities outside its recent historic range and seems to be spreading in a north-ward distribution.[47,48] Because it is often indistinguishable from other undifferentiated febrile illnesses in the tropics, the burden of murine typhus is likely vastly underestimated throughout the world.

Transitional Group Rickettsioses

Pathogenic rickettsial species in the transitional group include *R akari*, *R australis*, and *R felis* (see **Table 1**). *R akari*, the causative agent of rickettsialpox, has been recognized in New York City, other urban areas of the United States, Mexico, Ukraine, Croatia, and Turkey. The organism infects mice and their mites (*Liponyssoides sanguineus*).[49] The mites maintain the organism transovarially. *R australis* is the agent responsible for the illness called Queensland tick typhus and is transmitted by *Ixodes holocyclus* ticks along the eastern coast of Australia.[50] Disease attributed to *R felis* has been termed flea-borne spotted fever. The organism was originally described within a laboratory colony of cat fleas (*C felis*). These fleas are ubiquitously distributed throughout the world, and *R felis* has since been recognized as having a worldwide distribution.[51] The prevalence of *R felis* in cat fleas is often high and does not seem commensurate with the low burden of rickettsial disease in some areas.[52] The presence of *R felis* DNA has been increasingly reported within the bloodstream of febrile persons in sub-Saharan Africa, but it is also found in afebrile control individuals. It has been described from a variety of other sources, including nonhemophagous arthropods (book lice), and, in areas where book lice are prevalent, *R felis* has been detected from skin swabs of control persons. For these reasons, and the inconsistent serologic data to suggest that exposure elicits an immune response, the pathogenic potential of *R felis* has been questioned.[43] The detection of *R felis* DNA within various mosquito species and the experimental infection of *Anopheles gambiae* with *R felis* is curious, but its significance is yet to be elucidated.[53]

CLINICAL MANIFESTATIONS
Spotted Fever Group Rickettsioses

The SFG rickettsiae vary in pathogenicity and cause disease with a spectrum of severity ranging from a high case fatality rate (*R rickettsii*)[54] to those with mild manifestations (*R slovaca*).[32] Some SFG organisms may even cause seroconversion with little or no recognized illness. For the most part, pathogenic species cause an undifferentiated febrile illness that may mimic a variety of other syndromes,[55] especially in tropical areas where mosquito-borne illness and other infectious diseases are prevalent. Because of the increasing recognition of these pathogens throughout the world, the large and growing number of recognized species, and the varying degrees of disease, having a general sense of the clinical spectrum of illness is imperative for clinicians to recognize an SFG rickettsiosis.[1] Prominent symptoms include fever, headache, and myalgia. Although not a primary gastrointestinal illness, patients may have nausea, vomiting, and abdominal pain. This pattern has been especially noted in those with severe SFG rickettsioses, such as RMSF.[56]

The presence of rash is variable. It occurs in most patients with MSF and RMSF (97% and 90%, respectively), 46% in those with ATBF, and in only 2% with TIBOLA.[31,32,56–58] When present, rash is usually macular or maculopapular. In RMSF, the rash often starts on the wrists and ankles before appearing centrally on the trunk, but it may occur diffusely or start on the trunk. Although involvement of the palms and soles is often considered characteristic in RMSF, the finding is variable (36%–82%) and often a late manifestation.[56,57] A petechial rash is frequently noted in some SFG rickettsioses but occurs less frequently in others. In the case of ATBF and infection with *R parkeri*, papulovesicular and papulopustular rashes have been described in addition to the more typical maculopapular rash. An important cutaneous manifestation is an inoculation eschar or tache noir. Eschars are frequently found in some SFG rickettsioses. In ATBF and MSF, eschars occur in 95% and 72%, respectively.[31,58] Although eschars have been reported in RMSF, the finding is exceedingly rare or a manifestation of another SFG rickettsiosis (eg, *R parkeri* infection) occurring in an overlapping geographic location.[59] Multiple eschars are often seen in patients with ATBF, because the prevalence of *R africae* within ticks is high and multiple tick bites often occur.[31] Lymphadenopathy is sometimes noted in patients with RMSF (27%). In less severe SFG rickettsioses, regional lymphadenopathy of the nodes draining an inoculation eschar is more frequent. In the case of TIBOLA, probably the mildest spotted fever with the exception of asymptomatic seroconversion, symptoms are predominantly local. Manifestations include an eschar (usually on the head or neck), regional lymphadenopathy in up to 100%, alopecia surrounding the eschar, and asthenia. The constitutional symptoms of fever, headache, and rash occur in only 26%, 16%, and 2%, respectively.[32,33] Cases attributed to strains of *R raoultii* in China present with fever rather than the local symptoms typical of TIBOLA caused by *R raoultii* in Europe.[60]

In severe SFG rickettsioses, such as RMSF, pulmonary involvement may manifest as dyspnea, cough, or respiratory failure requiring ventilatory assistance; prerenal azotemia may lead to acute tubular necrosis and the need for hemodialysis; neurologic involvement may manifest as delirium, stupor, coma, and seizures; and gangrenous digits or extremities may complicate the course.[61] Glucose-6-phosphate dehydrogenase deficiency, alcoholism, older age, and use of sulfonamide antibiotics are risk factors for severe manifestations. In the postantibiotic era, the case fatality of RMSF is 4%[25] but is reported to be as high as 30% in Sonora, Mexico,[54] and 40% in Brazil. MSF is the second most severe SFG illness, with a case fatality rate of 2.5%.[28]

Typhus Group Rickettsioses

Typhus group rickettsioses (louse-borne epidemic typhus and murine typhus) are characterized by sudden onset of fever with accompanying headache and myalgias. Both diseases have a variable incidence of rash, the incidence of which is less often noted in patients with darkly pigmented skin.[36,62] Although an escharlike inoculation lesion has been described in a patient with murine typhus, eschar is otherwise not recognized as a manifestation of typhus group rickettsioses.[63] Gastrointestinal symptoms such as nausea and vomiting are noted in about half of patients.[36,62] Louse-borne typhus is more severe and is more often associated with neurologic manifestations (eg, delirium, seizures, stupor, and coma) than murine typhus. The case fatality rate of louse-borne typhus is 13%, but it has been reported as high as 50% in the harshest of conditions.[36] In contrast, flying squirrel–associated typhus and recrudescent typhus (Brill-Zinsser disease) are less severe and have never been attributed to a lethal case. Murine typhus has a case fatality rate of 0.4% overall and 4% in those severely ill enough to be hospitalized.[64,65]

Transitional Group Rickettsioses

Rickettsialpox is initially characterized by a papulovesicular lesion, which occurs within 2 days of the mite bite and progresses to an eschar with surrounding induration and edema. Constitutional symptoms such as fever, headache, and myalgias ensue 1 to 2 weeks after the initial lesion. In the days following the onset of systemic symptoms, a diffuse cutaneous eruption occurs in the form of macules, which evolve to papules to papulovesicles to crusted lesions.[49] The clinical presentation of

Queensland tick typhus is similar to the aforementioned SFG rickettsioses with maculopapular rash in 90% and eschar in up to 65% with associated regional lymphadenopathy.[50] Although more often mild, severe and fatal cases have been documented.[66] Flea-borne spotted fever also seems to have manifestations that are on the milder side of the clinical spectrum compared with other SFG rickettsioses. Rash has been reported in 75% and eschar in 13%.[67]

DIAGNOSIS

Recognition of compatible clinical symptoms and knowledge of the epidemiology are key to including a rickettsiosis in the differential diagnosis of an undifferentiated febrile illness. Historical details regarding exposure to potential vectors (ie, ticks, fleas, lice, and mites) should be elicited, but many people fail to recognize bites from these arthropods; they are small, often feed on inconspicuous areas of the body, and, in the case of ticks, are painless because of the production of antiinflammatory substances within tick saliva. Because many people fail to recall bites from the aforementioned vectors, historical details regarding travel, recreational activities, and occupation may give clues to whether a person has been in an environment that put them at risk for exposure to a potential rickettsial vector. Antibiotics should not be withheld while awaiting confirmatory laboratory testing.[68]

As with many other infectious diseases, the cultivation of an isolate from a patient is irrefutable evidence of infection, but, for the reasons herein discussed, techniques for the isolation of *Rickettsia* are rarely undertaken. Culture of SFG and typhus group rickettsiae may be performed on blood or tissue biopsy specimens but requires the use of cell culture techniques using an antibiotic-free medium.[69,70] Rickettsiae pose a risk to laboratory staff, because they can be aerosolized during manipulation and cause illness. Therefore, isolation techniques should be performed in a biosafety level 3 laboratory. Compared with more typical bacteria, it may take some time for detection of these organisms in culture. Furthermore, the administration of antibiotics before attempts at isolation decreases the yield of successful rickettsial growth.

The immunohistochemical detection of rickettsiae within skin biopsy specimens, taken from eschars or rash lesions, is a technique with the ability to confirm infection during the acute phase. The test is performed on formalin-fixed paraffin-embedded biopsy tissue. In addition to skin biopsies, it has been used to confirm rickettsial infection from tissues collected at autopsy.[2] The technique is not available in most clinical laboratories.

Serology is the mainstay of diagnosis, and the indirect immunofluorescence assay (IFA) is the serologic method of choice.[68] IFA uses fluorescein-labeled conjugate to detect serum antibodies bound to rickettsial antigens fixed on a slide. The method is superior to older serologic techniques (ie, complement fixation and latex agglutination) and far surpasses the Weil-Felix test, which is still used in some parts of the world despite its poor sensitivity and specificity. In the United States, IFA slides prepared with *R rickettsii* and *R typhi* antigen are available for the diagnosis of SFG and typhus group rickettsioses, respectively. Patients seldom have detectable antibodies during the first week of illness. The immunoglobulin (Ig) M isotype does not appear appreciably earlier than IgG and is less specific.[68,71] Therefore, IFA for the detection of IgG requires sera drawn during both the acute and convalescent stages of illness. Although a single reactive titer during illness may be suggestive of the diagnosis, confirmation requires seroconversion or a 4-fold increase in titer from acute-phase and convalescent-phase sera. Group-specific antigens are cross reactive. Therefore, serology is unable to offer a species-specific diagnosis without the use of cumbersome cross-absorption techniques, which are not available commercially.[72] However, this cross reactivity enables the serologic diagnosis of a rickettsiosis despite the numerous species and strains in nature.[73] When participating in the care of a traveler with a potential rickettsiosis, this cross reactivity is important, because some geographic areas have several endemic rickettsial species. Enzyme-linked immunosorbent assays are also commercially available for the diagnosis of SFG and typhus group rickettsioses but give more qualitative results (reactive vs nonreactive) rather than the titer reported with IFA.[68]

Amplification of rickettsial DNA by polymerase chain reaction (PCR) has been applied to the detection of several rickettsial species from peripheral blood, plasma, tissues (fresh frozen or paraffin embedded), and from swabs collected from the ulcerated base of eschars. A variety of genes have been targeted (citrate synthase, outer membrane protein A, outer membrane protein B, and the 17-kDa lipoprotein gene), but no gene target seems more effective than another.[74,75] Conventional, nested, and quantitative real-time PCR assays have been used. When rickettsial DNA is amplified using conventional or nested PCR techniques, sequencing can offer a species-specific diagnosis. When amplification is performed using certain primer sets, restriction fragment length polymorphism analysis can help identify the causal agent.[76] Real-time PCR has improved analytical sensitivity compared with conventional and nested PCR assays; it can detect fewer than 10 copies of genomic DNA per reaction.[74] Furthermore, with the use of species-specific probes, real-time PCR assays can diagnose to the species level without sequencing.[77] Despite the ability of PCR techniques to detect small quantities of DNA, the limited number of circulating rickettsiae hinders the clinical sensitivity of PCR when used on whole blood or serum. A recent review analyzed data available in the literature and reported a median sensitivity of 18%.[74] In people with RMSF, PCR is more often positive and with higher copy numbers in those with fatal outcomes.[78] PCR is much more useful when applied to rash or eschar biopsy specimens, for which it has a sensitivity of 48% to 92%. Swabbing the ulcerated base of an eschar with a saline-dipped sterile cotton swab is an effective method to detect the nucleic acids of *Rickettsia*.[79] Because PCR requires the expense of a thermocycler, reagents, and technical expertise, more inexpensive and easy-to-use nucleic amplification tests are desirable. The loop-mediated isothermal amplification assay is such a method and offers the ability to detect fewer than 100 copies of DNA per reaction.[80,81] Recombinase polymerase amplification assays are also inexpensive, with field applicability for use in resource-limited regions.[82] However, these methods are likely to have the aforementioned clinical limitations of PCR when used on peripheral blood specimens.

There is no available sensitive rapid point-of-care test for the diagnosis of rickettsioses. Considering the morbidity, mortality, loss of patient productivity, and associated health care costs related to delayed recognition of rickettsial diseases, such field-applicable diagnostic assays are much needed.[3,5,6]

TREATMENT

The most important aspect to timely and effective treatment of a rickettsial illness is clinical recognition. When a rickettsial illness is suspected or considered within reason, prompt empiric treatment with an effective antibiotic should administered.[4] It should be realized that many frequently prescribed antibiotics (eg, penicillins, cephalosporins, and sulfonamides) have no effect on rickettsiae. In the case of sulfonamides, such as trimethoprim-sulfamethoxazole, use has been associated with poor outcomes.[83]

The drug class of choice for all SFG and typhus group rickettsioses are the tetracyclines. Although there are few prospective trials evaluating antibiotic regimens for rickettsioses, and none specifically for RMSF, decades of clinical experience support the efficacy of tetracyclines.[68,83] In vitro, the minimum inhibitory concentration (MIC) of these agents to *Rickettsia* spp are 0.06 to 0.25 μg/mL.[84] With its improved tolerability and twice-daily dosing, doxycycline is the preferred agent of this class (**Table 2**).[68] Minocycline is also effective. Unlike their prototype congeners (eg, tetracycline hydrochloride), both doxycycline and minocycline are bioavailable in the presence of food, which ameliorates the gastrointestinal discomfort associated with the agents of this class. When critical illness or nausea and vomiting preclude oral administration, doxycycline should be given parenterally. Tetracycline has been associated with fatal hepatotoxicity and pancreatitis in pregnant women. It also deposits within the fetal skeleton and inhibits bone growth. These events seem not to occur in association with doxycycline.[85] Therefore, in the case of RMSF and other rickettsioses presenting with severe manifestations during pregnancy, the benefits of doxycycline outweigh the risks. Short and infrequent courses of tetracyclines, especially doxycycline, do not appreciably stain the developing permanent teeth of children.[86] Doxycycline is recommended for the treatment of children of all ages suspected of having RMSF or other severe rickettsioses.[68] Although true hypersensitivity to doxycycline seems to be infrequent, desensitization protocols are available for use in closely supervised settings such as the intensive care unit.[87,88]

Chloramphenicol has long been considered an effective alternative for the treatment of rickettsioses, including RMSF. The MICs of this agent for various species of *Rickettsia* range from 0.25 to 2.0 μg/mL. Although available in much of the world, chloramphenicol is not available in the oral form in the United States, and the parenteral formulation has become exceedingly difficult for hospitals to procure. In a retrospective study of RMSF, use of chloramphenicol was associated with a higher case fatality than in patients who took tetracyclines (7.6% vs 1.5%; odds ratio, 5.5; 95% confidence interval, 3.9–7.7).[89] In a retrospective study of various drug regimens for the treatment of murine typhus, patients who took chloramphenicol took longer to defervesce than those who took doxycycline (4.0 vs 2.9 days).[90] Where available, the severe adverse events associated with chloramphenicol should be considered before choosing the agent instead of doxycycline.

Fluoroquinolones have in vitro activity against SFG and typhus group *Rickettsia*. The MICs of ciprofloxacin and levofloxacin on various rickettsiae range from 0.25 to 1.0 μg/mL. Agents in this class have been studied prospectively in patients with milder presentations of MSF.[65] They seem to be effective in those with murine typhus, but, as with chloramphenicol, their use is associated with a longer time to defervesce compared with doxycycline (4.2 vs 2.9 days).[90] These agents can be considered an alternative for less severe SFG rickettsioses and murine typhus in the rare instances when doxycycline is contraindicated. The newer macrolides (ie, azithromycin and clarithromycin) have activity against organisms of both the spotted fever and typhus groups. Studies in children have shown that a 3-day course of azithromycin is as effective as a 5-day course of doxycycline in MSF. Clarithromycin has also been shown to be effective in MSF.[91] Otherwise, experience with these two agents is limited. Their use may be considered for mild rickettsioses during childhood or pregnancy. The successful use of rifampin has been reported in a patient with culture-confirmed ATBF.[92]

PREVENTION

There are no available vaccines for the prevention of SFG and typhus group rickettsioses. Avoidance of vectors with the use of repellents and protective clothing such as

Table 2
Treatment of rickettsial diseases

	Medication	Adult Dose	Pediatric Dose	Duration
First choice for RMSF and all other rickettsioses	Doxycycline oral or intravenous	100 mg twice daily	2.2 mg/kg (maximum 100 mg) twice daily	≥3 d after defervescence (minimum course 5–7 d)
Alternative for RMSF and all other rickettsioses[a]	Chloramphenicol oral or intravenous	500 mg every 6 h	12.5 mg/kg every 6 h	≥3 d after defervescence (minimum course 5–7 d)
Alternative for MSF and other less severe SFG rickettsioses	Oral fluoroquinolones — Ciprofloxacin	500 mg twice daily	Not recommended	5–7 d
	Levofloxacin	500 mg daily	Not recommended	5–7 d
	Oral macrolides — Clarithromycin	500 mg twice daily	7.5 mg/kg twice daily	7 d
	Azithromycin	500 mg daily	10 mg/kg daily	3 d
		500 mg × 1 then 250 mg daily	10 mg/kg × 1 then 5 mg/kg daily	5 d
Alternative for epidemic louse-borne typhus[b]	Short course oral doxycycline	200 mg once	—	—
Alternative for murine typhus	Oral fluoroquinolones — Ciprofloxacin	500 mg twice daily	Not recommended	5–7 d
	Levofloxacin	500 mg daily	Not recommended	5–7 d

[a] Chloramphenicol is inferior to doxycycline for RMSF. Its oral form is not available in the United States, and the parenteral form is difficult to procure.
[b] Only recommended if needed for mass treatment during an outbreak (relapses have been documented).

long socks to cover exposed skin is recommended. The use of permethrin-treated clothing is effective for the prevention of tick bites and lasts for at least 1 year on treated garments.[93] The use of DDT on rat harborages during the mid-1940s made a significant impact on the incidence of murine typhus in the United States and shows the effectiveness of vector control techniques in curtailing disease. On a smaller scale, vector control may play a role in the control of local outbreaks. During epidemics of louse-borne typhus, when conditions promote the proliferation of the body louse, washing blankets and clothing in hot water kills lice and their eggs. This washing is often not feasible during circumstances around a typhus epidemic. In such situations, the World Health Organization recommends mass treatment by compressed air dusting of permethrin on clothing.[94] In Arizona, Brazil, and Sonora, Mexico, where there is a high incidence of RMSF, the treatment of animals and the environment with acaricides has been shown to reduce the numbers of ticks and shows promise in reducing the burden of local disease.[19,95,96]

SUMMARY

Rickettsial diseases occur throughout the world and are associated with a variety of hematophagous arthropod vectors. They continue to emerge and remerge as important causes of febrile illness. Their clinical manifestations are largely undifferentiated and may range from a mild illness to one that is severe. Recognition of compatible signs and symptoms in the setting of the right epidemiology is key to the timely administration of empiric treatment and initiation of appropriate medical work-up.

ACKNOWLEDGMENTS

Lucas Blanton is supported by the Institute for Translational Sciences at the University of Texas Medical Branch, supported in part by a CTSA Mentored Career Development (KL2) Award (KL2TR001441) from the National Center for Advancing Translational Sciences, National Institutes of Health. The author thanks Dr. David H. Walker for his advice and thoughtful review.

REFERENCES

1. Parola P, Paddock CD, Socolovschi C, et al. Update on tick-borne rickettsioses around the world: a geographic approach. Clin Microbiol Rev 2013;26(4): 657–702.
2. Fang R, Blanton LS, Walker DH. Rickettsiae as emerging infectious agents. Clin Lab Med 2017;37(2):383–400.
3. Drexler NA, Yaglom H, Casal M, et al. Fatal Rocky Mountain spotted fever along the United States-Mexico Border, 2013-2016. Emerg Infect Dis 2017;23(10): 1621–6.
4. Regan JJ, Traeger MS, Humpherys D, et al. Risk factors for fatal outcome from Rocky Mountain spotted fever in a highly endemic area–Arizona, 2002-2011. Clin Infect Dis 2015;60(11):1659–66.
5. Drexler NA, Traeger MS, McQuiston JH, et al. Medical and indirect costs associated with a Rocky Mountain spotted fever epidemic in Arizona, 2002-2011. Am J Trop Med Hyg 2015;93(3):549–51.
6. Vohra RF, Walker DH, Blanton LS. Analysis of health-care charges in murine typhus: need for improved clinical recognition and diagnostics for acute disease. Am J Trop Med Hyg 2018;98(6):1594–8.

7. Rosenberg R, Lindsey NP, Fischer M, et al. Vital signs: Trends in reported vector-borne disease cases - United States and territories, 2004-2016. MMWR Morb Mortal Wkly Rep 2018;67(17):496–501.
8. Jensenius M, Han PV, Schlagenhauf P, et al. Acute and potentially life-threatening tropical diseases in western travelers–a GeoSentinel multicenter study, 1996-2011. Am J Trop Med Hyg 2013;88(2):397–404.
9. Raby E, Dyer JR. Endemic (murine) typhus in returned travelers from Asia, a case series: clues to early diagnosis and comparison with dengue. Am J Trop Med Hyg 2013;88(4):701–3.
10. Ocias LF, Jensen BB, Villumsen S, et al. Rickettsioses in Denmark: a retrospective survey of clinical features and travel history. Ticks Tick Borne Dis 2018;9(3): 573–9.
11. Jensenius M, Davis X, von Sonnenburg F, et al. Multicenter GeoSentinel analysis of rickettsial diseases in international travelers, 1996-2008. Emerg Infect Dis 2009;15(11):1791–8.
12. Yu X-J, Walker DH. Family I. Rickettsiaceae. In: Brenner DJ, Kreig NR, Stanley JT, editors. Bergey's manual of systematic bacteriology, vol. 2, 2nd edition. New York: Springer; 2005. p. 96–116.
13. Gillespie JJ, Williams K, Shukla M, et al. *Rickettsia* phylogenomics: unwinding the intricacies of obligate intracellular life. PLoS One 2008;3(4):e2018.
14. Mansueto P, Vitale G, Cascio A, et al. New insight into immunity and immunopathology of rickettsial diseases. Clin Dev Immunol 2012;2012:967852.
15. Harris EK, Verhoeve VI, Banajee KH, et al. Comparative vertical transmission of *Rickettsia* by *Dermacentor variabilis* and *Amblyomma maculatum*. Ticks Tick Borne Dis 2017;8(4):598–604.
16. Walker DH, Paddock CD, Dumler JS. Emerging and re-emerging tick-transmitted rickettsial and ehrlichial infections. Med Clin North Am 2008;92(6):1345–61, x.
17. Sakai RK, Costa FB, Ueno TE, et al. Experimental infection with *Rickettsia rickettsii* in an *Amblyomma dubitatum* tick colony, naturally infected by *Rickettsia bellii*. Ticks Tick Borne Dis 2014;5(6):917–23.
18. Labruna MB, Santos FC, Ogrzewalska M, et al. Genetic identification of rickettsial isolates from fatal cases of Brazilian spotted fever and comparison with *Rickettsia rickettsii* isolates from the American continents. J Clin Microbiol 2014;52(10): 3788–91.
19. Straily A, Drexler N, Cruz-Loustaunau D, et al. Notes from the field: community-based prevention of Rocky Mountain spotted fever – Sonora, Mexico, 2016. MMWR Morb Mortal Wkly Rep 2016;65(46):1302–3.
20. Tarragona EL, Soares JF, Costa FB, et al. Vectorial competence of *Amblyomma tonelliae* to transmit *Rickettsia rickettsii*. Med Vet Entomol 2016;30(4):410–5.
21. Padgett KA, Bonilla D, Eremeeva ME, et al. The Eco-epidemiology of Pacific Coast tick fever in California. PLoS Negl Trop Dis 2016;10(10):e0005020.
22. Herrick KL, Pena SA, Yaglom HD, et al. *Rickettsia parkeri* rickettsiosis, Arizona, USA. Emerg Infect Dis 2016;22(5):780–5.
23. Faccini-Martinez AA, Felix ML, Armua-Fernandez MT, et al. An autochthonous confirmed case of *Rickettsia parkeri* rickettsiosis in Uruguay. Ticks Tick Borne Dis 2018;9(3):718–9.
24. Drexler NA, Dahlgren FS, Heitman KN, et al. National surveillance of spotted fever group rickettsioses in the United States, 2008-2012. Am J Trop Med Hyg 2016; 94(1):26–34.
25. Walker DH. Changing dynamics of human-rickettsial interactions. Am J Trop Med Hyg 2016;94(1):3–4.

26. Dahlgren FS, Paddock CD, Springer YP, et al. Expanding Range of *Amblyomma americanum* and simultaneous changes in the epidemiology of spotted fever group rickettsiosis in the United States. Am J Trop Med Hyg 2016;94(1):35–42.

27. Levin ML, Killmaster LF, Zemtsova GE. Domestic dogs (*Canis familiaris*) as reservoir hosts for *Rickettsia conorii*. Vector Borne Zoonotic Dis 2012;12(1):28–33.

28. Herrador Z, Fernandez-Martinez A, Gomez-Barroso D, et al. Mediterranean spotted fever in Spain, 1997-2014: epidemiological situation based on hospitalization records. PLoS One 2017;12(3):e0174745.

29. Delord M, Socolovschi C, Parola P. Rickettsioses and Q fever in travelers (2004-2013). Travel Med Infect Dis 2014;12(5):443–58.

30. Zaharia M, Popescu CP, Florescu SA, et al. *Rickettsia massiliae* infection and SENLAT syndrome in Romania. Ticks Tick Borne Dis 2016;7(5):759–62.

31. Jensenius M, Fournier PE, Kelly P, et al. African tick bite fever. Lancet Infect Dis 2003;3(9):557–64.

32. Silva-Pinto A, de Lurdes Santos M, Sarmento A. Tick-borne lymphadenopathy, an emerging disease. Ticks Tick Borne Dis 2014;5(6):656–9.

33. Dubourg G, Socolovschi C, Del Giudice P, et al. Scalp eschar and neck lymphadenopathy after tick bite: an emerging syndrome with multiple causes. Eur J Clin Microbiol Infect Dis 2014;33(8):1449–56.

34. Burns JN, Acuna-Soto R, Stahle DW. Drought and epidemic typhus, central Mexico, 1655-1918. Emerg Infect Dis 2014;20(3):442–7.

35. Angelakis E, Bechah Y, Raoult D. The history of epidemic typhus. Microbiol Spectr 2016;4(4). https://doi.org/10.1128/microbiolspec.PoH-0010-2015.

36. Bechah Y, Capo C, Mege JL, et al. Epidemic typhus. Lancet Infect Dis 2008;8(7): 417–26.

37. Umulisa I, Omolo J, Muldoon KA, et al. A mixed outbreak of epidemic typhus fever and trench fever in a youth rehabilitation center: risk factors for illness from a case-control study, Rwanda, 2012. Am J Trop Med Hyg 2016;95(2):452–6.

38. Prusinski MA, White JL, Wong SJ, et al. Sylvatic typhus associated with flying squirrels (*Glaucomys volans*) in New York State, United States. Vector Borne Zoonotic Dis 2014;14(4):240–4.

39. Kuo CC, Wardrop N, Chang CT, et al. Significance of major international seaports in the distribution of murine typhus in Taiwan. PLoS Negl Trop Dis 2017;11(3): e0005430.

40. Bhengsri S, Baggett HC, Edouard S, et al. Sennetsu neorickettsiosis, spotted fever group, and typhus group rickettsioses in three provinces in Thailand. Am J Trop Med Hyg 2016;95(1):43–9.

41. Mayxay M, Sengvilaipaseuth O, Chanthongthip A, et al. Causes of fever in rural southern Laos. Am J Trop Med Hyg 2015;93(3):517–20.

42. Hamaguchi S, Cuong NC, Tra DT, et al. Clinical and epidemiological characteristics of scrub typhus and murine typhus among hospitalized patients with acute undifferentiated fever in northern Vietnam. Am J Trop Med Hyg 2015;92(5):972–8.

43. Blanton LS, Walker DH. Flea-borne rickettsioses and rickettsiae. Am J Trop Med Hyg 2017;96(1):53–6.

44. Russell EP. The strange career of DDT: experts, federal capacity, and environmentalism in World War II. Technol Cult 1999;40(4):770–96.

45. Blanton LS, Idowu BM, Tatsch TN, et al. Opossums and cat fleas: new insights in the ecology of murine typhus in Galveston, Texas. Am J Trop Med Hyg 2016; 95(2):457–61.

46. Maina AN, Fogarty C, Krueger L, et al. Rickettsial infections among *Ctenocephalides felis* and host animals during a flea-borne rickettsioses outbreak in Orange County, California. PLoS One 2016;11(8):e0160604.
47. Erickson T, da Silva J, Nolan MS, et al. Newly recognized pediatric cases of typhus group rickettsiosis, Houston, Texas, USA. Emerg Infect Dis 2017;23(12): 2068–71.
48. Murray KO, Evert N, Mayes B, et al. Typhus group rickettsiosis, Texas, USA, 2003-2013. Emerg Infect Dis 2017;23(4):645–8.
49. Kass EM, Szaniawski WK, Levy H, et al. Rickettsialpox in a New York City hospital, 1980 to 1989. N Engl J Med 1994;331(24):1612–7.
50. Stewart A, Armstrong M, Graves S, et al. *Rickettsia australis* and Queensland tick typhus: a rickettsial spotted fever group infection in Australia. Am J Trop Med Hyg 2017;97(1):24–9.
51. Brown LD, Macaluso KR. *Rickettsia felis*, an emerging flea-borne rickettsiosis. Curr Trop Med Rep 2016;3:27–39.
52. Billeter SA, Metzger ME. Limited evidence for *Rickettsia felis* as a cause of zoonotic flea-borne rickettsiosis in southern California. J Med Entomol 2017;54(1): 4–7.
53. Parola P, Musso D, Raoult D. *Rickettsia felis*: the next mosquito-borne outbreak? Lancet Infect Dis 2016;16(10):1112–3.
54. Alvarez-Hernandez G, Roldan JFG, Milan NSH, et al. Rocky Mountain spotted fever in Mexico: past, present, and future. Lancet Infect Dis 2017;17(6):e189–96.
55. Traeger MS, Regan JJ, Humpherys D, et al. Rocky Mountain spotted fever characterization and comparison to similar illnesses in a highly endemic area-Arizona, 2002-2011. Clin Infect Dis 2015;60(11):1650–8.
56. Helmick CG, Bernard KW, D'Angelo LJ. Rocky Mountain spotted fever: clinical, laboratory, and epidemiological features of 262 cases. J Infect Dis 1984; 150(4):480–8.
57. Kaplowitz LG, Fischer JJ, Sparling PF. Rocky Mountain spotted fever: a clinical dilemma. In: Remington JB, Swartz HN, editors. Current clinical topics in infectious diseases, vol. 2. New York: McGraw-Hill; 1981. p. 89–108.
58. Raoult D, Weiller PJ, Chagnon A, et al. Mediterranean spotted fever: clinical, laboratory and epidemiological features of 199 cases. Am J Trop Med Hyg 1986; 35(4):845–50.
59. Paddock CD, Finley RW, Wright CS, et al. *Rickettsia parkeri* rickettsiosis and its clinical distinction from Rocky Mountain spotted fever. Clin Infect Dis 2008; 47(9):1188–96.
60. Li H, Zhang PH, Huang Y, et al. Isolation and identification of *Rickettsia raoultii* in human cases: a surveillance study in 3 medical centers in China. Clin Infect Dis 2018;66(7):1109–15.
61. Archibald LK, Sexton DJ. Long-term sequelae of Rocky Mountain spotted fever. Clin Infect Dis 1995;20(5):1122–5.
62. Tsioutis C, Zafeiri M, Avramopoulos A, et al. Clinical and laboratory characteristics, epidemiology, and outcomes of murine typhus: a systematic review. Acta Trop 2017;166:16–24.
63. Blanton LS, Lea AS, Kelly BC, et al. An unusual cutaneous manifestation in a patient with murine typhus. Am J Trop Med Hyg 2015;93(6):1164–7.
64. Pieracci EG, Evert N, Drexler NA, et al. Fatal flea-borne typhus in Texas: a retrospective case series, 1985-2015. Am J Trop Med Hyg 2017;96(5):1088–93.
65. Dumler JS, Taylor JP, Walker DH. Clinical and laboratory features of murine typhus in south Texas, 1980 through 1987. JAMA 1991;266(10):1365–70.

66. Graves SR, Stenos J. Tick-borne infectious diseases in Australia. Med J Aust 2017;206(7):320–4.
67. Parola P. *Rickettsia felis*: from a rare disease in the USA to a common cause of fever in sub-Saharan Africa. Clin Microbiol Infect 2011;17(7):996–1000.
68. Biggs HM, Behravesh CB, Bradley KK, et al. Diagnosis and management of tick-borne rickettsial diseases: Rocky Mountain spotted fever and other spotted fever group rickettsioses, ehrlichioses, and anaplasmosis - United States. MMWR Recomm Rep 2016;65(2):1–44.
69. Segura F, Pons I, Pla J, et al. Shell-vial culture and real-time PCR applied to *Rickettsia typhi* and *Rickettsia felis* detection. World J Microbiol Biotechnol 2015; 31(11):1747–54.
70. Segura F, Pons I, Sanfeliu I, et al. Shell-vial culture, coupled with real-time PCR, applied to *Rickettsia conorii* and *Rickettsia massiliae*-Bar29 detection, improving the diagnosis of the Mediterranean spotted fever. Ticks Tick Borne Dis 2016;7(3): 457–61.
71. McQuiston JH, Wiedeman C, Singleton J, et al. Inadequacy of IgM antibody tests for diagnosis of Rocky Mountain spotted fever. Am J Trop Med Hyg 2014;91(4): 767–70.
72. Delisle J, Mendell NL, Stull-Lane A, et al. Human infections by multiple spotted fever group rickettsiae in Tennessee. Am J Trop Med Hyg 2016;94(6):1212–7.
73. Bizzini A, Peter O, Baud D, et al. Evaluation of a new serological test for the detection of anti-*Coxiella* and anti-*Rickettsia* antibodies. Microbes Infect 2015; 17(11–12):811–6.
74. Paris DH, Dumler JS. State of the art of diagnosis of rickettsial diseases: the use of blood specimens for diagnosis of scrub typhus, spotted fever group rickettsiosis, and murine typhus. Curr Opin Infect Dis 2016;29(5):433–9.
75. Portillo A, de Sousa R, Santibanez S, et al. Guidelines for the detection of *Rickettsia* spp. Vector Borne Zoonotic Dis 2017;17(1):23–32.
76. Peniche-Lara G, Zavala-Velazquez J, Dzul-Rosado K, et al. Simple method to differentiate among *Rickettsia* species. J Mol Microbiol Biotechnol 2013;23(3): 203–8.
77. Denison AM, Amin BD, Nicholson WL, et al. Detection of *Rickettsia rickettsii*, *Rickettsia parkeri*, and *Rickettsia akari* in skin biopsy specimens using a multiplex real-time polymerase chain reaction assay. Clin Infect Dis 2014;59(5):635–42.
78. Kato C, Chung I, Paddock C. Estimation of *Rickettsia rickettsii* copy number in the blood of patients with Rocky Mountain spotted fever suggests cyclic diurnal trends in bacteraemia. Clin Microbiol Infect 2016;22(4):394–6.
79. Morand A, Angelakis E, Ben Chaabane M, et al. Seek and Find! PCR analyses of skin infections in West-European travelers returning from abroad with an eschar. Travel Med Infect Dis 2018. [Epub ahead of print].
80. Hanaoka N, Matsutani M, Satoh M, et al. Development of a novel loop-mediated isothermal amplification (LAMP) assay for the detection of *Rickettsia* spp. Jpn J Infect Dis 2017;70(1):119–23.
81. Dittrich S, Castonguay-Vanier J, Moore CE, et al. Loop-mediated isothermal amplification for *Rickettsia typhi* (the causal agent of murine typhus): problems with diagnosis at the limit of detection. J Clin Microbiol 2014;52(3):832–8.
82. Chao CC, Belinskaya T, Zhang Z, et al. Development of recombinase polymerase amplification assays for detection of *Orientia tsutsugamushi* or *Rickettsia typhi*. PLoS Negl Trop Dis 2015;9(7):e0003884.

83. Dumler JS. Clinical disease: current treatment and new challenges. In: Palmer GH, Azad AF, editors. Intracellular pathogens II: Rickettsiales. Washington, DC: ASM Press; 2012. p. 1–39.

84. Rolain JM, Maurin M, Vestris G, et al. In vitro susceptibilities of 27 rickettsiae to 13 antimicrobials. Antimicrob Agents Chemother 1998;42(7):1537–41.

85. Cross R, Ling C, Day NP, et al. Revisiting doxycycline in pregnancy and early childhood–time to rebuild its reputation? Expert Opin Drug Saf 2016;15(3): 367–82.

86. Todd SR, Dahlgren FS, Traeger MS, et al. No visible dental staining in children treated with doxycycline for suspected Rocky Mountain spotted fever. J Pediatr 2015;166(5):1246–51.

87. Fernando SL, Hudson BJ. Rapid desensitization to doxycycline. Ann Allergy Asthma Immunol 2013;111(1):73–4.

88. Stollings JL, Chadha SN, Paul AM, et al. Doxycycline desensitization for a suspected case of ehrlichiosis. J Allergy Clin Immunol Pract 2014;2(1):103–4.

89. Holman RC, Paddock CD, Curns AT, et al. Analysis of risk factors for fatal Rocky Mountain spotted fever: evidence for superiority of tetracyclines for therapy. J Infect Dis 2001;184(11):1437–44.

90. Gikas A, Doukakis S, Pediaditis J, et al. Comparison of the effectiveness of five different antibiotic regimens on infection with *Rickettsia typhi*: therapeutic data from 87 cases. Am J Trop Med Hyg 2004;70(5):576–9.

91. Anton E, Munoz T, Traveria FJ, et al. Randomized trial of clarithromycin for Mediterranean spotted fever. Antimicrob Agents Chemother 2015;60(3):1642–5.

92. Strand A, Paddock CD, Rinehart AR, et al. African tick bite fever treated successfully with rifampin in a patient with doxycycline intolerance. Clin Infect Dis 2017; 65(9):1582–4.

93. Vaughn MF, Funkhouser SW, Lin FC, et al. Long-lasting permethrin impregnated uniforms: a randomized-controlled trial for tick bite prevention. Am J Prev Med 2014;46(5):473–80.

94. Epidemic typhus risk in Rwandan refugee camps. Wkly Epidemiol Rec 1994;69: 259.

95. Brites-Neto J, Nieri-Bastos FA, Brasil J, et al. Environmental infestation and rickettsial infection in ticks in an area endemic for Brazilian spotted fever. Rev Bras Parasitol Vet 2013;22(3):367–72.

96. Drexler N, Miller M, Gerding J, et al. Community-based control of the brown dog tick in a region with high rates of Rocky Mountain spotted fever, 2012-2013. PLoS One 2014;9(12):e112368.

Antimicrobial Resistance in the Tropics

Makeda Semret, MSc, MD, FRCP(C)[a],*, Louis-Patrick Haraoui, MD, MSc, FRCP(C)[b]

KEYWORDS

- Antimicrobial resistance • Antibiotics • Tropics • Travel • LMIC • ESBL
- Carbapenemase

KEY POINTS

- Antimicrobial resistance is on the rise and spreading rapidly worldwide.
- Low- and middle-income countries (LMICs), because of weak health systems, are particularly vulnerable to this increase.
- Population mobility further fuels the globalization of AMR, with travelers and migrants at significant risk of harboring drug-resistant organisms.

INTRODUCTION

Antimicrobial resistance (AMR) presents substantial challenges to the treatment of common infectious diseases. Currently AMR claims around 700,000 lives per year, but if current predictions hold true, it will surpass cancer as the leading cause of death and will be directly responsible for huge economic losses worldwide within the next 30 years.[1]

These apocalyptic predictions of a postantibiotic world have galvanized the global public health community and many governments toward efforts aimed at reducing overall antimicrobial consumption, and other strategies aligned with the World Health Organization's global action plan on AMR.[2]

Antibiotic resistance (the ability of a specific bacterium to survive in the presence of an antibiotic that was initially effective to treat infections caused by the bacterium, or

M. Semret holds a research grant awarded by the Joint Programming Initiative in Antimicrobial Resistance, and is supported by the Research Institute of McGill University Health Centre for work on antimicrobial resistance in Ethiopia. L.-P. Haraoui is funded by a Canadian Institutes of Health Research catalyst grant Global Governance of Antimicrobial Resistance in Conflicts. Conflicts of Interest: M. Semret has received in-kind support from Biomerieux for investigator-initiated research projects, but no consultancy or advisory fees. L.-P. Haraoui declares no conflicts of interest.
a Infectious Diseases and Medical Microbiology McGill University Health Centre, 1001, Boul Decarie Bloc E, E05.1616, Montreal, Quebec H4A3J1, Canada; b Department of Microbiology and Infectious Diseases, Faculty of Medicine and Health Sciences, Université de Sherbrooke, Office 200, 150 Place Charles-Le Moyne, Longueuil, Québec J4K 0A8, Canada
* Corresponding author.
E-mail address: Makeda.semret@mcgill.ca

Infect Dis Clin N Am 33 (2019) 231–245
https://doi.org/10.1016/j.idc.2018.10.009
id.theclinics.com
0891-5520/19/© 2018 Elsevier Inc. All rights reserved.

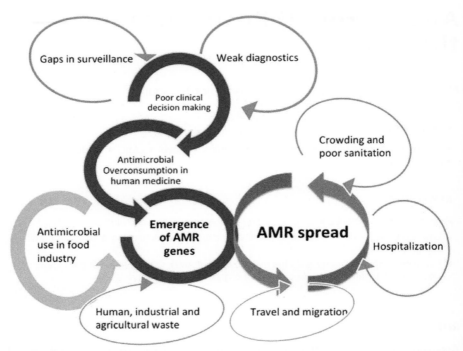

Fig. 1. Representation of the complex interplay between the many factors implicated in the emergence and spread of AMR.

the acquisition of a specific antibiotic resistance mechanism) was initially described mostly in association with hospital-associated infections in Europe and North America, but the epidemiology of antibiotic resistance has shifted in the past decade with the highest rates now reported from low- and middle-income countries (LMICs) in Asia, Africa, and the Middle East.[3] Furthermore, more than 90% of the mortality currently attributable to AMR occurs in regions that are already disproportionally burdened with infectious diseases, poor sanitary standards, reduced access to effective antimicrobials, and overall weak health infrastructures, essentially the very settings least able to afford it.[3,4]

The disparity in AMR occurrence in different regions of the world is linked in large part to variable consumption of antimicrobials for human medicine and the food industry. Dramatic increases in consumption of antibiotics have been reported for several LMICs in the last decade, with just a few countries responsible for three-quarters of the global growth in antibiotic use.[5,6] Meanwhile, every year, 2 billion people move across large geographic distances for business, leisure, resettlement, as refugees, asylum seekers, or migrant workers,[7] a proportion of which carry drug-resistant bacteria or mobile genetic elements with resistance genes, thereby contributing to the globalization of AMR (**Fig. 1**).[5,6]

In this review intended for clinicians, front-line health care workers, and members of the public health community, we provide an overview of the factors that contribute to the emergence, spread, and persistence of AMR, particularly antibiotic-resistance, in the tropics. We also address clinical implications of this emergent global crisis for migrants and travelers, using specific scenarios commonly encountered in those populations.

THE GLOBALIZATION OF ANTIMICROBIAL RESISTANCE

Resistance to antibiotics is acquired either through mutations on the bacterial chromosome, or, as is increasingly the case, on transmissible mobile genetic elements, such as plasmids. Selection pressure from antibiotic exposure provides a competitive advantage for the mutated bacteria; the resistant strains then multiply and spread to the environment or to other humans, either directly via person-to-person contact or indirectly via fomites and surfaces.

Antibiotic Selection Pressure Is Higher in the Tropics

Although the use of antibiotics for growth promotion of livestock has been banned in Europe and is in decline in North America, the relative importance of antibiotics in food production is variable in LMICs.[2] Estimates from China indicate that the animal agricultural sector accounts for 84% of the country's global antibiotic consumption, confirming that agricultural consumption of antibiotics significantly exceeds that of humans in that country.[8] Furthermore, influx of AMR genes from human and livestock wastewater, hospitals, and pharmaceutical plants is potentially more significant in LMICs where environmental legislation and enforcement of waste management regulations typically tend to be lax.[9]

India, China, and Pakistan are currently the largest consumers of antibiotics worldwide in terms of total tons of antibiotics, although their per capita usage remains lower than that of several wealthier nations. However, unlike the situation in high-income countries where overall antibiotic consumption has increased only modestly and rates of consumption per capita seem to be declining, the total antibiotic consumption and the rate per capita have dramatically increased in the past 15 years in LMICs, a phenomenon that correlates closely with growth in incomes and gross domestic product per capita.[10–13]

The increase in human consumption of antibiotics has been attributed, among several other factors, to policies and regulations on antibiotic prescribing in LMICs that tend to be generally less restrictive than in high-income countries: not only are more than two-thirds of all antibiotics sold without a prescription through the private sector, but also frequently dispensed by poorly qualified personnel, further compounding the issue of inappropriate use.[5,14]

Weak Diagnostic Infrastructure Impacts Clinical Decision-Making in Low- and Middle-Income Countries

Because LMICs face tremendous challenges in the provision and delivery of safe health care, funding priorities have tended to focus on specific devastating diseases, such as malaria, tuberculosis, or human immunodeficiency virus, rather than on comprehensive diagnostic infrastructure and clinical decision support systems for common bacterial infections. Most health care facilities in LMICs, especially in sub-Saharan Africa, lack the ability to perform even basic diagnostic testing to elucidate potential causes of fever let alone performing antibiotic susceptibility testing.[15–19] Furthermore, the successful roll-out of rapid diagnostic tests aimed at single pathogens, such as malaria, although reducing misuse of antimalarial treatment, might inadvertently lead to overuse of antibiotics for febrile patients in whom testing for malaria is negative. Several studies conducted in sub-Saharan Africa and Asia have demonstrated a wide range of pathogens implicated in febrile illnesses, only a minority of which should be treated with antibiotics.[20–25] Yet, the practice of treating almost all nonmalarial febrile illnesses with empiric antibiotics continues to be widespread, and clinicians operating in a diagnostic vacuum routinely must weigh the risks of possible bacterial sepsis with the relative ease of prescribing antibiotics.

Rates of Hospitalization, Hospital-Associated Infections, and Antimicrobial Resistance Are Increasing in Low- and Middle-Income Countries

Not only do LMICs shoulder the greatest global burden of malaria, human immunodeficiency virus, dengue, tuberculosis, typhoid fever, diarrheal illness, and respiratory infections,[20–25] but also rates of health care–associated or hospital-acquired infections (HAI) are at least three times higher than in high-income countries. Although still relatively undocumented, estimates show that at least 15% of hospitalized patients (and even higher proportions of those in intensive care unit [ICU], surgery, or neonatal units) develop HAIs in LMICs.[26,27] Chief among them are surgical site infections (SSI): patients in LMICs are at significantly greater risk of SSI than for comparable procedures in high-resource settings, and this despite, or perhaps because of, prolonged courses of preoperative and prophylactic antibiotics. Furthermore, antibiotic-resistant organisms are implicated in more than one-third of the SSI in LMICs.[28–30]

Surveillance and Monitoring of Antimicrobial Resistance Is Not in Place in Many Low- and Middle-Income Countries

The impact of weak diagnostic infrastructure is not limited to clinical care and decision-making in LMICs. By extension, adequate surveillance of AMR at regional or national levels is severely compromised because reference laboratories that are mandated to conduct integrated disease surveillance (and often the only ones sufficiently equipped to perform such testing) are distant from the point of care and lack connectivity with the facilities where patients are managed.[31,32] The result is that AMR surveillance remains fragmented and reliant on sporadic point prevalence surveys in many regions, with only a minority of LMICs providing up-to-date prospective epidemiologic intelligence on antibiotic resistance patterns at the regional level, further exacerbating difficulties in clinical and policy decisions on empiric antibiotic management.

Although variable, reviews of data from diverse sources reveal troubling trends of antibiotic resistance among bacteria commonly implicated in community-acquired and hospital-associated infections. In Africa, for example, studies published before 2013 suggested high prevalence of resistance to chloramphenicol, trimethoprim-sulfamethoxazole, and tetracycline for clinical gram-negative isolates, but most remained susceptible to third-generation cephalosporins and fluoroquinolones.[33,34] A clear shift has since been noted, with gram-negative organisms (from HAIs and from community infections) now highly resistant to third-generation cephalosporins and fluoroquinolones, whereas resistance to carbapenems is increasing.[34–39]

Population Mobility Can Fuel the Spread of Antimicrobial Resistance

About 2 billion persons move across large distances every year; in 2017, an estimated 258 million migrants, 26 million refugees/asylum seekers, and 1.5 billion tourists (of which 525 million traveled to LMICs) crossed international borders.[40,41] Furthermore, the growth of international travel is largely driven by Asian and African travel, which has more than doubled in the past 15 years.[42] Translating these travel and migration statistics into specific risk of spread and dispersal of AMR is challenging, but trajectories of multidrug-resistant (MDR) *Streptococcus pneumoniae* from South Africa to Europe and beyond, of drug-resistant gonorrhea from Asia to the Pacific and North America, and many other examples have been well described.[43,44] In recent years, the pace of AMR global spread has greatly accelerated with transmission of drug-resistance genes located on mobile genetic elements (rather than clonal spread of drug-resistant organisms), as was dramatically demonstrated with the New Delhi Metallo-beta-lactamase 1 (bla_{NDM-1}) gene from India and Pakistan to Europe and beyond[45]; the colistin-resistant (*mcr-1*) gene first found in gram-negative isolates from people and pigs in China in 2016, and identified in the United States that same year[46,47]; and many others.

Migration Is a Risk Factor for Acquiring Drug-Resistance En Route

Despite concerns that the migrant crisis could increase the burden of AMR in Europe and other high-income regions, there has so far been little (if any) transmission of AMR from migrant to host populations. A recent systematic review and meta-analysis assessing patterns of AMR migration to Europe suggests that migrants are actually more likely to acquire drug-resistance during their migration/transit or after arrival, than they are to spread it to the population of the host country. This was inferred from observations that migrants originating from different regions but with similar trajectories were colonized with the same microorganisms, and from clusters of recent transmission events unrelated to regions of origin or travel routes.[48–50] Inadequate sanitation and overcrowding either during transit or in refugee camps and detention centers likely foster an environment that is conducive to transmission of AMR among migrants, whereas onward transmission to the host populations is probably prevented by some degree of social segregation.

CLINICAL IMPLICATIONS: TRAVEL-ACQUIRED MULTIDRUG RESISTANCE

Many resistance genes of clinical relevance, such as those coding for extended-spectrum β-lactamase enzymes (ESBL-E) or for carbapenemases in enterobacteriacea (CPE) conferring resistance to most β-lactam antibiotics are found on plasmids. They are therefore able to spread rapidly from bacteria-to-bacteria within the intestinal tract, and from person-to-person via environmental or direct contact. Since the first strains of ESBL-E were reported in the 1980s in European hospitals, fecal carriage rates have remained low in Europe and America but skyrocketed in LMICs, suggesting that contaminated water and poor sanitary conditions play a major role in fecal-oral transmission.[51] According to current estimates, more than 1.1 billion community dwellers in Southeast Asia, 280 million in Western Pacific, and 110 million in Africa are carriers of ESBL-E.

Hospitalization Abroad Is a Major Risk Factor for Acquisition of Antimicrobial Resistance

Not surprisingly, a history of hospitalization during travel is a major risk factor for acquisition of AMR. Of the roughly 500 million travelers to LMICs, conservative estimates state that more than 1 million get hospitalized there, particularly the elderly, those with comorbidities, those visiting friends and relatives, or those on elective "medical tourism."[52,53] A recent study conducted in Finland demonstrated that more than half of patients hospitalized in the tropics (and more than three-quarters of those hospitalized in South Asia) were colonized with at least one drug-resistant pathogen on their return, and 11% developed a clinical drug-resistant infection within 1 month. Of note, patients hospitalized in Asia, sub-Saharan Africa, and Latin America were more likely to acquire ESBL-E, CPE, or methicillin-resistant *Staphylococcus aureus* (MRSA), but somewhat less likely to become carriers of vancomycin-resistant enterococci, MDR *Pseudomonas*, or drug-resistant *Acinetobacter* compared with those hospitalized in Europe, North America, or Oceania. The use of antimicrobials during the hospitalization and invasive procedures were independent risk factors for acquisition of AMR abroad.

Acinetobacter in Conflict Zones and Hospitals

Over the last 20 years, Acinetobacter sp, particularly Acinetobacter baumannii, has evolved from being an uncommon opportunistic pathogen to gaining worldwide attention as a major cause of MDR infections. Although its natural habitat is not well defined, reports of severe infections among soldiers injured during the Lebanese civil war and during Operation Iraqi Freedom linked acquisition of A baumannii with traumatic wounds, particularly in hot climates. Subsequent nosocomial spread of this pathogen is potentiated by its ability to rapidly acquire resistance determinants and to persist for extended periods of time in the hospital environment.[54,55] Carbapenem-resistant A baumannii (CRAB) infections among soldiers injured during Operation Iraqi Freedom increased from 12% at the beginning of the conflict in 2003 to 97.4% by 2011 (Personal communication from Dr Patrick McGann, 2018), largely because of production of a class of ß-lactamases called oxacillinases (particularly bla_{OXA-23}), and which have since been implicated in CRAB infections in ICU settings in South and Southeast Asia.[56] Several other relevant carbapenemase genes, including the bla_{NDM} metallo-beta-lactamase initially identified in Enterobacteriaceae in 2008,[57] have also emerged in hospital isolates of A baumannii in North Africa, China, India, and other countries.[58–60] Some analyses are in fact suggesting that bla_{NDM} is a "chimera" likely constructed in A baumannii rather than acquired from Enterobacteriacea.[61]

Although acquisition of CRAB seems to be less common than that of ESBL-E among travelers hospitalized in LMICs, soldiers and patients with extended stays in ICUs in the tropics remain at high risk of CRAB colonization and infection, notably hospital-associated pneumonia, nosocomial bloodstream infections, and wound infections with subsequent secondary transmission in the hospital setting.

Travel and Fecal Carriage of Drug-Resistant Enterobacteriacea

A growing body of evidence is showing that even without hospitalization, mere travel to LMICs is a major risk factor for acquisition of MDR Enterobacteriaceae. Several European studies comparing fecal samples of healthy travelers before and after travel have consistently reported that at least one-third acquire ESBL-E genes during their stay in regions where these are endemic, and can remain carriers for up to several months (median, 1 month) after returning, occasionally transmitting them to household members after their return.[62]

Major underlying risk factors for these acquisitions, besides "adventure" (outside of all-inclusive resorts) destinations in South and Southeast Asia, followed by Africa and South America, were occurrence of traveler's diarrhea (TD) and intake of antibiotics.[63–66] Among Finnish travelers, ESBL-E was acquired by 11% of those who did not experience TD and did not take antibiotics during travel, 21% of those who had TD but did not take antibiotics, and 37% of those who had TD and took antibiotics. The use of loperamide in combination with antibiotics for TD was associated with a greater risk for ESBL-E acquisition than antibiotics alone.[67]

Of the ESBL-E strains acquired in the tropics, coresistance to non-β-lactam antibiotics is frequent. Resistance to ciprofloxacin, tobramycin, and cotrimoxazole has been noted in 53%, 52%, 73% of travel-acquired ESBL-E strains, respectively[68]; among those who took fluoroquinolone for TD, coresistance to ciprofloxacin was noted in 95% of strains.

Of even greater concern, reports of acquisition of CPE by healthy travelers returning from Asia are emerging. The smaller number of cases precludes reliable assessment of specific risk factors, but many of these acquisitions occur in the absence of health care exposure abroad, suggesting increasing community transmission of CPE in some regions.[69–72]

Risk of Methicillin-Resistant Staphylococcus Aureus Colonization During Travel to the Tropics

S aureus is present in the nares of 30% of healthy individuals, and is a commensal and an opportunistic pathogen. This organism becomes MRSA via the acquisition of a mobile genetic element carrying the gene encoding resistance to most β-lactam antibiotics. MRSA can spread through direct skin-skin contact, or skin-fomite from an infected or colonized individual, within health care and within the community (community-acquired MRSA [CA-MRSA]). The latter often spreads through clonal expansion of specific strains genetically distinct from those circulating in hospitals, and is frequently equipped with additional virulence factors as the Panton-Valentine leukocidin cytotoxin.

Specific strains of MRSA, initially identified as continent-specific, have definitely spread via international travel.[73] Of note, several strains originated in North America (eg, USA300, USA400) and then spread globally, becoming the dominant clones in several tropical and subtropical regions,[74] signaling that travelers serve as vehicles for spread of drug-resistance in both directions. Older studies of MRSA cases imported into Sweden had estimated that the risk of acquiring MRSA was 59.4 per 1 million travelers after travel to the Middle East and North Africa, compared with 0.1 per million for travel to Nordic countries. Given the ubiquitous nature of this pathogen and that community prevalence is unknown for most of the tropics, estimating risk of acquisition for the healthy traveler is challenging. However, travelers with hospital exposure (including medical tourism) are clearly at significant risk, with MRSA being the second most common drug-resistant organism acquired during hospitalization abroad, after ESBL-E.[75–78]

APPROACH TO TREATMENT OF THE RECENT TRAVELER WITH SUSPECTED BACTERIAL INFECTION

After malaria, typhoid fever is the second most common cause of acute life-threatening tropical disease among returning travelers, whereas nontropical causes of fever, such as urinary and other bacterial infections, account for a substantial proportion of cases.[79–81] In the following section, we integrate current knowledge on the epidemiology of AMR in the tropics to provide a practical approach to initial antibiotic treatment of the returning traveler or migrant with a suspected bacterial infection.

Management of Typhoid Fever

MDR Salmonella enterica serovar Typhi (Salmonella typhi) was first reported in the late 1970s with isolates that were resistant to first-line treatments for typhoid fever at that time: ampicillin, trimethoprim-sulfamethoxazole, and chloramphenicol.[82] The genes associated with this MDR phenotype are generally associated with plasmids that can carry multiple resistance genes and disseminate, as is the case of S typhi H58, the haplotype that was the dominant clade in South and Southeast Asia in the past two decades and has now spread to parts of Africa and Oceania.[82] After the recommended initial treatment option in regions with MDR became fluoroquinolones, resistance emerged in the 1990s, leading to the recommendation to use third-generation cephalosporins for initial management of typhoid.[83] However since 2016, more than 300 cases of extensively drug-resistant (XDR) typhoid, which combine the MDR phenotype with resistance to quinolones and third-generation cephalosporins, have been reported out of Pakistan,[84] and sporadic cases have been identified elsewhere (most recently in Toronto Canada, related to travel to Pakistan). The emergent XDR clone harbors a large number of resistance determinants: those identified in MDR strains, and plasmids encoding ESBL genes likely acquired from widely distributed enteric bacteria.

Current therapeutic guidelines for typhoid suggest the use of quinolones for typhoid cases acquired outside of South and Southeast Asia, and third-generation cephalosporins for cases acquired in Asia. Given the spread of XDR in parts of Pakistan, one should consider treating cases acquired in South Asia (particularly Pakistan) initially with a carbapenem until susceptibility results are available. Clinical experience with carbapenems for typhoid fever is limited and at least one case report has shown persistence of S typhi bacteremia during meropenem monotherapy in a patient with XDR; in that individual, microbiologic and clinical cure was achieved only after combination with parenteral fosfomycin.[85]

Gram-Negative Sepsis in the Recent Traveler

Because a significant proportion of travelers carry ESBL-E strains for up to several months, empiric therapy for those with suspected bacterial sepsis should not rely on third- or fourth-generation cephalosporins, even in combination with fluoroquinolones or aminoglycosides given the high rates of coresistance to several classes of antimicrobials in these strains. Although the data are preliminary, combination β-lactamase-β-lactamase inhibitors may lead to higher mortality than treatment with carbapenems for ESBL-E sepsis, according to a recent randomized controlled trial.[86] In light of these data, it is prudent to recommend that empiric therapy in cases of suspected gram-negative sepsis after recent travel to the tropics should include a carbapenem. Given the potential for selection of carbapenem-resistant mutants during therapy, discontinuing the carbapenem as soon as an alternative has been identified through the microbiologic work-up and ensuring effective antimicrobial stewardship interventions is a critical aspect of the overall management of these patients.

Urinary Tract Infection in the Returning Traveler

Even in the absence of recent antibiotic treatment, empiric treatment of uncomplicated urinary tract infection (UTI) with cotrimoxazole or with ciprofloxacin in travelers returning from the tropics or in the newly arrived migrants carries a risk of treatment failure. Of note, susceptibility to nitrofurantoin seems to be conserved in many ESBL-E from the tropics (with only 2% of the strains noted to be resistant[87–89]), suggesting this agent might be the most useful treatment option for uncomplicated lower UTI among returning travelers. Urinary cultures and close clinical follow-up should be considered in all patients with suspected or confirmed UTI after recent travel to the tropics.

Gonorrhea in the Returning Traveler

Travelers are at increased risk of acquiring sexually transmitted infections (STIs), and a significant proportion of all STIs are acquired abroad; for example, 25% of gonorrhea cases reported over a 5-year period in four Northern European countries were acquired during travel.[87]

Resistance to sulfonamides, penicillins, tetracyclines, macrolides, fluoroquinolones, and early generation cephalosporins have long been widespread, and the main empiric monotherapy recommended for gonorrhea in many countries has been extended-spectrum cephalosporins. But reports of *in vitro* resistance and treatment failure to oral cefixime and more rarely to ceftriaxone have emerged.[88] According to the global Gonococcal Antimicrobial Surveillance Program, two-thirds of participating countries report that greater than 5% of their gonococcal isolates are resistant to extended-spectrum cephalosporins; resistance to azithromycin is reported in 81%, and resistance to ciprofloxacin in 97% of participating countries.[89] However, it should be noted that only 77 countries participate in this program, of which only nine are in Africa and six from Southeast Asia. Furthermore, because of significant technical variations in testing (antimicrobials tested and methods used), it is difficult to issue specific empiric treatment guidelines based on country of travel/acquisition. For cases potentially acquired in the tropics it is therefore prudent to avoid monotherapy with ciprofloxacin or oral cefixime in favor of dual therapy using parenteral ceftriaxone and azithromycin (even if chlamydia is not identified). Critically, because most cases are identified through nucleic acid amplification tests and lack antibiotic susceptibility results, patients with gonococcal disease should be closely followed with a test of cure 1 to 2 weeks after treatment, in addition to treatment of sexual partners and screening for other STIs.

Methicillin-Resistant Staphylococcus Aureus Infection in the Returning Traveler

Travelers and migrants may be at particular risk of MRSA acquisition because of reduced hygiene, increased sweating, and contact with contaminated surfaces or colonized/infected individuals. Once colonized with MRSA, they are also at higher risk of skin and soft tissue infections from wounds, insect bites, or other microtraumas causing breaches in the skin barrier.

Unlike the situation with hospital-acquired MRSA, nearly half of travelers who acquire CA-MRSA during their trip develop clinical infection (commonly skin and soft tissue infections, and more rarely, necrotizing pneumonia), which has important implications for therapy. Although most North-American CA-MRSA strains are susceptible to clindamycin, cotrimoxazole, and tetracyclines, little is known about susceptibilities of strains acquired in the tropics. For severe infections, empirical therapy should therefore include an agent with known predictable activity against MRSA, such as vancomycin. Most importantly pus and blood specimens for culture and susceptibility testing should be included in the routine evaluation and management of the returning traveler with a skin and soft tissue infection.

SUMMARY

Antibiotic resistance is increasing worldwide and is now one the biggest threats facing modern medicine. The causes are complex but central to this global crisis is the overconsumption of antibiotics. International travel predisposes to the acquisition of drug-resistant organisms, particularly ESBL-E and increasingly CPE, which have massively spread in the community of most of the tropics. Travelers should be advised that the risk of acquiring drug-resistant organisms is further exacerbated by the occurrence of diarrhea during travel, the intake of antibiotics, and travel to specific high-risk regions. They hence should be counseled on diarrhea prevention strategies, sanitary practices, and to limit use of antibiotics for specific clinical situations. Clinical evaluation of the febrile traveler in whom a bacterial infection is suspected should include careful consideration of the potential for a drug-resistant infection, and microbiologic screening and infection control precautions to limit spread of resistance determinants in hospitals.

ACKNOWLEDGMENTS

The authors thank Elena Guadagno for help with searching the published literature.

REFERENCES

1. O'Neill J. Antimicrobial resistance: tackling a crisis for the health and wealth of nations. 2014. Available at: https://amr-review.org/Publications.html.
2. World Health Organization. Global action plan on antimicrobial resistance. Geneva (Switzerland): World Health Organization; 2015.
3. World Health Organization. Antimicrobial resistance: global report on surveillance. Geneva (Switzerland): World Health Organization; 2014.
4. Laxminarayan R, Sridhar D, Blaser M, et al. Achieving global targets for antimicrobial resistance. Science 2016;353(6302):874–5.
5. Van Boeckel TP, Gandra S, Ashok A, et al. Global antibiotic consumption 2000 to 2010: an analysis of national pharmaceutical sales data. Lancet Infect Dis 2014; 14(8):742–50.
6. Laxminarayan R, Van Boeckel TP. The value of tracking antibiotic consumption. Lancet Infect Dis 2014;14(5):360–1.
7. MacPherson DW, Gushulak BD, Baine WB, et al. Population mobility, globalization, and antimicrobial drug resistance. Emerg Infect Dis 2009;15(11):1727–32.
8. Singer AC, Shaw H, Rhodes V, et al. Review of antimicrobial resistance in the environment and its relevance to environmental regulators. Front Microbiol 2016;7:1728.
9. Zhang QQ, Ying GG, Pan CG, et al. Comprehensive evaluation of antibiotics emission and fate in the river basins of China: source analysis, multimedia modeling, and linkage to bacterial resistance. Environ Sci Technol 2015;49(11): 6772–82.
10. Ji X, Shen Q, Liu F, et al. Antibiotic resistance gene abundances associated with antibiotics and heavy metals in animal manures and agricultural soils adjacent to feedlots in Shanghai, China. J Hazard Mater 2012;235-236:178–85.
11. Diwan V, Tamhankar AJ, Khandal RK, et al. Antibiotics and antibiotic-resistant bacteria in waters associated with a hospital in Ujjain, India. BMC Public Health 2010;10:414.
12. Robinson TP, Bu DP, Carrique-Mas J, et al. Antibiotic resistance is the quintessential One Health issue. Trans R Soc Trop Med Hyg 2016;110(7):377–80.
13. Adelowo OO, Muller J. Co-occurrence of multiple beta-lactamases and plasmid mediated quinolone resistance (PMQR) genes in Enterobacteriaceae from a polluted Nigerian wetland. Int J Med Microbiol 2016;306(8 Supplement 1):44–5.
14. Klein EY, Van Boeckel TP, Martinez EM, et al. Global increase and geographic convergence in antibiotic consumption between 2000 and 2015. Proc Natl Acad Sci U S A 2018;115(15):E3463–70.
15. World Health Organization. The world medicines situation. Geneva (Switzerland): World Health Organization; 2011.
16. Nguyen KV, Thi Do NT, Chandna A, et al. Antibiotic use and resistance in emerging economies: a situation analysis for Viet Nam. BMC Public Health 2013;13:1158.
17. Holloway K, Mathai E, Gray A, Community-Based Surveillance of Antimicrobial Use and Resistance in Resource-Constrained Settings Project Group. Surveillance of antimicrobial resistance in resource-constrained settings: experience from five pilot projects. Trop Med Int Health 2011;16(3):368–74.

18. Petti CA, Polage CR, Quinn TC, et al. Laboratory medicine in Africa: a barrier to effective health care. Clin Infect Dis 2006;42(3):377–82.
19. Nkengasong JN, Nsubuga P, Nwanyanwu O, et al. Laboratory systems and services are critical in global health: time to end the neglect? Am J Clin Pathol 2010; 134(3):368–73.
20. D'Acremont V, Kahama-Maro J, Swai N, et al. Reduction of anti-malarial consumption after rapid diagnostic tests implementation in Dar es Salaam: a before-after and cluster randomized controlled study. Malar J 2011;10:107.
21. D'Acremont V, Kilowoko M, Kyungu E, et al. Beyond malaria: causes of fever in outpatient Tanzanian children. N Engl J Med 2014;370(9):809–17.
22. Mayxay M, Castonguay-Vanier J, Chansamouth V, et al. Causes of non-malarial fever in Laos: a prospective study. Lancet Glob Health 2013;1(1):e46–54.
23. Maze MJ, Bassat Q, Feasey NA, et al. The epidemiology of febrile illness in sub-Saharan Africa: implications for diagnosis and management. Clin Microbiol Infect 2018;24(8):808–14.
24. Shrestha P, Roberts T, Homsana A, et al. Febrile illness in Asia: gaps in epidemiology, diagnosis and management for informing health policy. Clin Microbiol Infect 2018;24(8):815–26.
25. Acestor N, Cooksey R, Newton PN, et al. Mapping the aetiology of non-malarial febrile illness in Southeast Asia through a systematic review: terra incognita impairing treatment policies. PLoS One 2012;7(9):e44269.
26. Murray CJ, Vos T, Lozano R, et al. Disability-adjusted life years (DALYs) for 291 diseases and injuries in 21 regions, 1990-2010: a systematic analysis for the Global Burden of Disease Study 2010. Lancet 2012;380(9859):2197–223.
27. Allegranzi B, Bagheri Nejad S, Combescure C, et al. Burden of endemic health-care-associated infection in developing countries: systematic review and meta-analysis. Lancet 2011;377(9761):228–41.
28. Okeke IN, Laxminarayan R, Bhutta ZA, et al. Antimicrobial resistance in developing countries. Part I: recent trends and current status. Lancet Infect Dis 2005;5(8):481–93.
29. Bagheri Nejad S, Allegranzi B, Syed SB, et al. Health-care-associated infection in Africa: a systematic review. Bull World Health Organ 2011;89(10):757–65.
30. Collaborative G. Surgical site infection after gastrointestinal surgery in high-income, middle-income, and low-income countries: a prospective, international, multicentre cohort study. Lancet Infect Dis 2018;18(5):516–25.
31. Ombelet S, Ronat JB, Walsh T, et al. Clinical bacteriology in low-resource settings: today's solutions. Lancet Infect Dis 2018;18(8):e248–58.
32. Semret M, Ndao M, Jacobs J, et al. Point-of-care and point-of-'can': leveraging reference-laboratory capacity for integrated diagnosis of fever syndromes in the tropics. Clin Microbiol Infect 2018;24(8):836–44.
33. Leopold SJ, van Leth F, Tarekegn H, et al. Antimicrobial drug resistance among clinically relevant bacterial isolates in sub-Saharan Africa: a systematic review. J Antimicrob Chemother 2014;69(9):2337–53.
34. World Health Organization. Antimicrobial resistance: global report on surveillance. Geneva (Switzerland): World Health Organization; 2014. Available at: https://www.who.int/drugresistance/documents/surveillancereport/en/.
35. Tadesse BT, Ashley EA, Ongarello S, et al. Antimicrobial resistance in Africa: a systematic review. BMC Infect Dis 2017;17(1):616.
36. Le Doare K, Bielicki J, Heath PT, et al. Systematic review of antibiotic resistance rates among gram-negative bacteria in children with sepsis in resource-limited countries. J Pediatric Infect Dis Soc 2015;4(1):11–20.

37. Maina D, Revathi G, Nyerere K. Antimicrobial resistance patterns in ESBL producing *E. coli* and *K. pneumoniae* isolates in a private tertiary hospital, Kenya. Histopathology 2012;61:153–4.

38. Okoche D, Asiimwe BB, Katabazi FA, et al. Prevalence and characterization of carbapenem-resistant enterobacteriaceae isolated from Mulago National Referral Hospital, Uganda. PLoS One 2015;10(8):e0135745.

39. Agyepong N, Govinden U, Owusu-Ofori A, et al. Multidrug-resistant gram-negative bacterial infections in a teaching hospital in Ghana. Antimicrob Resist Infect Control 2018;7:37.

40. United Nations. International migration report. In: New York. Available at: http://www.un.org/en/development/desa/population/migration/publications/migrationreport/docs/MigrationReport2017_Highlights.pdf2017. Accessed June 15, 2018.

41. World Trade Organization. International tourism report. In. Washington, DC: The World Bank. Available at: https://data.worldbank.org/indicator/ST.INT.ARVL2017. Accessed June 15, 2018.

42. (UNWTO) UNWTO. Annual report. In. Available at: https://www.e-unwto.org/doi/book/10.18111/97892844198072017. Accessed June 15, 2018.

43. Reinert RR, Jacobs MR, Appelbaum PC, et al. Relationship between the original multiply resistant South African isolates of *Streptococcus pneumoniae* from 1977 to 1978 and contemporary international resistant clones. J Clin Microbiol 2005; 43(12):6035–41.

44. Sutrisna A, Soebjakto O, Wignall FS, et al. Increasing resistance to ciprofloxacin and other antibiotics in *Neisseria gonorrhoeae* from East Java and Papua, Indonesia, in 2004 - implications for treatment. Int J STD AIDS 2006;17(12): 810–2.

45. Kumarasamy KK, Toleman MA, Walsh TR, et al. Emergence of a new antibiotic resistance mechanism in India, Pakistan, and the UK: a molecular, biological, and epidemiological study. Lancet Infect Dis 2010;10(9):597–602.

46. Liu YY, Wang Y, Walsh TR, et al. Emergence of plasmid-mediated colistin resistance mechanism MCR-1 in animals and human beings in China: a microbiological and molecular biological study. Lancet Infect Dis 2016;16(2):161–8.

47. McGann P, Snesrud E, Maybank R, et al. *Escherichia coli* Harboring mcr-1 and blaCTX-M on a novel IncF plasmid: first report of mcr-1 in the United States. Antimicrob Agents Chemother 2016;60(7):4420–1.

48. Nellums LB, Thompson H, Holmes A, et al. Antimicrobial resistance among migrants in Europe: a systematic review and meta-analysis. Lancet Infect Dis 2018;18(7):796–811.

49. Angeletti S, Ceccarelli G, Vita S, et al. Unusual microorganisms and antimicrobial resistances in a group of Syrian migrants: sentinel surveillance data from an asylum seekers centre in Italy. Travel Med Infect Dis 2016;14(2):115–22.

50. Piso RJ, Käch R, Pop R, et al. A cross-sectional study of colonization rates with methicillin-resistant *Staphylococcus aureus* (MRSA) and extended-spectrum beta-lactamase (ESBL) and carbapenemase-producing enterobacteriaceae in four swiss refugee centres. PLoS One 2017;12(1):e0170251.

51. Woerther PL, Burdet C, Chachaty E, et al. Trends in human fecal carriage of extended-spectrum beta-lactamases in the community: toward the globalization of CTX-M. Clin Microbiol Rev 2013;26(4):744–58.

52. Siikamaki H, Kivela P, Fotopoulos M, et al. Illness and injury of travellers abroad: Finnish nationwide data from 2010 to 2012, with incidences in various regions of the world. Euro Surveill 2015;20(19):15–26.

53. Bacaner N, Stauffer B, Boulware DR, et al. Travel medicine considerations for North American immigrants visiting friends and relatives. JAMA 2004;291(23): 2856–64.

54. Scott P, Deye G, Srinivasan A, et al. An outbreak of multidrug-resistant *Acinetobacter baumannii-calcoaceticus* complex infection in the US military health care system associated with military operations in Iraq. Clin Infect Dis 2007; 44(12):1577–84.

55. Wong D, Nielsen TB, Bonomo RA, et al. Clinical and pathophysiological overview of acinetobacter infections: a century of challenges. Clin Microbiol Rev 2017; 30(1):409–47.

56. Hsu LY, Apisarnthanarak A, Khan E, et al. Carbapenem-resistant *Acinetobacter baumannii* and Enterobacteriaceae in South and Southeast Asia. Clin Microbiol Rev 2017;30(1):1–22.

57. Yong D, Toleman MA, Giske CG, et al. Characterization of a new metallo-beta-lactamase gene, bla(NDM-1), and a novel erythromycin esterase gene carried on a unique genetic structure in *Klebsiella pneumoniae* sequence type 14 from India. Antimicrob Agents Chemother 2009;53(12):5046–54.

58. Chen Y, Zhou Z, Jiang Y, et al. Emergence of NDM-1-producing *Acinetobacter baumannii* in China. J Antimicrob Chemother 2011;66(6):1255–9.

59. Jones LS, Toleman MA, Weeks JL, et al. Plasmid carriage of bla NDM-1 in clinical *Acinetobacter baumannii* isolates from India. Antimicrob Agents Chemother 2014;58(7):4211–3.

60. Boulanger A, Naas T, Fortineau N, et al. NDM-1-producing *Acinetobacter baumannii* from Algeria. Antimicrob Agents Chemother 2012;56(4):2214–5.

61. Toleman MA, Spencer J, Jones L, et al. blaNDM-1 is a chimera likely constructed in *Acinetobacter baumannii*. Antimicrob Agents Chemother 2012;56(5):2773–6.

62. Khawaja T, Kirveskari J, Johansson S, et al. Patients hospitalized abroad as importers of multiresistant bacteria-a cross-sectional study. Clin Microbiol Infect 2017;23(9):673.e1-8.

63. Arcilla MS, van Hattem JM, Haverkate MR, et al. Import and spread of extended-spectrum beta-lactamase-producing Enterobacteriaceae by international travellers (COMBAT study): a prospective, multicentre cohort study. Lancet Infect Dis 2017;17(1):78–85.

64. Ruppe E, Armand-Lefevre L, Estellat C, et al. High rate of acquisition but short duration of carriage of multidrug-resistant enterobacteriaceae after travel to the tropics. Clin Infect Dis 2015;61(4):593–600.

65. Tängdén T, Cars O, Melhus A, et al. Foreign travel is a major risk factor for colonization with *Escherichia coli* producing CTX-M-type extended-spectrum beta-lactamases: a prospective study with Swedish volunteers. Antimicrob Agents Chemother 2010;54(9):3564–8.

66. Hassing RJ, Alsma J, Arcilla MS, et al. International travel and acquisition of multidrug-resistant Enterobacteriaceae: a systematic review. Euro Surveill 2015; 20(47): pii 30074.

67. Kantele A, Lääveri T, Mero S, et al. Antimicrobials increase travelers' risk of colonization by extended-spectrum beta lactamase-producing Enterobacteriaceae. Clin Infect Dis 2015;60(6):837–46.

68. Kantele A, Mero S, Kirveskari J, et al. Increased risk for ESBL-producing bacteria from co-administration of loperamide and antimicrobial drugs for travelers' diarrhea. Emerg Infect Dis 2016;22(1):117–20.

69. Kantele A, Mero S, Kirveskari J, et al. Fluoroquinolone antibiotic users select fluoroquinolone-resistant ESBL-producing Enterobacteriaceae (ESBL-PE): data of a prospective traveller study. Travel Med Infect Dis 2017;16:23–30.

70. Ruppé E, Armand-Lefèvre L, Estellat C, et al. Acquisition of carbapenemase-producing Enterobacteriaceae by healthy travellers to India, France, February 2012 to March 2013. Euro Surveill 2014;19(14) [pii:20768].

71. van Hattem JM, Arcilla MS, Bootsma MC, et al. Prolonged carriage and potential onward transmission of carbapenemase-producing Enterobacteriaceae in Dutch travelers. Future Microbiol 2016;11:857–64.

72. Wi T, Lahra MM, Ndowa F, et al. Antimicrobial resistance in *Neisseria gonorrhoeae*: global surveillance and a call for international collaborative action. PLoS Med 2017;14(7):e1002344.

73. Zhou YP, Wilder-Smith A, Hsu LY. The role of international travel in the spread of methicillin-resistant *Staphylococcus aureus*. J Travel Med 2014;21(4):272–81.

74. Nimmo GR. USA300 abroad: global spread of a virulent strain of community-associated methicillin-resistant *Staphylococcus aureus*. Clin Microbiol Infect 2012;18(8):725–34.

75. Rogers BA, Aminzadeh Z, Hayashi Y, et al. Country-to-country transfer of patients and the risk of multi-resistant bacterial infection. Clin Infect Dis 2011;53(1):49–56.

76. Stenhem M, Ortqvist A, Ringberg H, et al. Imported methicillin-resistant *Staphylococcus aureus*, Sweden. Emerg Infect Dis 2010;16(2):189–96.

77. Ahmed-Bentley J, Chandran AU, Joffe AM, et al. Gram-negative bacteria that produce carbapenemases causing death attributed to recent foreign hospitalization. Antimicrob Agents Chemother 2013;57(7):3085–91.

78. Kaase M, Nordmann P, Wichelhaus TA, et al. NDM-2 carbapenemase in *Acinetobacter baumannii* from Egypt. J Antimicrob Chemother 2011;66(6):1260–2.

79. Bottieau E, Clerinx J, Schrooten W, et al. Etiology and outcome of fever after a stay in the tropics. Arch Intern Med 2006;166(15):1642–8.

80. Jensenius M, Han PV, Schlagenhauf P, et al. Acute and potentially life-threatening tropical diseases in western travelers: a GeoSentinel multicenter study, 1996-2011. Am J Trop Med Hyg 2013;88(2):397–404.

81. Thwaites GE, Day NPJ. Approach to fever in the returning traveler. N Engl J Med 2017;376(18):1798.

82. Crump JA, Sjölund-Karlsson M, Gordon MA, et al. Epidemiology, clinical presentation, laboratory diagnosis, antimicrobial resistance, and antimicrobial management of invasive salmonella infections. Clin Microbiol Rev 2015;28(4):901–37.

83. Wong VK, Baker S, Pickard DJ, et al. Phylogeographical analysis of the dominant multidrug-resistant H58 clade of *Salmonella typhi* identifies inter- and intracontinental transmission events. Nat Genet 2015;47(6):632–9.

84. Wain J, Hendriksen RS, Mikoleit ML, et al. Typhoid fever. Lancet 2015;385(9973):1136–45.

85. Klemm EJ, Shakoor S, Page AJ, et al. Emergence of an extensively drug-resistant salmonella enterica serovar typhi clone harboring a promiscuous plasmid encoding resistance to fluoroquinolones and third-generation cephalosporins. MBio 2018;9(1) [pii:e00105-18].

86. Harris PNA: Effect of piperacillin-tazobactam vs meropenem on 30-day mortality for patients with E coli or klebsiella pneumoniae bloodstream infection and ceftriaxone resistance: a randomized clinical trial. JAMA 2018;320(10):984–94.

87. Kleine CE, Schlabe S, Hischebeth GTR, et al. Successful therapy of a multidrug-resistant extended-spectrum beta-lactamase-producing and fluoroquinolone-resistant *Salmonella enterica* subspecies enterica serovar Typhi infection using

combination therapy of meropenem and fosfomycin. Clin Infect Dis 2017;65(10): 1754–6.

88. Beaute J, Cowan S, Hiltunen-Back E, et al. Travel-associated gonorrhoea in four Nordic countries, 2008 to 2013. Euro Surveill 2017;22(20) [pii:30537].

89. Unemo M, Shafer WM. Antimicrobial resistance in *Neisseria gonorrhoeae* in the 21st century: past, evolution, and future. Clin Microbiol Rev 2014;27(3):587–613.

Evidence-Based Clinical Management of Ebola Virus Disease and Epidemic Viral Hemorrhagic Fevers

Christophe Clément, MD[a,b], Neill K.J. Adhikari, MDCM, MSc[c,d], François Lamontagne, MD, MSc[d,e,*]

KEYWORDS

- Ebola virus disease • Viral hemorrhagic fever • Clinical management
- Evidence-based care

KEY POINTS

- The mortality of Ebola virus disease remains high, and opportunities to improve supportive care remain.
- Emerging technology enables rapid diagnosis in the field and monitoring of routine laboratory parameters, which may guide clinical management.
- Supportive care encompasses fluid resuscitation and correction of electrolyte disturbances. Early use of intravenous fluids is warranted in patients unable to drink. The net effect of nonspecific adjunctive treatments, such as antibiotics and antidiarrheal agents, is uncertain, and justification for their routine use decreases as diagnostic and therapeutic capacity increases.
- Currently recommended personal protective equipment impedes clinical management. More tolerable equipment or temperature control in Ebola treatment centers would enable longer presence at the patients' bedside.
- Despite numerous Ebola and Marburg fever outbreaks in the last 50 years, there is a dearth of documented clinical and biological data beyond patients' initial presentation. Proper data collection and medical record keeping remain high priorities.

Disclosure Statement: The authors have nothing to disclose.
[a] Intensive Care Unit, Polyclinique Bordeaux Nord Aquitaine, 15 rue Claude Boucher, Bordeaux 33000, France; [b] Intensive Care Unit, Mamoudzou Hospital, rue de l'Hôpital, Mayotte 97600, France; [c] Department of Critical Care Medicine, Sunnybrook Health Sciences Centre, 2075 Bayview Avenue, Toronto, Ontario M4N 3M5, Canada; [d] Interdepartmental Division of Critical Care, University of Toronto, 209 Victoria Street, 4th Floor, Room 411, Toronto, Ontario M5B 1T8, Canada; [e] Department of Medicine, Université de Sherbrooke, 300112e Avenue Nord, Sherbrooke, Québec J1H 5N4, Canada
* Corresponding author. Department of Internal Medicine, Centre Intégré Universitaire de Santé et Service Social-Estrie, 3001 12e avenue Nord, Sherbrooke, Québec J1H 5N4, Canada.
E-mail address: Francois.Lamontagne@usherbrooke.ca

Infect Dis Clin N Am 33 (2019) 247–264
https://doi.org/10.1016/j.idc.2018.10.013
0891-5520/19/© 2018 Elsevier Inc. All rights reserved.

id.theclinics.com

INTRODUCTION

The deadly 2014 to 2016 outbreak of Ebola virus disease (EVD) in West Africa underscored the severity of the threat posed by viral hemorrhagic fevers.[1] New outbreaks in the Democratic Republic of the Congo in 2018 further highlighted the pervasiveness of Ebola and other viruses, such as the Marburg and Lassa viruses, in certain regions of Africa.[2,3]

Outbreaks of viral hemorrhagic fevers caused by filoviruses have been identified since 1967, but the use of clinical or biological data collected over time remains limited. Although symptoms reported by patients on admission to Ebola treatment centers (ETCs) are described in several publications, objective data required to make clinical decisions, such as body temperature, blood pressure, heart rate, respiration rate, and fluid balance, have not been systematically collected over the entire clinical course. Similarly, limited data exist on derangements of electrolytes and acid-base balance, renal and hepatic function, and blood coagulation. Epidemiologic data suggesting a very poor prognosis for viral hemorrhagic fevers must be interpreted in light of historically limited clinical evaluation and management.

The prompt recognition and management of clinical, physiologic, and laboratory abnormalities on admission to an ETC should, in theory, improve outcomes. With this objective in mind, recommendations for basic clinical management for patients with EVD were created.[4] However, important clinical questions remain, and additional research would likely help future patients with viral hemorrhagic fevers. With the exception of emerging specific anti-Ebola treatments, this article addresses different aspects of the clinical management of viral hemorrhagic fevers, particularly on filoviruses, based on scientific evidence to the extent it exists. Broader considerations, such as epidemiology and modes of transmission, are addressed when they are likely to influence clinical decisions.

EPIDEMIOLOGY
Definitions

The generic term "viral hemorrhagic fevers" designates a group of viral diseases, some of which, such as Marburg fever and EVD, typically manifest as outbreaks. The most striking example remains the 2014 to 2016 outbreak of EVD in West Africa, which was widespread and deadly.[1] Certain other viral hemorrhagic fevers, such as Lassa fever, are mostly endemic, with sporadic outbreaks or significant upsurges, such as in Nigeria in 2018.[5] Viral hemorrhagic fevers that are mostly endemic are not discussed further.

Outbreaks of Filoviruses

Marburg fever is caused by a filovirus belonging to the Filoviridae family. Marburg fever was first described in 1967 when 2 outbreaks occurred simultaneously in Germany (Marburg and Frankfurt) and in Serbia (Belgrade).[6] These initial patients were infected by monkeys (*Cercopithecus aethiops*) imported from Uganda. Since then, approximately 10 outbreaks have occurred, each one infecting between 1 and 374 patients for an approximate total of 587 cases.

EVD is also caused by a filovirus belonging to the Filoviridae family and was first described in 1976 (**Tables 1** and **2**). There are 5 known species of this virus: *Zaire ebolavirus, Sudan ebolavirus, Tai Forest ebolavirus, Bundibugyo ebolavirus*, and *Reston ebolavirus*. Before 2014, 2387 cases had been recorded in African outbreaks, with a crude overall mortality of 67%.[7] Reston virus has been introduced several times through imported macaques from the Philippines to the United States and Italy.[8]

Table 1
Characteristics of viral hemorrhagic fevers

Family	Filoviridae		Arenaviridae			Bunyaviridae	
Genus	Filovirus	Filovirus	Tacaribe complex	Tacaribe complex	LCMV/Lassa complex	Nairovirus	Phlebovirus
Name	Ebola	Marburg	Junin	Machupo	Lassa	Crimean-Congo	Rift Valley
Geography	Africa	Africa	South America	South America	West Africa	Africa, Central Asia, Europe, Middle East	Africa, Yemen, Saudi Arabia
Host	Bats, monkeys	Bats, monkeys	Rodents (*Mastomys natalensis*)	Rodents	Rodents	Domestic and wild vertebrates	Ruminants
Vector	No	No	No	No	No	Tics (Hyalomma)	Mosquitoes (*Aedes* spp)
Incubation time (d)	2–21	2–21	7–14	9–15	5–21	3–14	2–6
Start	Sudden	Sudden	Progressive	Progressive	Progressive	Progressive	Sudden
Characteristics	Mortality (40%–90%) outbreaks	Mortality (30%–90%) outbreaks	Encephalitis	Encephalitis	Rare thrombocytopenia Low mortality (1%–2%)	Mortality 30%–50%	Mortality <10% Ocular involvement
Antiviral therapy	None has demonstrated efficacy	None	Ribavirin	?	Ribavirin	Ribavirin ineffective	Ribavirin

Abbreviation: LCMV, lymphocytic choriomeningitis virus.
Adapted from Tattevin P, Lagathu G, Revest R, et al. Les fièvres hémorragiques virales. Rev Francophone des Laboratoires 2016;480:72; with permission.

Table 2
Ebola outbreaks

Year	Country	Ebola virus species	Number of Cases	Number of Deaths	Mortality, %
Patients treated in Africa[a]					
2014	Democratic Republic of Congo	Zaire	66	49	74
2014	Senegal	Zaire	1	0	0
2014	Mali	Zaire	8	6	75
2014	Nigeria	Zaire	20	8	40
2014–2016[b]	Sierra Leone	Zaire	14,124*	3956*	28
2014–2016[b]	Liberia	Zaire	10,675*	4809*	45
2014–2016[b]	Guinea	Zaire	3811*	2543*	67
2012	Democratic Republic of Congo	Bundibugyo	57	29	51
2012	Uganda	Sudan	7	4	57
2012	Uganda	Sudan	24	17	71
2011	Uganda	Sudan	1	1	100
2008	Democratic Republic of Congo	Zaire	32	14	44
2007	Uganda	Bundibugyo	149	37	25
2007	Democratic Republic of Congo	Zaire	264	187	71
2005	Congo	Zaire	12	10	83

Year	Country	Species			
2004	Sudan	Sudan	17	7	41
2003 (Nov–Dec)	Congo	Zaire	35	29	83
2003 (Jan–Apr)	Congo	Zaire	143	128	90
2001–2002	Congo	Zaire	59	44	75
2001–2002	Gabon	Zaire	65	53	82
2000	Uganda	Sudan	425	224	53
1996	South Africa (ex-Gabon)	Zaire	1	1	100
1996 (Jul–Dec)	Gabon	Zaire	60	45	75
1996 (Jan–Apr)	Gabon	Zaire	31	21	68
1995	Democratic Republic of Congo	Zaire	315	254	81
1994	Côte d'Ivoire	Taï Forest	1	0	0
1994	Gabon	Zaire	52	31	60
1979	Sudan	Sudan	34	22	65
1977	Democratic Republic of Congo	Zaire	1	1	100
1976	Sudan	Sudan	284	151	53
1976	Democratic Republic of Congo	Zaire	318	280	88
Patients treated in Europe or North America[c]					
2014–2015	Zaire		27	5	18.5

* The '*' indicates 'includes suspect, probable, and confirmed cases'.
[a] From World Health Organization.[6]
[b] According to the World Health Organization, these numbers underestimate the reality in proportions that cannot be estimated.
[c] From Uyeki and colleagues.[9] Of note, some of the cases reported by Uyeki and colleagues may also be counted as African cases.

During the 2014 to 2016 outbreak in West Africa, there were 28,610 in West Africa, with an overall mortality of 39.5%.[7] During the same period, 27 patients were treated in Europe or in North America (overall mortality 18.5%).[9]

Although systematically higher than in Europe and in North America, mortalities reported in Africa vary widely. The reasons for this variation are not clear. There does not appear to be a consistent secular trend, given that outbreaks occurring in the 2000s were deadlier than some that occurred in the 1970s to 1980s. Part of this variation may be attributable to the viral species. Indeed, the Zaire ebolavirus species appears to be associated with higher mortality than the Sudan or Bundibugyo species.[10] Furthermore, variations in case definitions, surveillance systems, and clinical care also likely contributed to fluctuations in mortalities. For example, reporting mortality for both suspected and confirmed cases probably dilutes the mortality. During the 2014 to 2015 outbreak in West Africa, which was caused by a single species (*Zaire ebolavirus*), and using consistent definitions for suspect, probable, and confirmed cases, mortality was higher in Guinea (67%) than in Liberia (45%) and Sierra Leone (28%).[7] Within Sierra Leone, as an example, variation in mortality was apparent; for example, 74% of confirmed cases receiving care at an ETC early in the outbreak died,[11] much higher than the overall national mortality.

A better understanding of key prognostic factors requires virological confirmation of the diagnosis and improved collection of clinical and biological data on admission and during the entire clinical evolution in the ETC.

Modes of Transmission

In all likelihood, fruit bats of the Pteropodidae family are natural Ebola virus hosts.[8] Ebola is introduced into the human population through close contact with the blood, secretions, organs, or other bodily fluids of infected animals, such as chimpanzees, gorillas, bats, monkeys, forest antelope, or porcupines. Ebola then spreads through human-to-human transmission when mucous membranes come in contact with infected blood or other bodily fluids, which may contaminate surfaces and materials. Persistence of Ebola on environmental surfaces has been demonstrated in simulated conditions,[12] but is unlikely to be relevant in ETCs, where infection prevention and control procedures are followed.[13–15] Funeral rites during which family and friends are in direct contact with the body of the deceased likely played a critical role in the transmission of the Ebola virus in West Africa in 2014 to 2016.[16–18] Although concerns about the possibility of aerosolization of Ebola have been raised,[19] there have been no documented cases of airborne transmission.

CLINICAL FEATURES

Although outbreaks of Ebola viral hemorrhagic fever have afflicted Africa since 1976, clinical and biological descriptions of early epidemics remain extremely limited. Limitations in the clinical management of patients admitted to ETCs, which were primarily designed for quarantine rather than treatment, explain the emphasis on clinical status at presentation rather than subsequent evolution. Paradoxically, a more detailed description of clinical and laboratory evolution over time has emerged from case descriptions of a small number of patients treated outside of Africa in 1967[20] and in 2014 to 2016.[9] One review has highlighted the similarity between clinical presentations of EVD and of Marburg virus disease.[21] Given the dearth of clinical data reported since then, the following description encompasses the diseases caused by both viruses.

Symptoms Reported at Presentation

Clinical descriptions enumerate nonspecific symptoms of asthenia, fever, myalgia, headaches, vomiting, diarrhea, delirium, conjunctivitis, hiccups, and dyspnea.[22,23] Data collection relies on closed questions to which patients answer yes or no, but patients' precarious clinical states and frequent language barriers limit the reliability of these questionnaires. Although the relative frequency of individual symptoms varies, hemorrhagic manifestations appear to be uncommon. For example, Dickson and colleagues[22] report hemorrhagic symptoms in only 3 of the 44 patients in their cohort.

The absence of objective vital signs data, such as blood pressure, heart rate, and respiratory rate,[21] continues to be problematic in more recent descriptions of the 2014 to 2016 outbreak.[24,25] When collected, vital signs have been reported on admission only.[22–24] Accordingly, these observations are of limited utility to inform prognosis or to provide longitudinal and personalized care. In a prospective observational study of 118 patients with EVD, Hunt and colleagues[26] define 3 disease stages of severity according to clinical features on admission. Stage 3, characterized by the presence of shock (not defined), coma, hemorrhage, or organ failure, was associated with a significantly higher risk of death, but only a small number of patients (10%) met those criteria. Vernet and colleagues[27] adopted the same approach, obtaining similar results, based on symptoms reported by 97 patients with EVD. Only bleeding was a predictor of mortality, but it essentially constituted a premortem finding.

Laboratory Data

Close monitoring of objective physical signs and biological data during hospitalization is essential for early detection of potentially lethal but correctable complications. For example, vomiting and diarrhea in patients too weak to self-rehydrate led to hypovolemia and biochemical imbalances, as documented in 27 patients treated in Europe and North America in 2016.[9] Although obtained in a starkly different context, this clinical and laboratory characterization aligns with the data derived from African outbreaks. Recently, Hunt and colleagues[26] reported the results of biochemical analyses performed with a portable point-of-care device on 118 patients admitted to the Kerry Town ETC in Sierra Leone. Analyses conducted solely on admission were used to identify prognostic factors. Among this cohort, half of the patients presented with acute kidney injury (AKI), with increased levels of blood urea and creatinine. Although urine output was not evaluated, the investigators hypothesized that hypovolemia caused by dehydration was the predominant mechanism. Hemoconcentration, diagnosed in many patients, supported this hypothesis. Rhabdomyolysis was present in 83% of patients on admission, and in 100% of nonsurviving patients, likely contributing to the risk of AKI. In this study, the prognosis was independently associated with the severity of AKI on admission. Findings from a case series (n = 16) by Cournac and colleagues[23] echo the clinical importance of rhabdomyolysis; the investigators reported elevated creatine kinase (>1000 IU/L) in 59% of patients, and the severity of rhabdomyolysis was associated with mortality.[23]

Another very common biological abnormality observed during the 2014 to 2016 outbreak, as in previous epidemics, was an increase in liver transaminases.[21] Bilirubin was most often normal or low, and there were no symptoms associated with acute hepatocellular failure.[26–28] Admission electrolytes are typically only moderately abnormal, if at all. Although hypokalemia may be expected due to severe gastrointestinal losses, and hyperkalemia may be associated with AKI and metabolic acidosis,[26,27] electrolytes have not been measured over time. Repeated monitoring of electrolytes in critically ill patients is standard care and can be achieved even in resource-limited settings using point-of-care devices.[26,29]

DIAGNOSIS OF MARBURG AND EBOLA VIRUS INFECTIONS

The cornerstone of laboratory diagnosis of Ebola is a nucleic acid amplification test implemented by reverse transcriptase-polymerase chain reaction (RT-PCR); several kits are available and were implemented in mobile biocontainment laboratories.[30] These techniques have been limited by complexity (including the requirement for a continuous power supply), cost, and time required for specimen processing and analysis. Diagnostic properties may also degrade in new outbreak due to genomic drift.[31] More recently, a fully automated RT-PCR system (GeneXpert) showed comparable performance to standard RT-PCR, with much faster turnaround time and minimized need for specimen handling.[32] Both techniques provide an indirect measure of viral load, a strong prognostic variable,[27] by reporting the number of PCR cycles required to obtain a positive test result; the smaller the number of PCR cycles, the greater the viral load.[33]

Rapid tests that detect Ebola antigen are also available or under development and can be implemented in point-of-care testing platforms with results available in a few minutes. In addition to standard antigen capture enzyme-linked immunosorbent assay, other techniques (immunohistochemistry, lateral flow assay, fluorescent antibody) have also been developed.[30] Although antigen detection systems typically are positive 48 to 72 hours after RT-PCR, some evaluations have shown excellent sensitivity.[33,34] The antibody response to Ebola infection is too variable for use in acute diagnosis.

Although a comprehensive review of diagnostic modalities of VHF is beyond the scope of this article, this brief overview of evolving diagnostic modalities is relevant to the discussion of clinical management. Indeed, these recent advances have the potential to reduce the time to diagnosis and, therefore, the period of uncertainty during which suspect and probable cases are confined together in isolation. Moreover, early identification of cases should enable health workers to more rapidly allocate sparse resources to the patients who are most likely to benefit from them.

CLINICAL MANAGEMENT
Supportive Care

A crucial hypothesis of clinical management of viral hemorrhagic fevers is that mortality will be reduced when supportive care is delivered based on repeated evaluation of the patient's clinical, hemodynamic, and electrolyte status. Such care includes replacement for failing organs,[22,28] which "buys time" while the body's immune system forms antibody and clears the virus. Although many factors may have contributed to the lower mortality of patients repatriated to Europe and North America, it is plausible that part of this difference is attributable to the identification and effective correction of hypovolemia and biochemical disorders and use of organ-supporting care, such as renal replacement, vasopressors, and mechanical ventilation.[9] Similarly, as early as 2007, Bausch and colleagues[29] noted that during the only outbreak of Marburg fever (1967) occurring in countries (Germany and Yugoslavia) where supportive intensive care was possible, mortality was 22%, whereas it was more than 87% in Africa for the same condition several years later. Given these observations, several investigators exhort decision makers to focus on patient care, which may be achieved without jeopardizing the safety of health care providers.[29,35]

Failing to make this paradigm shift and ensure the delivery of life-sustaining therapies perpetuates the cycle of limited care, poor prognosis, and fear in the community of dying alone and untreated in an ETC. This paradigm shift occurred in certain ETCs during the 2014 to 2016 EVD outbreak in West Africa.[22,36] Supportive care interventions are not disease specific. Rather, they entail close and repeated monitoring of clinical signs (eg, heart rate, blood pressure, urine and stool output, oral intake of a sufficient quantity of oral rehydration solutions, capillary refill, mental status, respiratory rate, oxygen saturation, temperature) and laboratory disorders (eg, blood gases, sodium, potassium, blood urea nitrogen, creatinine, creatine kinase). Documentation of these physical signs and standard laboratory analyses for the entire duration of the stay in ETCs is crucial. Thus, it is impossible to dissociate quality of care from medical record keeping, and recent guidelines have also emphasized this connection.[4]

Accordingly, it is also essential to ensure that the necessary material resources and protocols are in place to collect clinical and laboratory information, record it, monitor it, and deliver care in response to correctable disorders that are detected. The availability of reliable point-of-care laboratory testing devices removed what was once an insurmountable technological barrier. However, it is conceivable that during an influx of patients, these analyses will not be possible without a considerable increase in the number of machines and of personnel dedicated to the analyses. Ideally, a fixed laboratory and dedicated staff should be able to operate adjacent to the high-risk zone with a window to the high-risk zone to receive samples, enabling the use of faster and more powerful machines that can process more samples in less time and at lower unit cost.[28]

When oral intake is insufficient, guidelines and expert opinion support parenteral fluid replacement.[4,37] Parenteral intake may require the placement of intraosseous needles in very dehydrated patients initially, followed by central venous catheters. Reluctance to install such venous access devices because of the danger to health care personnel has diminished since the recent outbreak of EVD in 2014. The feasibility and safety of installing central venous catheters in treatment centers have been reported.[22,36]

Advanced Replacement Therapy for Organ Failure

Implementation of advanced organ-supportive therapies (eg, renal replacement therapy, mechanical ventilation, vasopressor support) in areas where these interventions are not usually available is a matter of debate.[24] Until the 2014 outbreak of EVD, many did not consider this possibility due to the lack of resources in areas affected by most viral hemorrhagic fever outbreaks and because of the appalling prognosis reported in the literature, which led to claims of futility. The implementation of such techniques during the recent outbreak for patients transferred and treated in the United States or in Europe,[9] as well as in a small number of West African ETCs,[22,26,28] has led to calls for more widespread implementation.[35,38]

Associated Therapies

Antibiotics

Antibiotic therapy is advocated for patients with EVD in all expert recommendations.[4,37] Antibiotics are typically broad spectrum, such as third-generation cephalosporins or quinolones, and are intended to prevent bacterial translocation from the gut as EVD progresses. However, in the absence of the necessary laboratory facilities, this widespread practice during the 2014 to 2016 outbreak could not be supported by microbiologic evidence of bacterial infection. Such liberal use of broad-spectrum antibiotics in the context of a proven viral infection opposes efforts to use antibiotics more sparingly to reduce antibiotic resistance.[39] For patients with confirmed EVD by PCR, the value of empiric antimicrobials without evidence of a bacterial infection should be debated. Given that many areas have yet to implement a strategy to mitigate increasing rates of antibiotic resistance,[40] failure to do so may ultimately have dire consequences. Implementation of basic bacteriology using current technology,[41] notwithstanding the need to ensure laboratory personnel safety, would allow for reliable culture and sensitivity testing in ETCs and rational deescalation of initial empiric antibiotics in patients with negative cultures.

Antimalarials

The use of rapid diagnostic tests to detect *Plasmodium falciparum* should guide the prescription of antimalarials for curative purposes, although one study suggests that even with universal administration of antimalarials to patients in ETCs, initial parasitemia is associated with improved survival.[42] A complementary approach of mass community drug administration of antimalarials as part of a universal treatment program reduced the impact of patients presenting with febrile illness due to malaria when health care capacity was severely strained during the 2014 to 2016 West African outbreak, although the effect was attenuated after a few weeks.[43]

Antiemetic and antidiarrheal medications

The rationale for the use of antiemetic and antidiarrheal medications hinges on the assumption that they reduce the loss of fluids and electrolytes, which compounds the risk of death in situations where intensive monitoring and correction of losses are not possible.[44] However, enthusiasm for these interventions is tempered by the theoretic risk of slower pathogen clearance, bacterial overgrowth, and eventually, peritoneal translocation, despite the lack of published data supporting these concerns. In contrast to strategies aimed at restoring fluid volume and electrolytes, use of antiemetic and antidiarrheal medications should be considered in the context of clinical investigations.

Recovery

During the recent outbreak of EVD, patients were considered cured once clinical signs had resolved, provided that Ebola virus PCR was negative at least 3 days after disease onset. Current recommendations for discharge in surviving patients suggest 2 negative samples.[45] However, Ebola virus remains detectable by PCR for prolonged periods in certain bodily fluids, such as sperm,[46] breast milk,[47] cerebrospinal fluid,[48] and ocular aqueous humor.[49] Recent reports suggest that EVD may be sexually transmitted more than a year after clinical recovery.[50,51] In addition, a recent report described a household cluster of cases in 2015 that was most likely related to viral persistence or recrudescent disease in a postpartum woman who was presumed to have survived EVD 1 year previously.[52] In this context, recommendations are to advise male survivors to avoid sexual intercourse or use condoms for at least 3 months initially, and for a subsequent period guided by semen testing for Ebola virus.[37,53,54] During the postoutbreak period, clinicians and public health authorities must remain vigilant to new cases.

EQUIPMENT AND LOGISTICS
Personal Protective Equipment

One of the explanations for the gaps in care during the African outbreaks is that clinicians spent insufficient time providing bedside assessment and clinical care in the ETCs. At the height of the outbreak in November 2014, Chertow and colleagues[55] noted that direct contact between health care providers and patients in treatment centers was limited to 45 or 60 minutes, 2 or 3 times a day, due to the risk of heatstroke and dehydration associated with the personal protective equipment (PPE) worn by staff. Under these conditions, time spent with each patient did not exceed 1 to 2 minutes, on average.

Currently recommended PPE is summarized in **Table 3**, and posters of recommended donning and doffing procedures are available.[56] A principal means of transmission of infection from patient to clinician occurs during PPE removal, although this can be reduced (but not eliminated) by education efforts.[57] Simulation studies have shown moderate thermal strain with 1 hour in conventional PPE in simulated West African climate conditions.[58] In addition, simulation using Ebola PPE even in European room temperature conditions shows that providers perceive advanced medical procedures to be more complicated, more stressful, and less comfortable compared to standard protection.[59] Whether variations of PPE can make medical care for extended periods in ETCs more feasible, by increasing comfort and decreasing heat strain, while maintaining safety, requires urgent study. In addition, whether air-conditioned ETCs would allow for standard Ebola PPE to be worn for longer periods in the high-risk zone and thus for more intensive care to be delivered has not been studied, although clinical experience from one ETC in Sierra Leone the latter part of the West African outbreak suggests this to be the case (Ref.[60] and see Fig. 2 in Ref.[28]).

Data Collection and Transfer

The challenges associated with the collection and transmission of clinical data outside the high-risk zone also contributed to gaps in clinical management. Paper-based data collection materials cannot easily be removed from the high-risk zone. Approximate solutions (eg, photographs of a paper sheet held at arm's length by a health care provider) should be replaced by more reliable, long-term solutions. Buhler and colleagues[61] created an inventory of the various possible methods by surveying 40 health care providers who had been involved in prior Ebola or Marburg virus outbreaks. Among the most promising options are wired or wireless computer networks that only require one computer or mobile device inside the contaminated zone that communicates with the outside.

Functionality of Ebola Treatment Centers

ETCs serve 2 purposes: to stop transmission of Ebola in a community by isolating patients and to provide a safe environment for the provision of high-quality clinical care. To accomplish these objectives, engineering controls are needed that divide the ETC into zones and direct the flow of patients and staff (**Figs. 1** and **2**). The entire ETC is separated from the outside world while maintaining the ability of ambulatory patients to safely visit with family members across plastic mesh fences that allow for visual contact and conversation. Within the ETC, the green zone is a low-contamination risk zone with space for staff meetings, staff toilets and showers, preparation of chlorine, laundering and drying of reusable materials, pharmacy, and equipment storage. The red zone is at high risk for contamination and has space for patient care (suspected, probable, confirmed cases), patient toilets and showers, waste disposal (including sharps), management of infectious waste, and a morgue for deceased patients. Movement of patients is one way from the triage area to the suspect ward, then to the confirmed ward, and then outside the ETC after passing through a dedicated shower. Access to the red zone for clinical staff is also unidirectional; staff must enter via the PPE donning area and exit via the PPE doffing area. Staff movement is from the lowest to

Table 3
Recommended personal protective equipment for Ebola

Recommendation	Strength of Recommendation	Quality of Evidence of Effectiveness of Preventing Filovirus Transmission to Health Workers
The mucous membranes of eyes, mouth, and nose should be completely covered by PPE	Strong	High-quality evidence for protecting mucous membranes compared with no protection
Use either a face shield or goggles	Strong	Very low-quality evidence comparing face shields and goggles
Use a fluid-resistant medical or surgical mask with a structured design that does not collapse against the mouth (eg, duckbill or cup shape)	Strong	Low-quality evidence comparing medical or surgical mask with particulate respirator
Use a fluid-resistant particulate respirator during procedures that generate aerosols of body fluids	Strong	Moderate-quality evidence, when evidence on protection against other pathogens during aerosol-generating procedures is also considered
Use double gloves	Strong	Moderate-quality evidence comparing double gloves to single gloves
Nitrile gloves are preferred over latex gloves	Strong	Moderate-quality evidence on health worker tolerance of nitrile gloves compared with latex gloves
Use protective body wear in addition to regular on duty clothing (eg, surgical scrubs)	Strong	High-quality evidence for using protective body wear compared with not using protection, based on accumulated evidence from other infections with similar modes of transmission
The choice of PPE for covering clothing should be either a disposable gown and apron, or a disposable coverall and apron; the gown and the coverall should be made of fabric that has been tested for resistance to penetration by blood and other body fluids or by blood-borne pathogens	Conditional	Very low-quality evidence comparing gowns and coveralls
The choice of apron should be, in order of preference: • A disposable, waterproof apron • If disposable aprons are not available, heavy-duty, reusable waterproof aprons may be used, provided that they are appropriately cleaned and disinfected between patients	Strong	Very low-quality evidence comparing disposable and reusable aprons

(continued on next page)

Table 3 (continued)		
Recommendation	Strength of Recommendation	Quality of Evidence of Effectiveness of Preventing Filovirus Transmission to Health Workers
Use waterproof boots (eg, rubber or gum boots)	Strong	Very low-quality evidence comparing boots with closed shoes with or without shoe covers
Use a head cover that covers head and neck	Conditional	Low-quality evidence comparing head covers with no head cover
It is suggested that the head cover is separate from the gown or coverall, so that it can be removed separately	Conditional	Low-quality evidence comparing different types of head covers

From Personal protective equipment for use in a filovirus disease outbreak: rapid advice guideline. Geneva (Switzerland): World Health Organization; 2016. p. xiii; with permission.

highest risk areas, that is, starting in the suspect ward and then moving to the probable ward, confirmed ward (these 2 may be combined), and waste management area or morgue (if needed). The ETC has 4 exits: one for staff to the green zone (exit after PPE removal, hand hygiene, and cleaning and disinfection) and 3 for patients. A suspect patient who tests negative for Ebola exits after a shower but without passing through the confirmed ward; deceased patients exit through the morgue; and recovered probable and confirmed patients exit after taking a shower.

Improved ETC engineering may simultaneously enhance quality of patient care and health care worker safety. Air-conditioned ETCs may allow for more intensive clinical care while maintaining the thermal comfort of patients and clinicians. Alternatively, individual patient care rooms made of transparent plastic and air conditioned, such as the "Biosecure Emergency Care Unit for Outbreaks" developed by one non-governmental organization,[62] may allow for easier monitoring of multiple patients and delivery of some medical care by health care workers not in full PPE, who access the patient via plastic-lined portholes.

Ebola Treatment Centers Staffing and Policies

ETC operations hinge on the complementary expertise of numerous staff members. The ideal clinical team includes doctors, nurses, psychologists, and social support staff. In addition, the infection prevention and control team includes a clinical specialist, cleaners, hygienists, and a water and sanitation specialist. Support staff includes specialists in logistics, coordination, laundry, and safe burial. Additional nonclinical staff experts in epidemiology, data management, and research may also be present.

Clinicians (nurses, clinical officers, physicians) should be organized into shifts of approximately 8 hours according to context and workload, with the objective of providing clinical coverage 24 hours per day and a ratio of 1 clinician per 4 or fewer patients to enable adequate clinical contact with patients. During a shift, the number and duration of visits should be guided by patient requirements. Clinicians should always be paired in the red zone so that adherence to infection prevention and control

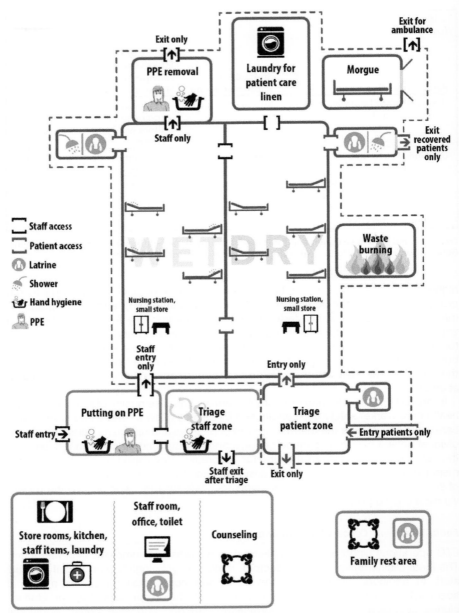

Fig. 1. Sample architecture of an ETC. (*From* Manual for the care and management of patients in Ebola care units/community care centres: interim emergency guidance. Geneva (Switzerland): World Health Organization; 2015. p. 4; with permission.)

practices is ensured and for assistance during tasks (for example, intravenous cannula insertion). Similar to a medical ward, regular rounds should take place in the green zone to conduct handover between shifts, develop plans for the day, and prioritize care for the sickest patients.

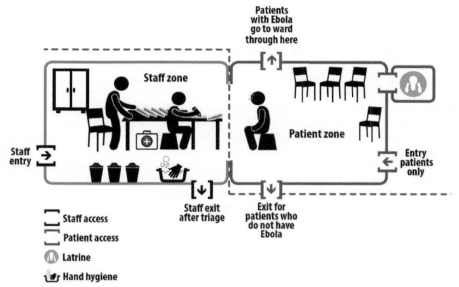

Fig. 2. Sample layout of a triage area. (*From* Manual for the care and management of patients in Ebola care units/community care centres: interim emergency guidance. Geneva (Switzerland): World Health Organization; 2015. p. 5; with permission.)

Policies should promote the safety and well-being of ETC staff, including training for the provision of supportive care, regular training on PPE donning and doffing, scheduled days off and sufficient salary so that there is no temptation to work simultaneously in non-ETC facilities, and a nonblame culture whereby sick clinicians are promptly evaluated and cared for as needed, while still receiving a salary.

REFERENCES

1. WHO Ebola Response Team, Agua-Agum J, Allegranzi B, Ariyarajah A, et al. After Ebola in west africa–unpredictable risks, preventable epidemics. N Engl J Med 2016;375(6):587–96.
2. Ebola Outbreak Epidemiology Team. Outbreak of Ebola virus disease in the democratic republic of the congo, april-may, 2018: An epidemiological study. Lancet 2018;392(10143):213–21.
3. Nakkazi E. Dr congo Ebola virus outbreak: responding in a conflict zone. Lancet 2018;392(10148):623.
4. Lamontagne F, Fowler RA, Adhikari NK, et al. Evidence-based guidelines for supportive care of patients with Ebola virus disease. Lancet 2018; 391(10121):700–8.
5. Roberts L. Nigeria hit by unprecedented lassa fever outbreak. Science 2018; 359(6381):1201–2.
6. Siegert R, Shu HL, Slenczka W, et al. On the etiology of an unknown human infection originating from monkeys [german]. Dtsch Med Wochenschr 1967;92(51): 2341–3.

7. Ebola virus disease: key facts. World Health Organization. Available at: http://www.who.int/news-room/fact-sheets/detail/ebola-virus-disease. Accessed July 30, 2018.

8. Feldmann H, Geisbert TW. Ebola haemorrhagic fever. Lancet 2011;377(9768):849–62.

9. Uyeki TM, Mehta AK, Davey RT Jr, et al. Clinical management of Ebola virus disease in the united states and europe. N Engl J Med 2016;374(7):636–46.

10. Bannister B. Viral haemorrhagic fevers imported into non-endemic countries: risk assessment and management. Br Med Bull 2010;95(1):193–225.

11. Schieffelin JS, Shaffer JG, Goba A, et al. Clinical illness and outcomes in patients with Ebola in sierra leone. N Engl J Med 2014;371(22):2092–100.

12. Fischer R, Judson S, Miazgowicz K, et al. Ebola virus stability on surfaces and in fluids in simulated outbreak environments. Emerg Infect Dis 2015;21(7):1243–6.

13. Bausch DG, Towner JS, Dowell SF, et al. Assessment of the risk of Ebola virus transmission from bodily fluids and fomites. J Infect Dis 2007;196(Suppl 2):S142–7.

14. Vetter P, Fischer WA 2nd, Schibler M, et al. Ebola virus shedding and transmission: Review of current evidence. J Infect Dis 2016;214(suppl 3):S177–84.

15. Poliquin PG, Vogt F, Kasztura M, et al. Environmental contamination and persistence of Ebola virus RNA in an Ebola treatment center. J Infect Dis 2016;214(suppl 3):S145–52.

16. Curran KG, Gibson JJ, Marke D, et al. Cluster of Ebola virus disease linked to a single funeral - moyamba district, sierra leone, 2014. MMWR Morb Mortal Wkly Rep 2016;65(8):202–5.

17. International Ebola Response Team, Agua-Agum J, Ariyarajah A, Aylward B, et al. Exposure patterns driving Ebola transmission in west africa: a retrospective observational study. PLoS Med 2016;13(11):e1002170.

18. Victory KR, Coronado F, Ifono SO, et al, Centers for Disease Control and Prevention (CDC). Ebola transmission linked to a single traditional funeral ceremony - kissidougou, guinea, december, 2014-january 2015. MMWR Morb Mortal Wkly Rep 2015;64(14):386–8.

19. Jones RM, Brosseau LM. Aerosol transmission of infectious disease. J Occup Environ Med 2015;57(5):501–8.

20. Martini GA. Marburg virus disease. Clinical syndrome. In: Martini GA, Siegert R, editors. Marburg virus disease. Berlin Heidelberg: Springer-Verlag; 1971. p. 1–9.

21. Kortepeter MG, Bausch DG, Bray M. Basic clinical and laboratory features of filoviral hemorrhagic fever. J Infect Dis 2011;204(Suppl 3):S810–6.

22. Dickson SJ, Clay KA, Adam M, et al. Enhanced case management can be delivered for patients with evd in africa: Experience from a uk military ebola treatment centre in sierra leone. J Infect 2018;76(4):383–92.

23. Cournac JM, Karkowski L, Bordes J, et al. Rhabdomyolysis in Ebola virus disease. Results of an observational study in a treatment center in guinea. Clin Infect Dis 2016;62(1):19–23.

24. Bah EI, Lamah MC, Fletcher T, et al. Clinical presentation of patients with Ebola virus disease in conakry, guinea. N Engl J Med 2015;372(1):40–7.

25. Lamontagne F, Clement C, Fletcher T, et al. Doing today's work superbly well–treating ebola with current tools. N Engl J Med 2014;371(17):1565–6.

26. Hunt L, Gupta-Wright A, Simms V, et al. Clinical presentation, biochemical, and haematological parameters and their association with outcome in patients with Ebola virus disease: an observational cohort study. Lancet Infect Dis 2015;15(11):1292–9.

27. Vernet MA, Reynard S, Fizet A, et al. Clinical, virological, and biological parameters associated with outcomes of Ebola virus infection in macenta, guinea. JCI Insight 2017;2(6):e88864.

28. Leligdowicz A, Fischer WA 2nd, Uyeki TM, et al. Ebola virus disease and critical illness. Crit Care 2016;20(1):217.

29. Bausch DG, Feldmann H, Geisbert TW, et al. Outbreaks of filovirus hemorrhagic fever: Time to refocus on the patient. J Infect Dis 2007;196(Suppl 2):S136–41.

30. Coarsey CT, Esiobu N, Narayanan R, et al. Strategies in Ebola virus disease (evd) diagnostics at the point of care. Crit Rev Microbiol 2017;43(6):779–98.

31. Sozhamannan S, Holland MY, Hall AT, et al. Evaluation of signature erosion in Ebola virus due to genomic drift and its impact on the performance of diagnostic assays. Viruses 2015;7(6):3130–54.

32. Semper AE, Broadhurst MJ, Richards J, et al. Performance of the genexpert Ebola assay for diagnosis of Ebola virus disease in sierra leone: a field evaluation study. PLoS Med 2016;13(3):e1001980.

33. Merens A, Bigaillon C, Delaune D. Ebola virus disease: Biological and diagnostic evolution from 2014 to 2017. Med Mal Infect 2018;48(2):83–94.

34. Broadhurst MJ, Kelly JD, Miller A, et al. Reebov antigen rapid test kit for point-of-care and laboratory-based testing for Ebola virus disease: a field validation study. Lancet 2015;386(9996):867–74.

35. Murthy S, Ebola Clinical Care authors group. Ebola and provision of critical care. Lancet 2015;385(9976):1392–3.

36. Rees PS, Lamb LE, Nicholson-Roberts TC, et al. Safety and feasibility of a strategy of early central venous catheter insertion in a deployed uk military Ebola virus disease treatment unit. Intensive Care Med 2015;41(5):735–43.

37. Clinical management of patients with viral haemorrhagic fever: a pocket guide for the front-line health worker. Geneva (Switzerland): World Health Organization; 2016.

38. Brown C, Kreuels B, Baker P, et al. Ebola and provision of critical care. Lancet 2015;385(9976):1392.

39. Global action plan on antimicrobial resistance. Geneva (Switzerland): World Health Organization; 2015.

40. Essack SY, Desta AT, Abotsi RE, et al. Antimicrobial resistance in the who african region: current status and roadmap for action. J Public Health (Oxf) 2017;39(1):8–13.

41. Ombelet S, Ronat JB, Walsh T, et al. Clinical bacteriology in low-resource settings: today's solutions. Lancet Infect Dis 2018;18(8):e248–58.

42. Rosenke K, Adjemian J, Munster VJ, et al. Plasmodium parasitemia associated with increased survival in Ebola virus-infected patients. Clin Infect Dis 2016;63(8):1026–33.

43. Aregawi M, Smith SJ, Sillah-Kanu M, et al. Impact of the mass drug administration for malaria in response to the Ebola outbreak in sierra leone. Malar J 2016;15:480.

44. Chertow DS, Uyeki TM, DuPont HL. Loperamide therapy for voluminous diarrhea in Ebola virus disease. J Infect Dis 2015;211(7):1036–7.

45. World Health Organization. Module 4b: clinical care in designated Ebola treatment centres (etc). Ebola: clinical management of Ebola virus disease. 2018. Available at: https://openwho.org/courses/ebola-clinical-management. Accessed September 16, 2018.

46. Deen GF, Broutet N, Xu W, et al. Ebola RNA persistence in semen of Ebola virus disease survivors - final report. N Engl J Med 2017;377(15):1428–37.

47. Sissoko D, Keita M, Diallo B, et al. Ebola virus persistence in breast milk after no reported illness: a likely source of virus transmission from mother to child. Clin Infect Dis 2017;64(4):513–6.

48. Jacobs M, Rodger A, Bell DJ, et al. Late Ebola virus relapse causing meningoencephalitis: a case report. Lancet 2016;388(10043):498–503.

49. Varkey JB, Shantha JG, Crozier I, et al. Persistence of Ebola virus in ocular fluid during convalescence. N Engl J Med 2015;372(25):2423–7.

50. Mate SE, Kugelman JR, Nyenswah TG, et al. Molecular evidence of sexual transmission of Ebola virus. N Engl J Med 2015;373(25):2448–54.

51. Diallo B, Sissoko D, Loman NJ, et al. Resurgence of Ebola virus disease in guinea linked to a survivor with virus persistence in seminal fluid for more than 500 days. Clin Infect Dis 2016;63(10):1353–6.

52. Dokubo EK, Wendland A, Mate SE, et al. Persistence of Ebola virus after the end of widespread transmission in liberia: an outbreak report. Lancet Infect Dis 2018; 18(9):1015–24.

53. Soka MJ, Choi MJ, Baller A, et al. Prevention of sexual transmission of Ebola in liberia through a national semen testing and counselling programme for survivors: an analysis of Ebola virus RNA results and behavioural data. Lancet Glob Health 2016;4(10):e736–43.

54. Clinical care for survivors of Ebola virus disease: interim guidance. Geneva (Switzerland): World Health Organization; 2016.

55. Chertow DS, Kleine C, Edwards JK, et al. Ebola virus disease in west africa–clinical manifestations and management. N Engl J Med 2014;371(22):2054–7.

56. How to put on and how to remove personal protective equipment - posters. Geneva (Switzerland): World Health Organization; 2015.

57. Tomas ME, Kundrapu S, Thota P, et al. Contamination of health care personnel during removal of personal protective equipment. JAMA Intern Med 2015; 175(12):1904–10.

58. Grelot L, Koulibaly F, Maugey N, et al. Moderate thermal strain in healthcare workers wearing personal protective equipment during treatment and care activities in the context of the 2014 Ebola virus disease outbreak. J Infect Dis 2016; 213(9):1462–5.

59. Grillet G, Marjanovic N, Diverrez JM, et al. Intensive care medical procedures are more complicated, more stressful, and less comfortable with Ebola personal protective equipment: a simulation study. J Infect 2015;71(6):703–6.

60. Langer M, Portella G, Finazzi S, et al. Intensive care support and clinical outcomes of patients with Ebola virus disease (EVD) in west africa. Intensive Care Med 2018;44(8):1266–75.

61. Buhler S, Roddy P, Nolte E, et al. Clinical documentation and data transfer from Ebola and marburg virus disease wards in outbreak settings: health care workers' experiences and preferences. Viruses 2014;6(2):927–37.

62. Cube, the biosecure emergency care unit. Available at: https://www.alima-ngo. org/fr/alima-cube. Accessed September 15, 2018.

Migration Medicine

Christina Greenaway, MD, MSc[a,b,c,*],
Francesco Castelli, MD, FRCP (Lond), FFTM RCPS (Glasg), FESCMID[d,e]

KEYWORDS

- Migration • Infectious diseases • Screening • Health promotion

KEY POINTS

- Migration is increasing, and practitioners need to be aware of the unique health needs of this population.
- The prevalence of infectious diseases among migrants varies and generally mirrors that of their countries of origin but is modified by the circumstance of migration, presence of pre-arrival screening programs and post arrival access to health care.
- Take all opportunities to screen migrants at risk for latent infections and update routine vaccines in all age groups.
- Be aware of "rare and tropical infections" related to migration and return travel.

INTRODUCTION

Human migration is rising globally and has increased substantially in recent years, resulting in movement of microbes to new geographic regions. This trend has implications for the health of migrant populations and receiving country health practitioners and health systems. The number of migrants has reached unprecedented levels, with 258 million people or 3.6% of the world's population living outside their country of birth in 2017, a number that has tripled since the 1970s[1] (**Fig. 1**). The number of forced migrants has also increased to 68 million people, the highest recorded number since World War II. Forced migration is driven primarily by growing global inequities,

The authors are responsible for the choice and presentation of views contained in this article and for opinions expressed therein, which are not necessarily those of UNESCO and do not commit the Organization.

[a] Division of Infectious Diseases, Jewish General Hospital, Room E0057, 3755 Côte Ste-Catherine Road, Montreal, Quebec H3T 1E2, Canada; [b] Centre for Clinical Epidemiology, Lady Davis Institute for Medical Research, 3755 Côte Ste-Catherine Road, Montreal, Quebec H3T 1E2, Canada; [c] J.D. MacLean Center for Tropical Diseases at McGill, McGill University Health Centre, Glen Site, 1001 Décarie Boulevard, Montreal, Quebec H4A 3J1, Canada; [d] University Department of Infectious and Tropical Diseases, University of Brescia and ASST Spedali Civili, Piazza del Mercato, 15, Lombardy, Brescia 25121, Italy; [e] UNESCO Chair "Training and Empowering Human Resources for Health Development in Resource-Limited Countries", University of Brescia, Brescia, Italy
* Corresponding author. Division of Infectious Diseases, Jewish General Hospital, Room E0057, 3755 Côte Ste-Catherine Road, Montreal, Quebec H3T 1E2, Canada.
E-mail address: ca.greenaway@mcgill.ca

Infect Dis Clin N Am 33 (2019) 265–287
https://doi.org/10.1016/j.idc.2018.10.014
0891-5520/19/© 2018 Elsevier Inc. All rights reserved.

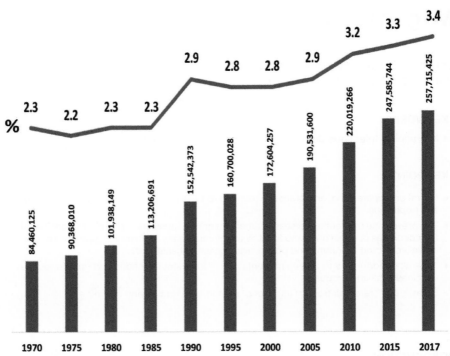

Fig. 1. Number and percent of international migrants between 1970 and 2017. The bar graph shows the total number of international migrants. (*From* United Nations 19 September, 2016; Pages https://refugeesmigrants.un.org/ declaration on 27 June 2018 Agenda items 13 and 117. ©2018 United Nations. Used with the permission of the United Nations.)

escalating human conflicts, and natural disasters.[2] Human mobility is not a new phenomenon because people have been migrating for centuries to seek out a better life for themselves and their families. Several different "push-and-pull" factors interact to drive migration flows, including socioeconomic, political, environmental economic, and individual factors.[3] As a result, migrants comprise a large proportion of the populations in high-income countries, most of whom originate from low- and middle-income countries.[4] In Organization for Economic Co-operation and Development countries, 13% of the population is foreign born. Some countries have even larger proportions of migrants, including Switzerland (30%), Australia (28%), and Canada (23%)[4] (**Figs. 2** and **3**). The recent increase in forced migration, particularly into Europe in 2015 and 2016, overwhelmed the social and health systems and has propelled this issue to the highest level of international discourse, resulting in a global focus on migrant health issues.[2,5,6]

According to the International Organization for Migration, a migrant is "any person who is moving or has moved across an international border or within a state away from his/her habitual place of residence, regardless of (1) the person's legal status; (2) whether the movement is voluntary or involuntary; (3) what the causes of the movement are; or (4) what the length of stay is."[7] A distinction is generally made between short-term or temporary migration vs long-term or permanent migration, the latter referring to those who have changed their country of residence for a duration

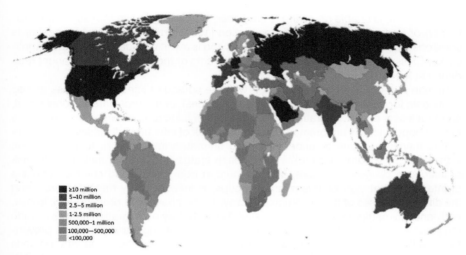

Fig. 2. Total number of migrants living in receiving countries. (*From* United Nations 19 September, 2016; Pages https://refugeesmigrants.un.org/ declaration on 27 June 2018 Agenda items 13 and 117. ©2018 United Nations. Used with the permission of the United Nations.)

of 1 year or more.[8] Migrants fall into 2 broad categories: (1) economic migrants moving for work opportunities or family reunification, and (2) forced migrants, including asylum seekers and refugees. A refugee is a person who, "*owing to a well-founded fear of persecution for reasons of race, religion, nationality, membership of a particular social group or political opinions, is outside the country of his*

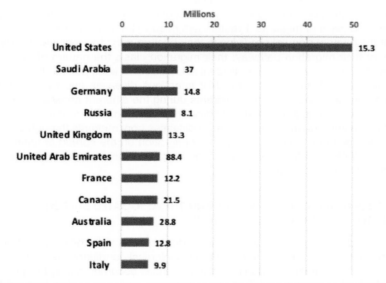

Fig. 3. Number of migrants in million in the top 10 migrant receiving countries. (*Data from* United Nations 19 September, 2016; Pages https://refugeesmigrants.un.org/. Declaration on 27 June 2018, Agenda items 13 and 117.)

nationality and is unable or, owing to such fear, is unwilling to avail himself of the protection of that country" (Geneva Convention [1951, Art. 1A]). An asylum seeker is someone who has applied for refugee status and is awaiting a decision on their application.[7] This review focuses on long-term migrants or those seeking permanent residence in host countries.

Human mobility has been associated with the spread of infectious disease across continents for centuries due to exploration, conquest, commerce, international travel, and to a lesser extent, migration.[9] Transmission of infectious diseases from migrants to host populations is uncommon. The greatest risk of infectious diseases is to the migrants themselves due to undetected and untreated infections or to transmission within their own communities.[10,11] The health status of migrants, including the risk of infectious disease exposure, and the burden from undetected chronic sequelae of infections that vary across migrant groups, is influenced by many factors along the different phases of the migration pathway. These phases are premigration, transit, early and late settlement, and return travel (**Table 1**). Key premigration factors include the prevalence of infectious diseases in the countries of origin and access to preventive health care, such as vaccination. The circumstances of how and why persons migrated may increase the risk of exposure to infectious diseases during transit. Critical postmigration factors that influence migrant health include entitlement to health care and accessibility to and responsiveness of health practitioners and host health care systems to the cultural and linguistic needs of migrants. In addition, socioeconomic factors, risk behaviors after arrival, presence of medical comorbidities, and the immune status of the individual as well as reexposure during travel to their countries of origin also play a role.[12,13] Migrants often have better initial health status compared with host populations, a term known as the "healthy immigrant effect." This effect is primarily because the act of migration requires those involved to be in good health.[12,14] Certain subgroups of migrants, such as refugees, asylum seekers, those without status, and those with low income, are particularly vulnerable and are at increased risk for deteriorating health status after arrival.[12]

The composition of migrants in each host country varies by the patterns of source countries and class of migrants. Practitioners need to be aware of the local epidemiology of the migrant populations living in their host country; this includes the circumstances of their migration pathway, their migration class, the pattern of diseases in their countries of origin, and the individual risk factors for each patient. In this review, the authors describe the most prevalent infectious diseases and their associated burden among immunocompetent migrants during the different phases of migration, with implications for health screening and health promotion. They also address the potential for transmission of certain infectious diseases from migrants through blood and from organ donation. Finally, the impact of migration on the spread of antimicrobial resistance (AMR) and the potential role of migrants in the reintroduction of vector borne diseases will be addressed.

PREVALENCE OF INFECTIOUS DISEASES AND THE ASSOCIATED BURDEN OF UNDETECTED AND UNTREATED INFECTIONS

On arrival and in reception areas, infectious diseases are not a health priority for migrants because traumatic, obstetric, and psychological conditions are more frequent concerns.[11,15] The most common infectious diseases occurring during this period are gastrointestinal or respiratory infections or diseases such as scabies, that are transmitted through having lived in crowded, unhygienic conditions.[11] The key infectious diseases to be considered for screening among migrants are discussed.

Table 1
Risk factors for infectious disease exposure and or due to undetected chronic infections at the different stages of the migration pathway

Migration Phase	Risk Factors for Infectious Disease Exposure and Increased or Decreased Disease Burden	Infectious Disease
Pre-arrival	• Epidemiology of infectious diseases in countries of origin • Lack of adequate sanitation • Lack of access to preventive health care and vaccination • Cultural practices (female genital mutilation, ritual scarification, tattoos, etc.) • Lifestyle (bathing in contaminated fresh water, etc.)	TB, HBV and HCV, HIV, HTLV-I, Strongyloidiasis, Schistosomiasis, Chagas disease, Malaria, VPD
Transit	• Physical or sexual violence (irregular migration or human trafficking) • Mode and conditions of transport and detention • Crowded unhygienic living conditions	HBV, HCV, HIV, STIs, TB, Scabies, VPD

Early arrival: Reception centers and refugee camps	• Crowded unhygienic living conditions in reception camps
	• Barriers in access to health care due to:
	  ○ Variable entitlement to health care
	  ○ Lack of linguistically or culturally adapted health system
	  ○ Stigma, fear of deportation
		Respiratory infections, Gastrointestinal infections, Scabies, VPD, TB

Late Settlement	• Prior screening in pre-arrival screening programs
	• Presence/absence of post-arrival health screening programs or routine update of vaccinations in host country
	• Risk behaviors (alcohol, drug use, sexual contacts, etc.)
	• Barriers in access to health care due to:
	  ○ Variable entitlement to health care
	  ○ Lack of linguistically or culturally adapted health system
	  ○ Stigma
		Active TB and Latent TB, Chronic HBV and HCV infections and associated ESLD and HCC, HIV, Strongyloidiasis, Schistosomiasis, Chagas disease, Other parasitic infections, VPD

(continued on next page)

Table 1 (continued)		
Migration Phase	**Risk Factors for Infectious Disease Exposure and Increased or Decreased Disease Burden**	**Infectious Disease**
Return travel to visit friends and relatives (VFRs)	• Misperception of health risks during return travel • Lack of vaccinations or malaria chemoprophylaxis due to lack of seeking pre-travel advice or financial barriers to uptake • Increase risk of re-exposure due to proximity to local population, sexual activity, or use of medical care in destination country • Increased risk of infections in children born in host country	Malaria, Typhoid fever, Hepatitis A, TB, HBV, STIs, HIV

Abbreviations: ESLD, end stage liver disease; HBV, hepatitis B virus; HCC, hepatocellular carcinoma; HCV, hepatitis C virus; HTLV-I human T-cell lymphotropic virus; STIs, sexually transmitted infections; TB, tuberculosis; VPD, vaccine preventable diseases.

TUBERCULOSIS

The foreign-born population makes up an increasing and disproportionate number of all tuberculosis (TB) cases in high-income, low TB incidence (<10 cases/100,000 population) countries and challenge TB control efforts in these countries.[16] Migrants make up more than half of all TB cases in most low TB incidence countries and have TB incidence rates that are several fold higher than that in host populations.[16,17] Most of these cases are due to reactivation of latent tuberculosis infection (LTBI) acquired in the patients' countries of origin.[16] The strongest predictors for the development of active TB in immigrant populations are TB incidence in their countries of origin, immigration category, the presence of underlying medical comorbidities, and the time since arrival in host countries.[18] The rate of active TB among migrants is highest in the first year of arrival and is similar to that in their countries of origin.[18–20] Refugees have higher rates of TB compared with other migrants. The higher TB rates in refugees may be due to an increased risk of recent TB exposure while living in crowded conditions in their countries of origin, during transit, or while incarcerated or in detention. The presence of factors such as undernutrition or human immunodeficiency virus (HIV) coinfection (resulting from violence or sexual exploitation) increases the risk of the development of active TB.[17] After arrival in host countries, some migrants may be excluded from health services or be fearful of accessing services due to their legal status. Migrants are also at risk for drug-resistant TB, contributing to most (73%–95%) drug-resistance cases in low TB incidence countries.[21–23] Cases of multi-drug-resistant tuberculosis (MDR-TB) among migrants are usually imported, and disease rates reflect that in their countries of origin; however, poor compliance with treatment after arrival is also a driver of MDR-TB.[24] Prearrival active TB screening programs with a chest radiograph and the treatment of those found to have active disease before arrival are routinely performed on migrants coming to the United States, Canada, Australia, and the United Kingdom and may benefit TB control in host countries.[16] An evaluation of the American program demonstrated that detecting prevalent active TB before arrival reduced TB notification rates among migrants in the first years after arrival.[25] Travel back to endemic countries is also an important risk factor for active TB in migrants. One-fifth of TB cases among Asian migrants in the United Kingdom were attributed to a recent trip to Asia, and 56% of TB cases among Moroccans living in the Netherlands were attributable to recent travel to Morocco.[26,27]

The risk of TB remains elevated throughout a migrant's lifetime and more than one-half of all TB cases among migrants occur 5 or more years after their arrival.[28] Providing targeted latent TB screening and treatment to those at highest risk will therefore be critical to achieving the World Health Organization (WHO) TB elimination goals. There are numerous challenges to implementing these programs due to the large pool of migrants with LTBI (a small proportion of whom will develop active TB), long latent TB treatments, and a weak cascade of care.[28,29] Only 14.8% of migrants eligible for TB screening actually complete latent TB therapy due to losses at each step along the care continuum (screening, initiating therapy, and treatment completion).[29] LTBI screening using a tuberculin skin test (TST) or an interferon-gamma release assay (IGRA), soon after arrival, for migrants originating from high TB-incidence countries and ensuring treatment completion will be key to achieving TB elimination in low TB incidence countries (**Table 2**).[28]

Table 2
Suggested screening tests for health assessment of migrant populations

Health Condition	Suggested Screening/Assessment
Infectious diseases	
Latent TB	Screen migrants from high TB endemic countries with a TST or an IGRA as soon as possible after arrival
HBV	Screen all originating from a region with ≥2% HBsAg prevalence for infection and immunity for HBsAg, anti-HBc (if available), and anti-HBs Provide all nonimmune children with HBV vaccine and, if possible, all nonimmune adults
HCV	Screen all individuals with risk factors for HCV infection and those originating from a region with ≥2% HCV seroprevalence
HIV	At a minimum, screen individuals originating from a country with a prevalence of ≥1% or if presence of risk factors for HIV Some countries suggest screening all migrants
Sexually transmitted infections	Urine for chlamydia, gonorrhea, and syphilis serology if presence of risk factors and for unaccompanied minors
Strongyloidiasis	Screen with serology individuals at risk from endemic tropical countries
Schistosomiasis	Screen with serology individuals at risk from Africa or other endemic countries
Chagas disease	Migrants originating from Latin America, particularly children, women of reproductive age, and those with symptoms
Vaccine-preventable diseases	Provide vaccines to appropriate age groups according to locally accepted schedules
Varicella vaccine	Varicella serology if negative/unclear history and >13 y of age; offer varicella vaccine if nonimmune Vaccinate children as per routine host country vaccination schedule

VIRAL HEPATITIS

Undetected and untreated imported cases of hepatitis B (HBV) and hepatitis C (HCV) among migrants born in endemic countries are an important yet underappreciated contributor to the growing morbidity and mortality from viral hepatitis in high-income, low-prevalence countries. Migrants born in intermediate and high viral hepatitis prevalence counties are approximately 10- to 12-fold and 1.5- to 2-fold more likely to be infected with chronic HBV (6% vs 0.5%–1%) and HCV (2% vs 1%), respectively, than host populations and have prevalence of infection reflecting that in their countries of origin.[30–32] As a consequence, immigrants account for up to 50% or more of all cases of HBV and 15% to 80% of all cases of HCV in low-prevalence countries.[32,33] Approximately one-third of persons with chronic HBV and HCV will die from complications of their disease after a more than 30-year asymptomatic period, unless they are detected early and provided with appropriately timed antiviral therapy.[33,34] Migrants have a 2- to 4-fold higher rate of dying from hepatocellular carcinoma compared with host populations.[35,36] The higher rate of death is likely due to the long delay to HBV diagnosis (mean 6 years), HCV diagnosis (mean 10 years), and HCV treatment (mean 15 years) after arrival.[37–39] Despite the availability of effective therapies, less than half of all HBV and HCV cases are diagnosed and less than 30% are treated, due to numerous barriers.[33,40,41] The decreasing cost of HCV treatment and the availability of pangenotypic therapy make HCV elimination possible.[42] As part of the WHO strategy to eliminate viral hepatitis by 2035, it is recommended that individuals originating from a country with an HBV or HCV prevalence of $\geq$2% be screened for these diseases, which includes many migrants living in low-incidence countries. Those found to be positive should be linked to care and treatment.[34,43] Children should be screened for immunity for HBV and vaccinated if nonimmune.[34] Consider screening migrants of all ages originating from countries with HBsAg $\geq$2% for HBV immunity and vaccinate those found to be nonimmune; however, this is less cost-effective than vaccinating children.[44]

HUMAN IMMUNODEFICIENCY VIRUS

Prevalence of HIV infection is highest among migrants from high HIV prevalence countries and those with typical risk factors for disease acquisition.[45] On premigration HIV screening in 634,958 persons before arrival in Canada, the overall HIV prevalence was low (0.15%). The highest risk group was Sub-Saharan African refugees who accounted for 67% of cases and had a prevalence ranging from 3.3% to 4.3%.[46] The risk of HIV acquisition continues after arrival as demonstrated in a study in the United Kingdom, which found that 33% of Sub-Saharan African migrants acquired HIV after arrival, highlighting the need for continued targeted HIV prevention efforts in at-risk migrant communities and the provision of appropriate treatment to infected individuals.[47] In Europe, approximately 70% of HIV cases among migrants were acquired after migration and occurred primarily in migrants with high-risk factors, such as intravenous drug use or among men who have sex with men.[48,49] African-born women are a particularly vulnerable group and have a 12 times higher risk of HIV infection compared with women of the host population and may have acquired HIV before or after arrival.[50] Some countries recommend screening all migrants for HIV.[51] Other countries recommend screening all adult and adolescent new immigrants from countries where HIV prevalence is greater than 1%, and among children at risk, such as unaccompanied minors.[45] Important challenges in addressing HIV among the migrant population are overcoming the stigma associated with an HIV diagnosis, increasing screening uptake, and securing access to antiretroviral treatment for those who tested positive, regardless of their legal status.[50,52] Migrants are at risk for other sexually transmitted infections that may have been acquired in the country of origin or during travel (often following sexual violence, especially for women) or in the destination country when there is ongoing high-risk behaviors.[11,53]

VACCINE-PREVENTABLE DISEASES

Adult and child migrants may be more susceptible to several vaccine-preventable diseases, such as measles, mumps, rubella, and tetanus, as compared with host populations.[54–57] Nonimmunity to vaccine-preventable diseases among migrants may be due to several factors including underimmunization in their countries of origin, lack of having vaccinations updated after arrival in host countries, or vaccine hesitancy after arrival.[56,58–61] Global immunization coverage ranges widely (47%–85%) with large variation between geographic regions.[62] Migrant children have lower immunity than adults.[54,56] Large numbers of susceptible migrants may lead to decreased herd immunity and outbreaks which may be associated with negative disease-associated outcomes. Outbreaks of measles have been documented in newly arrived migrants in refugee camps in Europe facilitated by nonimmune individuals living together in crowded conditions. Significant vaccination gaps among migrants due to vaccine hesitancy after arrival are highlighted by recent outbreaks of measles among the Somali population who had been living in the United States for many years. Low vaccination uptake over several years occurred due to concerns that the increased rate of autism in the community was related to measles vaccine. Controlling the outbreak and increasing vaccine rates required considerable effort and work with the Somali community in a linguistically and culturally sensitive manner.[60,61] The consequences of undervaccination is also illustrated by several outbreaks of rubella and documented cases of congenital rubella due to low rubella immunity among migrant women.[55,63–65] Ensuring high vaccination coverage is a key priority in high-income countries, but important gaps remain. Providing vaccinations for migrants has been a particular problem with the large movement of migrants into Europe in 2015 and 2016.[58] The high mobility of these migrants without vaccination records challenged the vaccination process, especially when multiple appointments were required.[56] Vaccine gaps among adolescents and adults may exist when children are the priority of national vaccination policies, and other age groups are excluded from initiatives to assess immunization status or from catch-up vaccinations.[58] Age-appropriate vaccinations should be offered to migrants without delay regardless of legal status according to the local immunization schedule of the host country. Attention should be paid to potential vaccine gaps in all age groups, including adults.

Varicella is an important infection in migrants because a large proportion of adolescents and adults (15%–30%) born in tropical countries are susceptible to varicella due to different transmission dynamics and the lack of varicella vaccination programs in most of these countries.[66] Non-immunity to varicella in older age groups is important because adults are more likely to develop severe varicella and to be hospitalized and to die from varicella as compared with children. The most cost-effective approach is to provide vaccination for adolescents (>13 years of age), to screen adults from tropical countries for varicella antibodies, and to provide vaccine if nonimmune.[67]

PARASITIC INFECTIONS

Migrants originating from tropical and subtropical areas are commonly affected by chronic helminthiasis that may go undetected for long periods due to the lack of clinical symptoms. *Strongyloides* is a ubiquitous parasite found in tropical and sub-tropical countries with prevalence reported to be between 10% and 40%.[68] It is a unique parasite because it persists in the host for a lifetime due to autoinfection. It is often asymptomatic in immunocompetent hosts or may cause mild symptoms. Strongyloidiasis can result in life-threatening disseminated disease in immunocompromised hosts, particularly in those receiving corticosteroid therapy, those with transplant-related immunosuppression, patients with hematologic malignancies, and those with coinfection with human T-cell lymphotropic virus-1 (HTLV-1). The immunosuppression associated with these conditions permits massive larval proliferation (hyperinfection) and dissemination to multiple organs, with case fatality rates exceeding 50%.[69] In a systematic review, the overall seroprevalence of strongyloidiasis among migrants living in low endemic countries was 12·2% (95% confidence interval 9.0%–15.9%) with risk occurring in migrants from all endemic regions irrespective of age, sex, and immigrant class.[70] The screening test of choice is detection of antibodies in serum; however, sensitivity of this test decreases with immunosuppression, highlighting the importance of early screening and treatment.[71] Screening should to be offered to all immunosuppressed migrants and all immunocompetent migrants originating from high-risk countries or in the presence of eosinophilia.[72]

Schistosomiasis is a parasitic infection that is present in many countries, but 90% of the global burden of the 207 million infected persons live in Africa.[73] Focal areas of infection also occur in Asia, North Africa, the Middle East, and South America; however, successful mass treatment initiatives have greatly interrupted infection transmission in these regions.[74] *Schistosomes* infect humans through freshwater exposure. Infection may remain active for years leading to long-term complications that occur due to the host immune response to the *schistosome* eggs. Chronic inflammation from species such as *Schistosomiasis mansoni* is associated with fibrosis in the hepatointestinal system, whereas *Schistosomiasis hematobium* is tropic to the urogenital system and is associated with bladder neoplasia. Results from a systematic review of schistosomiasis among migrants living in nonendemic countries found that the prevalence of schistosomiasis among migrants is similar to that of their countries of origin.[70] Sub-Saharan African migrants had the highest seroprevalence [25% (17.5%-33.3%)]. Serologic tests are the diagnostic test of choice for schistosomiasis in migrants, but they overestimate active infection because they do not distinguish between current and past infection.[75] A recent report of several cases of *S hematobium* diagnosed among African migrants living in Italy highlights the importance of recognizing this disease, and screening those at risk, and providing treatment to those found to be positive.[76]

Chagas disease resulting from *Trypanosoma cruzi* infection is endemic in Latin America, with the highest prevalence in Bolivia, Argentina, Paraguay, Ecuador, El Salvador, and Guatemala.[77] International migration has contributed to the spread of the disease from rural Latin America to nonendemic countries with an estimated 300,000 infected persons in the United States and 68,000 to 120,000 infected persons in Europe.[78,79] A total of 4.2% of Latin American migrants in Europe have Chagas disease; however, only 10% are diagnosed.[79] The highest risk group is Bolivian migrants, who have a seroprevalence of 18%. Other migrant groups are also at substantial risk, including those from El Salvador (5.6%), Paraguay (5.5%), Nicaragua (4.6%), and Honduras (3.7%). Chagas disease is transmitted via by Triatominae vectors, vertically from mother to child, through blood transfusion, via organ transplantation, or orally through ingestion of contaminated food.[77] Infected persons remain asymptomatic for 30 or more years. Approximately one-third of infected people will develop cardiac or gastrointestinal pathology. The earlier in the course of the disease and the younger the age at treatment, the more effective treatment is. Antiparasitic treatment is effective in curing those with congenital infection (>95%), those with acute infection (70%–80%), and adolescents (60%–94%).[77] Screening for Chagas disease among Latin American migrants from endemic countries is cost-effective and is particularly important for pregnant women and women of child-bearing age to prevent congenital infection. Screening and treatment of children and adolescents is important due to high treatment efficacy.[80,81]

Malaria in nonendemic countries occurs mainly among migrants who travel back to their countries of origin to visit friends and relatives (VFR).[82,83] Unlike travelers, VFRs spend a longer time in endemic areas, mingle closely with the local population, and are less likely to seek pretravel medical advice and chemoprophylaxis.[83] Decreased uptake of pretravel advice is due to several factors, including urgent last minute trips, decreased risk perception driven by cultural beliefs, or limited access to preventive health services.[84] The pretravel visit provides an opportunity for health promotion and risk reduction through a culturally and linguistically tailored approach. A minority of malaria cases are imported at the time of arrival. Recently arrived migrants from endemic areas however, may have asymptomatic malaria and serve as a potential reservoir for autochthonous malaria, an issue that is addressed later in this article.

Migrants are at increased risk for other neglected parasitic diseases, such as cysticercosis and leishmaniasis. In high-income countries, most cases of neurocysticercosis are imported by migrants.[85] In the United States, 62% of reported cases of fatal cysticercosis occurred among migrants from Mexico. In Europe, 61% of all cases of neurocysticercosis occurred among migrants, most of whom were from Latin America.[86,87] Almost all cases of imported leishmaniasis are due to cutaneous leishmaniasis (CL) and occur among travelers and migrants.[88–90] The Syrian conflict and the movement of large numbers of refugees associated with it have led to a significant increase in the number of cases diagnosed in the region as well as imported CL cases into nonendemic regions in Europe and North America.[89,91]

TRANSMISSION OF LATENT INFECTIONS BY BLOOD OR ORGAN DONATION

Asymptomatic latent infections such as TB, viral hepatitis, HIV, and selected parasitic infections are prevalent in many migrants. These infections may reactivate many years after migration for both physiologic (aging) and iatrogenic reasons (immunosuppressive drugs).[92] Donors with latent infections may represent a risk for the recipients of blood transfusions or organ transplantation. A careful assessment for latent infections among donors and recipients should be done routinely prior to transplantation. Recommendations to screen solid organ donors from endemic areas have recently been published and are summarized in **Table 3**.[93]

ORGAN TRANSPLANTATION

Evidence of transmission of *Strongyloides stercoralis*,[94] *Plasmodium* spp,[95] *T cruzi*,[96] HTLV-I,[97] and other geographically limited infections through organ transplantation has been reported. Chronic *S stercoralis* infection is of particular importance in transplantation medicine due to systemic involvement such that any transplanted organ from an infected donor may be affected (liver, kidney, heart, or pancreas).[98–102] The resulting infection in the transplanted recipient is usually severe, with hyperinfection occurring due to post transplant immunosuppressive therapy. Several reports of *Schistosoma* spp–infected liver and renal grafts have been published with few clinical consequences when the infestation has been promptly diagnosed and treated before

Table 3
Specific screening for latent infections among migrants who are solid organ transplant donors/recipients or blood donors

Disease	Candidates for Screening	Geographic Considerations	Available Tests
Viral diseases			
HTLV-I	SOT-D, BD	Latin America, Caribbean, Africa, Japan	Serology
Mycobacterial diseases			
TB	SOT-R, SOT-D	Any area	TST/IGRA
Protozoan diseases			
T cruzi	SOT-R, SOT-D, BD	Latin America	Serology
Plasmodium spp	SOT-R, SOT-D, BD	Malaria areas	Serology, PCR
Leishmania spp	SOT-R, SOT-D	Endemic areas	Serology, PCR
Helminthic diseases			
Strongyloides	SOT-R, SOT-D	Endemic areas	Serology/stool microscopy
Schistosoma spp	SOT-R, SOT-D	Endemic areas	Serology, stool or urine microscopy

Abbreviations: BD, blood donor; HTLV-I, human T-cell lymphotropic virus; IGRA, interferon gamma release assay; PCR, polymerase chain reaction; SOT-D, solid organ transplant donor; SOT-R, solid organ transplant recipient; TB, tuberculosis; TST, tuberculin skin test.

surgery.[103,104] It has been suggested that patients with a known history of schistosomiasis can be considered for liver donation or kidney donation as a life-saving measure if no alternative exists.[105,106] Other chronic latent helminthiasis, such as clonorchiasis (endemic in East Asia), cysticercosis, Wuchereria bancrofti filariasis, and echinococcosis, may cause graft-related infections, although there have only been a few reported cases.[107–110]

The main risk for protozoan-associated infection in the transplantation setting is American trypanosomiasis (Chagas disease).[78,79] The infection may undergo a chronic phase, and parasites may be asymptomatically present for decades in specific organs (in particular, heart and the intestine, but also kidneys and liver) and may be transmitted to the organ recipient. Pretransplant treatment of the infected donor may be considered if no other alternative exists.[96] T cruzi–infected recipients may also reactivate latent infection during the posttransplant immunosuppression phase, in particular, affecting the heart. Asymptomatic carriage of malaria that can persist for as long as 13 years may also result in organ-mediated transmission of malaria from an individual who has spent a significant amount of time in endemic areas.[95] Screening the migrant donor before transplant with a molecular technique to detect low-level parasitemia is advisable. Transmission of visceral leishmaniasis from a latently infected organ migrant donor has rarely been reported.[93] Transmission of organ-related TB has also been variably reported, leading to severe disseminated infections in the immunosuppressed recipients and has also led to secondary cases.[111,112]

BLOOD TRANSFUSIONS

Screening blood has considerably improved the safety of blood transfusion, with greater than a 1000-fold decrease in the risk of HIV, HBV, and HCV transmission via blood transfusion as compared to before screening.[113] Transfusion of blood products is also a well-known way to transmit malaria. At least 100 cases of transfusion associated malaria have been described in nonendemic areas with most donors being migrants from endemic areas.[114] Plasmodia species including *Plasmodium falciparum* have been demonstrated to persist for as long as 13 years in asymptomatic carriers.[115] This evidence supports screening donors who have lived in *P falciparum* malaria endemic areas including resettled migrants from endemic area who have lived in host countries for many years. The adoption of serologic screening for migrants or travelers who lived in malaria endemic areas has proved to be effective, although this practice has led to discarding a significant number of serologically positive (but parasitologically negative) blood units.[116] *T cruzi* infection may also be transmitted via blood transfusion from a chronically infected donor. In nonendemic areas, selective serologic screening may avoid such risk while minimizing the loss of donations.[117,118] HTLV-I is an important potentially blood-transmissible virus that requires specific blood screening policies in nonendemic countries.[119]

ANTIMICROBIAL RESISTANCE AMONG MIGRANTS AND IMPACT ON EMERGENCE AND SPREAD

Antimicrobial resistance (AMR) and multi-drug-resistant organisms (MDRO) are increasing and have spread globally due inappropriate use of antibiotics, industrialization, and population movement.[120,121] Human mobility, primarily due to travelers and to a lesser extent to migrants, has played a role in the emergence and importation of antimicrobial drug resistance by linking regions of marked health disparities.[122] There is evidence of increased prevalence of AMR and MDRO in migrants and refugees compared with local populations.[123,124] In special vulnerable groups such as refugees, the precarious and often unhygienic conditions of the journey and crowded camps or settlements are drivers of the spread of AMR.[125] In a German study, hospitalized refugees were found to have a 4-fold higher prevalence of colonization (60.8% vs 16.7%) with multi-drug-resistant gram-negative bacteria, including extended-spectrum beta-lactamase (ESBL)-producing *Escherichia coli* (23% vs 4.9%) and ESBL-producing *Klebsiella pneumoniae* (4.2% vs 0.8%), compared with the hospitalized host population.[126] In addition, methicillin-resistant *Staphylococcus aureus* (MRSA) was also found at higher rates in hospitalized refugees compared with local populations (5.6% vs 1.2%).[126] These findings were consistent across Europe where there was 10-fold higher prevalence of MRSA among refugees and asylum seekers compared with general populations in Switzerland and the Netherlands.[127,128] Screening for AMR and MDRO would not be relevant or feasible to do routinely on arrival; however, screening for AMR among migrants admitted to hospital is a prudent approach.[129]

IMPACT OF MIGRATION ON THE RISK FOR POTENTIAL REINTRODUCTION OF VECTOR-BORNE DISEASES

Migrant populations may harbor microorganisms that are potentially transmittable by vectors present in the destination countries and raises the possibility of (re)introduction of vector-borne diseases in these settings. Climate change facilitates the transmission potential through shortening the pathogen life cycle in vectors and expanding the seasonal range of vectors' activity in temperate areas.[130]

Vectors of malaria are present in the United States and Europe and in many non-malarious Asian regions.[131] Sporadic autochthonous *Plasmodium vivax* malaria cases have been reported in Europe and the United States.[132,133] A small outbreak of *P vivax* in Greece was found to be epidemiologically linked to infected migrants.[134]

Apart from rare outbreaks, however, the permanent reintroduction of *P vivax* in temperate nonendemic countries would require large population movements from endemic areas.[135] It has been shown that a substantial proportion of migrants from Sub-Saharan Africa harbor *P falciparum* parasites[136]; however, the competence of local *Anopheles* vector to transmit *P falciparum* malaria in Europe and North America has been debated. The recent possible local transmission from an infected migrant in France where *Anopheles maculipennis s.l.* and *Anopheles claviger s.s.* mosquitoes have been detected[137] raises the issue of the need to screen and treat migrants before or after immigration as is done in certain countries. Refugees arriving in the United States are provided presumptive malarial treatment prior to departure whereas refugees in Australia are screened for malaria after arrival and those found to be positive are treated.[51,138] Migrants diagnosed with falciparum malaria and living in vector-competent regions of northern Australia are given a single dose of antigametocidal primaquine in addition to treatment of active infection. The rationale for this is to eliminate the human reservoir of sexual forms of malaria and decrease the risk of infecting local mosquitoes. The administration of a single dose of primaquine (25 mg/kg) has proven to be effective in reducing gametocyte carrier rates in *P falciparum* patients in West Africa.[139]

There is also the potential risk of re-introduction of selected arboviral infections (Dengue, Chikungunya, and Zika virus) from infected migrants living in countries such as the United States and Mediterranean European countires where the Aedes albopictus vector is present. The epidemics of dengue that occurred in the Portuguese islands of Madeira in 2012 to 2013 are linked to Venezula.[140] Local sporadic dengue transmission (by *Ae albopictus* mosquito) has been reported in nonendemic areas of Europe and the United States.[141,142] The specific role of migration in these specific cases however has not been ascertained. The 2 extensive outbreaks of Chikungunya that occurred in Italy in 2007 and 2017,[143] together with sporadic autochthonous cases in North America and Europe, are good examples of the possible threat of (re)introduction of vector-borne infections following human mobility. In the 2007 Italian epidemic, the importation of the virus from India by a low symptomatic VFR was presumed.[144] The recent epidemic of *Zika* virus, a flavivirus mainly transmitted by *Aedes aegypti*, in Brazil and other Latin American countries has also raised the concern that secondary locally acquired cases could occur in nonendemic countries where other competent vectors exist.[145]

There is also the potential for transmission of infections in non-endemic settings through competent intermediate hosts in the environment. An example of this is the outbreaks of autochthonous urogenital schistosomiasis that occurred in Corsica, France.[146] There is evidence that this schistosomiasis strain has now become endemic in Corsica.[147]

SCREENING AND PROMOTING HEALTH AMONG MIGRANTS

Identifying infectious diseases early is important because it mitigates adverse clinical outcomes and in some instances onward transmission. The burden of infectious disease among migrants after arrival in high-income countries is due to lack of systematic screening and vaccination programs as well as barriers in accessing health care. Barriers accessing health care occur at the patient, practitioner, and health system levels.[148,149] On an individual or patient level, disease-related stigma, poverty, discrimination, and linguistic and cultural challenges may lead to low disease diagnosis and treatment uptake.[148] Provider level barriers, such as limited knowledge of migrants' health needs, and communication difficulties may be problematic. At the policy and health system level, there is a lack of (1) universal entitlement to health care, (2) routine screening or health promotion programs in most settings and (3) interpreters to ensure adequate communication. Successful models of care are ones that are linguistically and culturally adapted and where screening is integrated, with several infections being addressed at the same time.[28,150]

SUMMARY

The globalizing mobile world requires that all practitioners be aware of the health needs of the migrant population, because they will likely encounter migrants in their practices. Health care providers will need to be aware of the geographic distribution of disease and risk factors for specific infectious diseases. They must be aware of "rare and tropical infections" related to migration and return travel, and that migrants may harbor multi-resistant organisms that have important implications for hospital infection control practices. Immunocompromised migrants and potential organ transplantation donors and recipients must also be appropriately screened for latent infections to prevent transmission to others, or reactivation during immunosuppression. Health care workers can promote the health of the migrant population through screening for highly prevalent asymptomatic latent infections and updating vaccinations during any health encounter. Screening for infectious diseases however will only be effective if linkage to care and treatment are ensured.

REFERENCES

1. International Organization for Migration. World migration report 2018. Geneva (Switzerland): IOM, The UN Migration Agency; 2018.
2. United Nations High Commissioners for Refugees (UNHCR). The Global Report 2017. Geneva, Switzerland. Available at: http://reporting.unhcr.org/sites/default/files/gr2017/pdf/GR2017_English_Full_lowres.pdf. Accessed June 29, 2018.
3. Castelli F. Drivers of migration: why do people move. J Travel Med 2018;25(1): 1–7.
4. OECD 2018;Pages. OECD Publishing at Available at: https://www.oecd-ilibrary. org/social-issues-migration-health/international-migration-outlook-2018_migr_ outlook-2018-en. Accessed July 30, 2018.
5. United Nations 19 September, 2016. Available at: https://refugeesmigrants.un. org/declaration. Accessed June 27, 2018. Agenda items 13 and 117.
6. World Health Organization. Promoting the health of refugees and migrants. Framework of priorities and guiding principles to promote the health of refugees and migrants. Geneva (Switzerland): World Health Organization; 2017.
7. International Organization for Migration 2018. 2018. Available at: https://www. iom.int/key-migration-terms. Accessed June 30, 2018.
8. United Nations 2018. Available at: https://refugeesmigrants.un.org/definitions. Accessed June 30, 2018.
9. Greenaway C, Gushulak B. Pandemics, migration and global health security. In: Bourbeau P, editor. Handbook on migration and security. Cheltenham (United Kingdom): Edward Elgar Publishing; 2017. p. 316–38.
10. Sandgren A, Sañé Schepisi M, Sotgiu G, et al. Tuberculosis transmission between foreign- and native-born populations in the EU/EEA: a systematic review. Eur Respir J 2014;43(4):1159–71.
11. Castelli F, Sulis G. Migration and infectious diseases. Clin Microbiol Infect 2017; 23(5):283–9.

12. Gushulak BD, Pottie K, Hatcher Roberts J, et al. Migration and health in Canada: health in the global village. CMAJ 2011;183(12):E952–8.

13. Zimmerman C, Kiss L, Hossain M. Migration and health: a framework for 21st century policy-making. PLoS Med 2011;8(5):e1001034.

14. Rechel B, Mladovsky P, Ingleby D, et al. Migration and health in an increasingly diverse Europe. Lancet 2013;381(9873):1235–45.

15. Pavli A, Maltezou H. Health problems of newly arrived migrants and refugees in Europe. J Travel Med 2017;24(4):1–8.

16. Pareek M, Greenaway C, Noori T, et al. The impact of migration on tuberculosis epidemiology and control in high-income countries: a review. BMC Med 2016; 14:48.

17. Lönnroth K, Mor Z, Erkens C, et al. Tuberculosis in migrants in low-incidence countries: epidemiology and intervention entry points. Int J Tuberc Lung Dis 2017;21(6):624–37.

18. Greenaway C, Sandoe A, Vissandjee B, et al. Tuberculosis: evidence review for newly arriving immigrants and refugees. Can Med Assoc J 2011;183(12): E939–51.

19. Greenaway C, Pareek M, Abou Chakra CN, et al. The effectiveness and cost-effectiveness of screening for active tuberculosis among migrants in the EU/EEA: a systematic review. Euro Surveill 2018;23(14):5–18.

20. Ronald LA, Campbell JR, Balshaw RF, et al. Demographic predictors of active tuberculosis in people migrating to British Columbia, Canada: a retrospective cohort study. CMAJ 2018;190(8):E209–16.

21. European Centre for Disease Prevention and Control/WHO Regional Office for Europe. Tuberculosis surveillance and monitoring in Europe 2017. Stockholm (Sweden): European Centre for Disease Prevention and Control; 2017.

22. Centers for Disease Control and Prevention. Reported tuberculosis in the United States. Atlanta (GA): CDC; 2016.

23. Gallant V, Vachon J, Siu W. Tuberculosis drug resistance in Canada: 2006–2016. Can Commun Dis Rep 2017;43(11):236–41.

24. Hargreaves S, Lonnroth K, Nellums LB, et al. Multidrug-resistant tuberculosis and migration to Europe. Clin Microbiol Infect 2017;23(3):141–6.

25. Liu Y, Posey DL, Cetron MS, et al. Effect of a culture-based screening algorithm on tuberculosis incidence in immigrants and refugees bound for the United States: a population-based cross-sectional study. Ann Intern Med 2015; 162(6):420–8.

26. Kik S, Mensen M, Beltman M, et al. Risk of travelling to the country of origin for tuberculosis among immigrants living in a low-incidence country. Int J Tuberc Lung Dis 2011;15:38–43.

27. McCarthy O. Asian immigrant tuberculosis—the effect of visiting Asia. Br J Dis Chest 1984;78:248–53.

28. Greenaway C, Pareek M, Abou Chakra CN, et al. The effectiveness and cost-effectiveness of screening for latent tuberculosis among migrants in the EU/EEA: a systematic review. Euro Surveill 2018;23(14):1–21.

29. Alsdurf H, Hill PC, Matteelli A, et al. The cascade of care in diagnosis and treatment of latent tuberculosis infection: a systematic review and meta-analysis. Lancet Infect Dis 2016;16(11):1269–78.

30. Rossi C, Shrier I, Marshall L, et al. Seroprevalence of chronic hepatitis B virus infection and prior immunity in immigrants and refugees: a systematic review and meta-analysis. PLoS One 2012;7(9):e44611.

31. Greenaway C, Ma AT, Kloda LA, et al. The seroprevalence of hepatitis C antibodies in immigrants and refugees from intermediate and high endemic countries: a systematic review and meta-analysis. PloS One 2015;10(11):e0141715.

32. European Centre for Disease Prevention and Control Epidemiological assessment of hepatitis B and C among migrants in the EU/EEA. Stockholm (Sweden): ECDC; 2016.

33. Canadian Liver Foundation. Liver disease in Canada: a crisis in the making. Markham (Ontario): Canadian Liver Foundation; 2013.

34. WHO. Global hepatitis report. Geneva (Switzerland): World Health Organization; 2017.

35. DesMeules M, Gold J, McDermott S, et al. Disparities in mortality patterns among Canadian immigrants and refugees, 1980–1998: results of a national cohort study. J Immigr Health 2005;7(4):211–32.

36. McDermott S, Desmeules M, Lewis R, et al. Cancer incidence among Canadian immigrants, 1980-1998: results from a national cohort study. J Immigr Minor Health 2011;13(1):15–26.

37. Ngoma A, Allard R, Cox J, et al. A population-based cohort study of acute and chronic hepatitis B infection in the immigrant and non-immigrant populations in Quebec, Canada. Poster presentation at the 15th Conference of the International Society of Travel Medicine, Barcelona, Spain, May 14–18, 2017.

38. Greenaway C, Azoulay L, Allard R, et al. A population-based study of chronic hepatitis C in immigrants and non-immigrants in Quebec, Canada. BMC Infect Dis 2017;17(1):140.

39. Cooper CL, Thavorn K, Damian E, et al. Hepatitis C virus infection outcomes among immigrants to Canada: a retrospective cohort analysis. Ann Hepatol 2017;16(5):720–6.

40. McMahon BJ. Editorial Commentary: sliding Down the cascade of care for chronic hepatitis B virus infection. Clin Infect Dis 2016;63(9):1209–11.

41. Polaris Observatory Collaborators. Global prevalence, treatment, and prevention of hepatitis B virus infection in 2016: a modelling study. Lancet Gastroenterol Hepatol 2018;3(6):383–403.

42. Marshall AD, Pawlotsky JM, Lazarus JV, et al. The removal of DAA restrictions in Europe - one step closer to eliminating HCV as a major public health threat. J Hepatol 2018;69(5):1188–96.

43. World Health Organization. Guidelines on hepatitis B and C testing. Geneva (Switzerland): WHO; 2017.

44. Rossi C, Schwartzman K, Oxlade O, et al. Hepatitis B screening and vaccination strategies for newly arrived adult canadian immigrants and refugees: a cost-effectiveness analysis. PloS one 2013;8(10):e78548.

45. Pottie K, Greenaway C, Feightner J, et al. Evidence-based clinical guidelines for immigrants and refugees. CMAJ 2011;183(12):E824–925.

46. Zencovich M, Kennedy K, MacPherson DW, et al. Immigration medical screening and HIV infection in Canada. Int J STD AIDS 2006;17(12):813–6.

47. Rice BD, Elford J, Yin Z, et al. A new method to assign country of HIV infection among heterosexuals born abroad and diagnosed with HIV. AIDS 2012;26(15):1961–6.

48. Alvarez-Del Arco D, Fakoya I, Thomadakis C, et al. High levels of postmigration HIV acquisition within nine European countries. AIDS 2017;31(14):1979–88.

49. Fakoya I, Alvarez-del Arco D, Woode-Owusu M, et al. A systematic review of post-migration acquisition of HIV among migrants from countries with

generalised HIV epidemics living in Europe: mplications for effectively managing HIV prevention programmes and policy. BMC Public Health 2015;15:561.

50. Okoro ON, Whitson SO. HIV risk and barriers to care for African-born immigrant women: a sociocultural outlook. Int J Womens Health 2017;9:421–9.

51. Chaves N, Paxton G, Biggs B, et al. Recommendations for comprehensive post-arrival health assessment for people from refugee-like backgrounds. Australasian Society for Infectious Diseases; 2016.

52. Deblonde J, Sasse A, Del Amo J, et al. Restricted access to antiretroviral treatment for undocumented migrants: a bottle neck to control the HIV epidemic in the EU/EEA. BMC Public Health 2015;15:1228.

53. Freedman J. Sexual and gender-based violence against refugee women: a hidden aspect of the refugee "crisis". Reprod Health Matters 2016;24(47):18–26.

54. Barnett E, Christiansen D, Figueira M. Seroprevalence of measles, rubella, and varicella in refugees. Clin Infect Dis 2002;35(4):403–8.

55. Greenaway C, Dongier P, Boivin J, et al. SUsceptibility to measles, mumps, and rubella in newly arrived adult immigrants and refugees. Ann Intern Med 2007;146(1):20–4.

56. Mipatrini D, Stefanelli P, Severoni S, et al. Vaccinations in migrants and refugees: a challenge for European health systems. A systematic review of current scientific evidence. Pathog Glob Health 2017;111(2):59–68.

57. Freidl GS, Tostmann A, Curvers M, et al. Immunity against measles, mumps, rubella, varicella, diphtheria, tetanus, polio, hepatitis A and hepatitis B among adult asylum seekers in the Netherlands, 2016. Vaccine 2018;36(12):1664–72.

58. De Vito E, Parente P, de Waure C, et al. A review of evidence on equitable delivery, access and utilization of immunization services for migrants and refugees in the WHO European Region. Health Evidence Network (HEN) synthesis report 53. Copenhagen (Denmark): WHO Regional Office for Europe; 2017.

59. Hargreaves S, Nellums LB, Ramsay M, et al. Who is responsible for the vaccination of migrants in Europe? Lancet 2018;391(10132):1752–4.

60. Hall V, Banerjee E, Kenyon C, et al. Measles outbreak - Minnesota April-May 2017. MMWR Morb Mortal Wkly Rep 2017;66(27):713–7.

61. Bahta L, Ashkir A. Addressing MMR vaccine resistance in Minnesota's Somali Community. Minn Med 2015;98(10):33–6.

62. World Health Organisation. Global Vaccine Action Plan, Monitoring, Evaluation & Accountability Secretariat Annual Report 2016. Geneva (Switzerland): World Health Organization; 2016.

63. Red de Vigilancia Epidemiológica de la Comunidad de Madrid C. Outbreak of rubella in the madrid region, spain, 2005. Weekly releases (1997–2007) 2005;10(27):2742.

64. Danovaro-Holliday M, LeBaron CW, Allensworth C, et al. A large rubella outbreak with spread from the workplace to the community. JAMA 2000;284(21):2733–9.

65. Reef SE, Frey TK, Theall K, et al. The changing epidemiology of rubella in the 1990s: On the verge of elimination and new challenges for control and prevention. JAMA 2002;287(4):464–72.

66. Greenaway C, Boivin JF, Cnossen S, et al. Risk factors for susceptibility to varicella in newly arrived adult migrants in Canada. Epidemiol Infect 2014;142(8):1695–707.

67. Merrett P, Schwartzman K, Rivest P, et al. Strategies to prevent varicella among newly arrived adult immigrants and refugees: a cost-effectiveness analysis. Clin Infect Dis 2007;44(8):1040–8.

68. Schar F, Trostdorf U, Giardina F, et al. Strongyloides stercoralis: global distribution and risk factors. PLoS Negl Trop Dis 2013;7(7):e2288.
69. Buonfrate D, Requena-Mendez A, Angheben A, et al. Severe strongyloidiasis: a systematic review of case reports. BMC Infect Dis 2013;13:78.
70. Asundi A, Beliavsky A, Liu X, et al. Prevalence of strongyloidiasis and schistosomiasis among migrants: a systematic review and meta-analysis. Lancet Glob Health, in press.
71. Requena-Mendez A, Chiodini P, Bisoffi Z, et al. The laboratory diagnosis and follow up of strongyloidiasis: a systematic review. PLoS Negl Trop Dis 2013; 7(1):e2002.
72. Requena-Mendez A, Buonfrate D, Gomez-Junyent J, et al. Evidence-based guidelines for screening and management of strongyloidiasis in non-endemic countries. Am J Trop Med Hyg 2017;97(3):645–52.
73. World Health Organization. 2017. Available at: http://www.who.int/mediacentre/factsheets/fs115/en/. Accessed December 26, 2017.
74. Colley DG, Bustinduy AL, Secor WE, et al. Human schistosomiasis. Lancet 2014;383(9936):2253–64.
75. Weerakoon KG, Gobert GN, Cai P, et al. Advances in the diagnosis of human schistosomiasis. Clin Microbiol Rev 2015;28(4):939–67.
76. Riccardi N, Nosenzo F, Peraldo F, et al. Increasing prevalence of genitourinary schistosomiasis in Europe in the Migrant Era: Neglected no more? PLoS Negl Trop Dis 2017;11(3):e0005237.
77. Pérez-Molina JA, Molina I. Chagas disease. Lancet 2018;391(10115):82–94.
78. Bern C, Kjos S, Yabsley MJ, et al. Trypanosoma cruzi and chagas' disease in the United States. Clin Microbiol Rev 2011;24(4):655–81.
79. Requena-Mendez A, Aldasoro E, de Lazzari E, et al. Prevalence of Chagas disease in Latin-American migrants living in Europe: a systematic review and meta-analysis. PLoS Negl Trop Dis 2015;9(2):e0003540.
80. Sicuri E, Munoz J, Pinazo MJ, et al. Economic evaluation of Chagas disease screening of pregnant Latin American women and of their infants in a non endemic area. Acta Trop 2011;118(2):110–7.
81. Requena-Méndez A, Bussion S, Aldasoro E, et al. Cost-effectiveness of Chagas disease screening in Latin American migrants at primary health-care centres in Europe: a Markov model analysis. Lancet Glob Health 2017;5(4):e439–47.
82. Leder K, Torresi J, Libman MD, et al. GeoSentinel surveillance of illness in returned travelers, 2007-2011. Ann Intern Med 2013;158(6):456–68.
83. Angelo KM, Libman M, Caumes E, et al. Malaria after international travel: a GeoSentinel analysis, 2003-2016. Malar J 2017;16(1):293.
84. Heywood AE, Zwar N. Improving access and provision of pre-travel healthcare for travellers visiting friends and relatives: a review of the evidence. J Travel Med 2018;25(1):1–8.
85. Schantz PM, Wilkins PP, Tsang VCW. Immigrants, imaging and immunoblots: the emergence of neurocysticercosis as a significant public health problem. In: Scheld WM, Craig W, Hughes JM, editors. Emerging infections 2. Washington, DC: ASM Press; 1998.
86. Laranjo-Gonzalez M, Devleesschauwer B, Trevisan C, et al. Epidemiology of taeniosis/cysticercosis in Europe, a systematic review: Western Europe. Parasit Vectors 2017;10(1):349.
87. Sorvillo FJ, DeGiorgio C, Waterman SH. Deaths from cysticercosis, United States. Emerg Infect Dis 2007;13(2):230–5.

88. Pavli A, Maltezou HC. Leishmaniasis, an emerging infection in travelers. Int J Infect Dis 2010;14(12):e1032–9.

89. Isenring E, Fehr J, Gültekin N, et al. Infectious disease profiles of Syrian and Eritrean migrants presenting in Europe: a systematic review. Travel Med Infect Dis 2018;25:65–76.

90. Stark D, van Hal S, Lee R, et al. Leishmaniasis, an emerging imported infection: report of 20 cases from Australia. J Travel Med 2008;15(5):351–4.

91. Bradshaw S, Litvinov IV. Dermal leishmaniasis in a 25-year-old Syrian refugee. CMAJ 2017;189(45):E1397.

92. Bartalesi F, Scire C, Requena-Mendez A, et al. Recommendations for infectious disease screening in migrants to Western Europe with inflammatory arthropathies before starting biologic agents. Results from a multidisciplinary task force of four European societies (SIR, SER, SIMET, SEMTSI) facing the largest impact of the flow of migrants today. Clin Exp Rheumatol 2017;35(5):752–65.

93. Clemente WT, Pierrotti LC, Abdala E, et al. Recommendations for management of endemic diseases and travel medicine in solid-organ transplant recipients and donors: Latin America. Transplantation 2018;102(2):193–208.

94. Cooper AJR, Dholakia S, Holland CV, et al. Helminths in organ transplantation. Lancet Infect Dis 2017;17(6):e166–76.

95. Menichetti F, Bindi ML, Tascini C, et al. Fever, mental impairment, acute anemia, and renal failure in patient undergoing orthotopic liver transplantation: post-transplantation malaria. Liver Transpl 2006;12(4):674–6.

96. Pierrotti LC, Carvalho NB, Amorin JP, et al. Chagas disease recommendations for solid-organ transplant recipients and donors. Transplantation 2018;102(2S Suppl 2):S1–7.

97. Gallo RC, Willems L, Hasegawa H, Global Virus Network's Task Force on HTLV-1. Screening transplant donors for HTLV-1 and -2. Blood 2016;128(26):3029–31.

98. Ben-Youssef R, Baron P, Edson F, et al. Stronglyoides stercoralis infection from pancreas allograft: case report. Transplantation 2005;80(7):997–8.

99. Brügemann J, Kampinga GA, Riezebos-Brilman A, et al. Two donor-related infections in a heart transplant recipient: one common, the other a tropical surprise. J Heart Lung Transplant 2010;29(12):1433–7.

100. Hamilton KW, Abt PL, Rosenbach MA, et al. Donor-derived Strongyloides stercoralis infections in renal transplant recipients. Transplantation 2011;91(9):1019–24.

101. Rodriguez-Hernandez MJ, Ruiz-Perez-Pipaon M, Canas E, et al. Strongyloides stercoralis hyperinfection transmitted by liver allograft in a transplant recipient. Am J Transplant 2009;9(11):2637–40.

102. Chokkalingam Mani B, Mathur M, Clauss H, et al. Strongyloides stercoralis and Organ Transplantation. Case Rep Transplant 2013;2013:549038.

103. Mahmoud KM, Sobh MA, El-Agroudy AE, et al. Impact of schistosomiasis on patient and graft outcome after renal transplantation: 10 years' follow-up. Nephrol Dial Transplant 2001;16(11):2214–21.

104. Patel RA, Cummings OW, Mangus RS, et al. Incidental schistosomiasis in transplant liver: a case report and review of the literature. J Transplant Technol Res 2015;5:150.

105. Kayler LK, Rudich SM, Merion RM. Orthotopic liver transplantation from a donor with a history of schistosomiasis. Transplant Proc 2003;35(8):2974–6.

106. Shokeir AA. Renal transplantation: the impact of schistosomiasis. BJU Int 2001;88(9):915–20.

107. Capobianco I, Frank M, Königsrainer A, et al. Liver fluke-infested graft used for living-donor liver transplantation: case report and review of the literature. Transpl Infect Dis 2015;17(6):880–5.
108. Eris C, Akbulut S, Sakcak I, et al. Liver transplant with a marginal donor graft containing a hydatid cyst–a case report. Transplant Proc 2013;45(2):828–30.
109. Gupta RK, Jain M. Renal transplantation: potential source of microfilarial transmission. Transplant Proc 1998;30(8):4320–1.
110. Purvey S, Lu K, Mukkamalla SK, et al. Conservative management of neurocysticercosis in a patient with hematopoietic stem cell transplantation: a case report and review. Transpl Infect Dis 2015;17(3):456–62.
111. Freytag I, Bucher J, Schoenberg M, et al. Donor-derived tuberculosis in an anesthetist after short-term exposure : an old demon transplanted from the past to the present. Anaesthesist 2016;65(5):363–5.
112. Jensen TO, Darley DR, Goeman EE, et al. Donor-derived tuberculosis (TB): isoniazid-resistant TB transmitted from a lung transplant donor with inadequately treated latent infection. Transpl Infect Dis 2016;18(5):782–4.
113. Seghatchian J, Putter JS. Pathogen inactivation of whole blood and red cell components: an overview of concept, design, developments, criteria of acceptability and storage lesion. Transfus Apher Sci 2013;49(2):357–63.
114. Verra F, Angheben A, Martello E, et al. A systematic review of transfusion-transmitted malaria in non-endemic areas. Malar J 2018;17(1):36.
115. Ashley EA, White NJ. The duration of Plasmodium falciparum infections. Malar J 2014;13:500.
116. Grande R, Petrini G, Silvani I, et al. Immunological testing for malaria and blood donor deferral: the experience of the Ca' Granda Polyclinic Hospital in Milan. Blood Transfus 2011;9(2):162–6.
117. Kitchen AD, Hewitt PE, Chiodini PL. The early implementation of Trypanosoma cruzi antibody screening of donors and donations within England: preempting a problem. Transfusion 2012;52(9):1931–9.
118. Niederhauser C, Gottschalk J, Tinguely C. Selective testing of at-risk blood donors for trypanosoma cruzi and plasmodium spp. in Switzerland. Transfus Med Hemother 2016;43(3):169–76.
119. de Mendoza C, Caballero E, Aguilera A, et al. Human T-lymphotropic virus type 1 infection and disease in Spain. AIDS 2017;31(12):1653–63.
120. Hawkey PM, Jones AM. The changing epidemiology of resistance. J Antimicrob Chemother 2009;64(Suppl 1):i3–10.
121. MacPherson DW, Gushulak BD, Baine WB, et al. Population mobility, globalization, and antimicrobial drug resistance. Emerg Infect Dis 2009;15(11):1727–32.
122. World Health Organisation. Antimicrobial resistance global report on surveillance. Geneva (Switzerland): World Health Organization; 2014.
123. Piper Jenks N, Pardos de la Gandara M, D'Orazio BM, et al. Differences in prevalence of community-associated MRSA and MSSA among U.S. and non-U.S. born populations in six New York Community Health Centers. Travel Med Infect Dis 2016;14(6):551–60.
124. Maltezou HC, Theodoridou M, Daikos GL. Antimicrobial resistance and the current refugee crisis. J Glob Antimicrob Resist 2017;10:75–9.
125. de Smalen AW, Ghorab H, Abd El Ghany M, et al. Refugees and antimicrobial resistance: a systematic review. Travel Med Infect Dis 2017;15:23–8.
126. Reinheimer C, Kempf VA, Gottig S, et al. Multidrug-resistant organisms detected in refugee patients admitted to a University Hospital, Germany June December 2015. Euro Surveill 2016;21(2):1–5.

127. Piso RJ, Kach R, Pop R, et al. A Cross-Sectional Study of Colonization Rates with Methicillin-Resistant Staphylococcus aureus (MRSA) and Extended-Spectrum Beta-Lactamase (ESBL) and Carbapenemase-Producing Enterobacteriaceae in Four Swiss Refugee Centres. PLoS One 2017;12(1):e0170251.
128. Ravensbergen SJ, Berends M, Stienstra Y, et al. High prevalence of MRSA and ESBL among asylum seekers in the Netherlands. PLoS One 2017;12(4): e0176481.
129. Seybold U, Wagener J, Jung J, et al. Multidrug-resistant organisms among refugees in Germany: we need evidence-based care, not fear-based screening. J Hosp Infect 2016;92(3):229–31.
130. Semenza JC, Suk JE. Vector-borne diseases and climate change: a European perspective. FEMS Microbiol Lett 2018;365(2):1–9.
131. Piperaki ET, Daikos GL. Malaria in Europe: emerging threat or minor nuisance? Clin Microbiol Infect 2016;22(6):487–93.
132. Romi R, Boccolini D, Menegon M, et al. Probable autochthonous introduced malaria cases in Italy in 2009-2011 and the risk of local vector-borne transmission. Euro Surveill 2012;17(48) [pii:20325].
133. Sunstrum J, Elliott LJ, Barat LM, et al. Probable autochthonous Plasmodium vivax malaria transmission in Michigan: case report and epidemiological investigation. Am J Trop Med Hyg 2001;65(6):949–53.
134. Danis K, Baka A, Lenglet A, et al. Autochthonous Plasmodium vivax malaria in Greece, 2011. Euro Surveill 2011;16(42) [pii:19993].
135. Petersen E, Severini C, Picot S. Plasmodium vivax malaria: a re-emerging threat for temperate climate zones? Travel Med Infect Dis 2013;11(1):51–9.
136. Marangi M, Di Tullio R, Mens PF, et al. Prevalence of Plasmodium spp. in malaria asymptomatic African migrants assessed by nucleic acid sequence based amplification. Malar J 2009;8:12.
137. European Centre for Disease Prevention and Control. Multiple reports of locally-acquired malaria infections in the EU – 20 September 2017. Stockholm (Sweden): ECDC; 2017.
138. Centers for Disease Control and Prevention. Overseas refugee health guidelines: malaria. Atlanta (GA): CDC; 2012.
139. Tine RC, Sylla K, Faye BT, et al. Safety and efficacy of adding a single low dose of primaquine to the treatment of adult patients with plasmodium falciparum malaria in senegal, to reduce gametocyte carriage: a randomized controlled trial. Clin Infect Dis 2017;65(4):535–43.
140. Wilder-Smith A, Quam M, Sessions O, et al. The 2012 dengue outbreak in Madeira: exploring the origins. Euro Surveill 2014;19(8):20718.
141. Messenger AM, Barr KL, Weppelmann TA, et al. Serological evidence of ongoing transmission of dengue virus in permanent residents of Key West, Florida. Vector Borne Zoonotic Dis 2014;14(11):783–7.
142. Succo T, Noel H, Nikolay B, et al. Dengue serosurvey after a 2-month long outbreak in Nimes, France, 2015: was there more than met the eye? Euro Surveill 2018;23(23):1–10.
143. Rezza G. Chikungunya is back in Italy: 2007-2017. J Travel Med 2018;25(1):1–4.
144. Rezza G, Nicoletti L, Angelini R, et al. Infection with chikungunya virus in Italy: an outbreak in a temperate region. Lancet 2007;370(9602):1840–6.
145. Main BJ, Nicholson J, Winokur OC, et al. Vector competence of Aedes aegypti, Culex tarsalis, and Culex quinquefasciatus from California for Zika virus. PLoS Negl Trop Dis 2018;12(6):e0006524.

146. Boissier J, Grech-Angelini S, Webster BL, et al. Outbreak of urogenital schisto-somiasis in Corsica (France): an epidemiological case study. Lancet Infect Dis 2016;16(8):971–9.
147. Berry A, Fillaux J, Martin-Blondel G, et al. Evidence for a permanent presence of schistosomiasis in Corsica, France, 2015. Euro Surveill 2016;21(1):1–4.
148. Seedat F, Hargreaves S, Nellums LB, et al. How effective are approaches to migrant screening for infectious diseases in Europe? A systematic review. Lancet Infect Dis 2018;18(9):e259–71.
149. Ahmed S, Shommu NS, Rumana N, et al. Barriers to access of primary health-care by immigrant populations in Canada: a literature review. J Immigr Minor Health 2016;18(6):1522–40.
150. Pareek M, Noori T, Hargreaves S, et al. Linkage to care is important and neces-sary when identifying infections in migrants. Int J Environ Res Public Health 2018;15(7) [pii:E1550].

Moving?

Make sure your subscription moves with you!

To notify us of your new address, find your **Clinics Account Number** (located on your mailing label above your name), and contact customer service at:

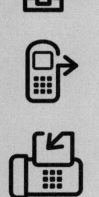

Email: journalscustomerservice-usa@elsevier.com

800-654-2452 (subscribers in the U.S. & Canada)
314-447-8871 (subscribers outside of the U.S. & Canada)

Fax number: 314-447-8029

Elsevier Health Sciences Division
Subscription Customer Service
3251 Riverport Lane
Maryland Heights, MO 63043

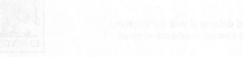

Printed and bound by CPI Group (UK) Ltd, Croydon, CR0 4YY

08/05/2025

01864741-0001